Ethical Issues
In Death and Dying

ETHICAL ISSUES IN DEATH AND DYING

Edited by

TOM L. BEAUCHAMP
SEYMOUR PERLIN

PRENTICE-HALL, INC., Englewood Cliffs, New Jersey 07632

Library of Congress Cataloging in Publication Data
Main entry under title:

Ethical issues in death and dying.

Bibliography: p.
1. Terminal care—Moral and religious aspects
—Addresses, essays, lectures. 2. Death—
Addresses, essays, lectures. 3. Right to die—
Addresses, essays, lectures. 4. Death—Proof
and certification—Addresses, essays, lectures.
5. Suicide—Addresses, essays, lectures.
I. Beauchamp, Tom L. II. Perlin, Seymour.
R726.E77   1978   174'.2   77-25179
ISBN   0-13-290114-5

Printed in the United States of America

10   9   8   7   6   5   4   3   2

PRENTICE-HALL INTERNATIONAL, INC., *London*
PRENTICE-HALL OF AUSTRALIA PTY. LIMITED, *Sydney*
PRENTICE-HALL OF CANADA, LTD., *Toronto*
PRENTICE-HALL OF INDIA PRIVATE LIMITED, *New Delhi*
PRENTICE-HALL OF JAPAN, INC., *Tokyo*
PRENTICE-HALL OF SOUTHEAST ASIA PTE. LTD., *Singapore*
WHITEHALL BOOKS LIMITED, *Wellington, New Zealand*

CONTENTS

48249

v

PREFACE

The authors and editors of this volume believe that many judgments made *in* and *about* the treatment of the dying are in fundamental respects ethical judgments. Related beliefs about suicide and the significance of death similarly incorporate an ethical dimension. This book is not, however, simply an anthology of ethical judgments and attitudes about death and dying. It is a book about unresolved controversies, and each author attempts to show the importance of critical analysis and ethical theory for the resolution of some important contemporary controversy. The way we decide such ethical problems, and the public policies we adopt as reflections of our answers, will directly affect the lives of us all. It is important for this reason that all major perspectives on the issues be presented, and we have specifically arranged the essays in an order which incorporates different perspectives. Even when there is no direct debate—as there often is —authors who present widely divergent viewpoints have been selected.

We have attempted to provide readings that are free of the technical jargon of a particular discipline, but which introduce controlled and sustained argument. Of course, some readings are more difficult than others, some are more philosophical than others, and some are more medical than others. Those who use the book as a text would, for this reason, be advised to select articles at the appropriate level. We are confident that the book can be used in this way for courses in several different fields. The editors are themselves from different fields, and many hours were spent in arranging the book so that it retained a usable interdisciplinary format.

Somewhat because of its interdisciplinary orientation, several features are introduced to make it a teachable book. Analytical introductions begin each chapter, and transitional explanations, which link each article to its successor, are provided. Each chapter concludes with a selected bibliography intended to guide the reader in further research. These bibliographies contain readings, other bibliographies, and encyclopedia references. There also is a bibliography at the end of the book which lists important sources on topics in death and dying not covered by our chapters. Finally, the editors have taken considerable editorial license in deleting from the readings passages which they consider either too technical or too difficult for use in the classroom.

Many individuals have contributed to the development and improvement of this book. We are indebted especially to our colleagues at both the Kennedy Institute, Georgetown University, and the George Washington University Medical School for many comments that led to alterations in earlier drafts. We are especially grateful for the original manuscripts, published here for the first time, by H. Tristram Engelhardt, Jr., Peter Black, and Robert Schwager. William Bruce Pitt contributed valuable bibliographical assistance, and Mary Baker was the driving organizational force without which the book would have been considerably delayed.

TOM L. BEAUCHAMP

SEYMOUR PERLIN

Ethical Issues
In Death and Dying

THE DEFINITION
AND DETERMINATION
OF DEATH

INTRODUCTION

Until recently the problem of defining death seemed to most lay and medical persons quite straightforward: death occurs if and only if there is a total cessation of respiration and blood flow. In the last few years the definition of death has been complicated by two developments in biomedical technology. First, various artificial devices have been created that sustain respiration and heartbeat indefinitely, even though there is no significant activity in the brain. Despite the artificially induced presence of vital signs, it has seemed to many that such persons are dead, not alive. Yet if they are dead, it is only too obvious that the traditional heart-lung criteria of death are of questionable adequacy. Second, various forms of transplant surgery have been developed that require well-preserved human organs. This situation creates pressure to declare a person dead at the earliest possible moment. On the other hand, there is equal reason to be cautious in declaring that a patient is truly dead, so that organs are not removed from the living.

The history of this problem dates from the late 1950s, when physicians in Europe and the United States were confronted with a clinical situation in which patients' hearts would beat spontaneously, but respiration was exclusively mechanical and no brain activity was discernible. Their major physiological functions were otherwise intact. These patients were comatose, where the coma was sufficiently deep from severe trauma (mechanical injury) or cerebral anoxia (absence of oxygen) that they could not breathe for themselves. They were also medically hopeless, since recovery was impossible. Yet in the traditional sense they were alive.

In this setting an Ad Hoc Committee of the Harvard Medical School, whose proposals are reprinted in this chapter, was formed with the purpose of more adequately defining death. Because the committee included members from fields other than medicine, and because they skillfully synthesized previous proposals, their criteria—published in 1968—gained widespread acceptance. Most transplantation units and a great many hospitals have adopted the Harvard criteria or closely related ones. Underlying all versions of the criteria is a basic assumption: Irreparable brain damage that is more or less total to the whole brain is a physical point beyond which the return of patients to *spontaneous,* respirator-independent bodily activity is impossible. They also seem to share the conviction—which is backed by some empirical evidence—that cardiac death shortly and inevitably follows such brain damage.

The Harvard Committee Report specifically lists four criteria of death: (1) unreceptivity and unresponsivity, (2) no spontaneous muscular movements or spontaneous breathing, (3) no reflexes, and (4) flat EEG (electroencephalogram). More than any other single document, this Report has established a framework within which the controversy over redefining death can take place. It has been widely criticized, as we shall see in this chapter, but no other document has been as influential on policy formulation.

Philosophical and Medical Problems

In discussing the nature of death, some writers tend to focus on the death of the human person, others on the death of the physical organism. This possibility of two different foci raises the important preliminary philosophical question: When questions about human death are raised, what sort of human entity are we attempting to determine to be alive or dead?

Philosophical Theories. We have seen that a human body that is alive by traditional criteria could be dead by some brain-death criterion. However, when we are determining whether some individual is dead, it can make a difference whether what is at issue is the death of a whole *body,* a *brain,* or a *person.* It could be said, without contradiction, that a comatose individual's *body* is alive (because all biological activities are intact), but that the *person* is dead (because all psychological activity has irreversibly ceased). Whether a "body" or a "person" or a "brain" is dead or alive further depends on a prior definition of these quite different terms, including a *theory* of the essential properties of a body or a person or a brain. These definitions in turn incline one toward a particular concept of death. If, for example, it is believed that rationality is essential to being a person, then when there is an irreversible loss of rationality there is also an irreversible loss of personhood. In some theories this loss would be sufficient to declare death, even if other vital signs were present. The Harvard Committee seems at times to say that if a person lapses into irreversible coma he is *at that point dead*—yet the judgment of death, as distinct from the judgment of irreversible coma, presupposes a philosophical theory concerning the loss at that point of essential properties. It remains a matter of philosophical controversy precisely what entity—body, brain, or person—should rightly be declared dead.

Medical Theories. Once the philosophical preliminaries are settled, medical problems concerning the criteria necessary and sufficient for death remain. There are several possible points of disagreement with the traditional emphasis on irreversible loss of respiratory and circulatory functioning. The main objections to the traditional view center on the lack of attention to the importance of brain functioning. For this reason the debate over updating the definition of death is often referred to as the "brain-death" issue, though the spinal cord may receive as much attention as the brain. Criteria suggested as necessary and sufficient for death include unresponsiveness, apnea (cessation of spontaneous breathing), absence of cephalic reflexes, flat EEG, pupil dilation, and absence of cerebral blood flow. There is considerable medical controversy over whether such lists are better or worse than the Harvard criteria. It should be noted that some of the items on such lists are criteria of *death,* whereas others are criteria for the *determination that death has occurred.* For example, the first three Harvard criteria seem to be criteria of death (any body satisfying these three criteria *is* dead), while the last criterion (EEG) is a confirmatory one used to ascertain that death has in fact occurred (the final criterion *confirms* that the body is dead). This distinction between death and the determination that death has occurred is a vital one often ignored in the literature on defining death.

Legal and Ethical Problems

The lack of an adequate definition of death in state laws has recently raised legal problems closely connected to the philosophical and medical ones. In an interesting case in New York, a woman was clubbed into a comatose condition by an attacker. Later she was removed from an artificial respirator by a doctor. The lawyer defending the accused argued that the doctor's action, not that of the accused, had caused the woman's death. The lawyer argued that she was alive when the doctor shut down the respirator, whereas the doctor maintained she was dead at that point. The doctor's appeal was to some form of brain-death criterion. Many sensational cases like this one, especially those involving possible premature removal of organs, have led both doctors and legislators to conclude that laws must be updated in accordance with an updated definition of death. Many states in the United States are currently considering "brain-death" legislation.

Kansas, the first state to enact a new law on the subject, took the compromise route of allowing the use by doctors of *either* of two alternative definitions of death, one based on heart-lung functioning and the other on brain functioning. Considerable controversy has emerged over such a legislative strategy. Some have argued that two definitions will almost certainly result in chaotic conditions in court, while others have maintained that a judicial remedy would be preferable to a legislative remedy. At present, conditions in courts and in legislatures seem unsettled. We shall probably see in the immediate future the enactment of several different proposals, perhaps corresponding to some of the many ideas about definition presented in the readings in this chapter.

Ethical as well as medical and legal problems are involved in these attempts to revise current definitions of death. It will become ever more tempting to declare persons dead as quickly as possible in order to harvest and transplant vital human organs. While everyone is opposed to the premature removal of organs from the living, the question of prematurity is ambiguous to the extent that a definition of death is ambiguous. In uncertain definitional situations, it becomes imperative to ask at what point it is morally acceptable to remove human organs. (It is even possible that the point might on some occasions be justifiably drawn *prior* to death.) This problem is further confused by the fact that the physician may or may not have the patient's consent. But the larger and most critical point is that *definitional* problems of death often cannot be discussed apart from *moral* considerations.

Dr. Peter Black, a neurosurgeon who has also done graduate work in and published articles in philosophy, surveys the past and current situation with regard to medical aspects of the definition of death. He explains how the modern problems have emerged and outlines the current options, explicating the medical problems that must be considered in any attempt to provide an adequate definition of death. He argues the interesting theses that "tradition, rather than clear clinical or pathological data, will [in the future probably] have determined our use of the term 'brain death'" and that whether respirators can be turned off will in the end "depend at least as much on our social needs as on our medical knowledge."

Peter McL. Black

DEFINITIONS OF BRAIN DEATH *

The problem of defining death is becoming more pressing in our society. The discussion of brain death is an important adjunct to this concern. This paper outlines the physiological basis for brain death, the historical development of the brain death concept, the present state of our definitions, and the direction future concepts may take.

THE PHYSIOLOGICAL FOUNDATIONS OF BRAIN DEATH

Human breathing is a complicated process, controlled both by voluntary and by involuntary mechanisms. The most fundamental areas of control seem to be in the brain stem, the part of the brain involved in many reflex activities. If these areas are destroyed, signals to begin or to end a respiratory effort fail and breathing ceases. Normally this means death of the heart. Sometimes, however, respiration can be artificially sustained. For example, during anesthesia a paralyzing agent is often used, and complete control of breathing is taken over by a machine or an anesthetist. Also, in some kinds of drug overdose or poisoning, the brain stem centers are suppressed only temporarily and breathing can be sustained until these centers function again. Life can be maintained by artificially sustained breathing in the absence of brain function because the heart beat has its own intrinsic rhythm. Unlike breathing muscles, heart muscle is so arranged that its rhythmic contraction continues as long as it has adequate oxygen and fluid to bathe in. The brain acts as a modulator of heart action: as we get excited, for example, our heart speeds up. But the brain is not necessary for heart action, at least for many days. As long as respiration continues, the heart will be able to beat.

Therefore there exists the possibility that without a functioning brain or brain stem, a body could still be kept breathing and its heart would continue to beat. As long as oxygenation and circulation were adequate, there would exist a living, or at least functioning, heart in a body with a dead, or at least not functioning, brain.

This possibility has been well known to experimental physiologists as a so-called "heart-lung preparation" in animals. Its existence in medical

* Original Manuscript commissioned for this volume. Copyright © Peter Black, 1977.

practice, however, is a recent phenomenon. Only in the last twenty years have physicians been able to design and use respirators capable of keeping a patient breathing in adequate fashion for many days without requiring the cumbersome apparatus of an iron lung. The widespread use of such respirators has led to the problem of how to act toward a body with living heart but dead brain.

THE HISTORY OF BRAIN DEATH

The explicit idea of brain death came out of work by French neurologists in the early 1950s. Mollaret and Goulon discussed "grades of coma," progressively deepening until "coma dépassé," a state without movement, spontaneous breathing, reflex activity, or regulation of temperature.[1] Essentially this was a state approaching conventional death except for the presence of a beating heart kept alive by artificially controlled lungs.

This state began to receive increasing attention. In 1967 a group of Harvard University scholars and physicians proposed the following "criteria for the determination of brain death": [2]

1. Unreceptivity and unresponsivity—no response even to painful stimuli like strong pinching.
2. No movements after observation by a physician for an hour continuously, and no breathing after three minutes off the respirator.
3. No reflexes, including brain stem reflexes. Pupils fixed and dilated.
4. A "flat" electroencephalogram (EEG). This is considered "of great confirmatory value" if technically adequate.
5. All of these tests repeated at least 24 hours later with no change.
6. Two conditions must be excluded: hypothermia, and central nervous system depression by drugs such as barbiturates.

These are essentially attempts to formulate criteria that would show that no brain function is present. The complete lack of movement or of responsiveness to stimuli indicates that the cortex is not functioning. The isoelectric or "flat" EEG helps to confirm this. The lack of so called "brain stem" reflexes indicates that the brain stem is also not working at all. Thus the lack of pupil change when a bright light is shone in the eye; the lack of eye movement when the head is turned or ice water is irrigated in one ear; the lack of coughing or gagging with manipulation at the back of the throat; the loss of the basic stimulus to breathe—these indicate a serious loss of even minimal function, for they are thought to be fundamental reflexes in the nervous system underlying the most rudimentary human life. The Ad Hoc Committee criteria first demand proof that a state of deep coma exists. They then demand a demonstration that this coma is irreversible: first, by excluding the known reversible causes of deep coma such as drug overdosage and low body temperature; second, by repeating all tests 24 hours later in order to detect any changes in the state of the patient. The Ad Hoc Committee provided a standard for criteria to be used in determining brain death.

Over the next few years these criteria became widely accepted in North America. In Europe, however, slightly different guidelines were used, involving an emphasis on brain circulation rather than EEG.

There are good historical reasons for the importance of the EEG in the diagnosis of brain death in the United States. Electroencephalographers were among the earliest to wrestle with the clinical problem of brain death. Much of the work of the Ad Hoc Committee was based on a paper by Silverman and his associates on the reliability of "electrocerebral silence" in predicting brain death. This group showed that in 3009 cases, no patient in whom drug overdosage or hypothermia was excluded survived once one "flat" EEG was obtained.[3] Since then, however, there have been isolated reports of survival after "flat" EEGs in certain rare circumstances.[4] The technical adequacy of the EEG tracing is unclear in some of these cases, and in others the remaining Harvard criteria were not met.

Time has supported the adequacy of the Harvard criteria in predicting irreversible coma and a state of widespread brain destruction on post-mortem examination. There is perhaps a self-fulfilling tendency in such predictions; after a while, patients fulfilling criteria for brain death may not receive aggressive measures to keep the heart beating. Most critics of these criteria, however, have argued that they are too strict rather than too lenient. They exclude a significant number of patients who are irreversibly comatose and will go on to die, but are not by these guidelines "brain dead."

The Harvard criteria rely partly on the EEG to show brain inactivity. Another approach to assessing brain inactivity involves demonstration that there is no circulation to the brain. This approach has been adopted in many European countries. When a patient fulfills certain clinical criteria and has an isoelectric EEG, the next step is arteriography.[5] This is a test in which the brain circulation is outlined by dye in the arteries and veins. In brain death there is no brain circulation. The brain cells swell because of lack of oxygen and nutrients and ultimately cut off all blood flow. The arteriogram shows that no blood at all enters the brain.

This test has the advantage that it shows an irreversible state. Further, it does so in a short period of time—usually about thirty minutes of angiogram time. No survivors have been reported after the demonstration of complete lack of circulation in the brain. The arteriogram is therefore more accurate than the EEG. However, the arteriogram test is more cumbersome than the EEG, and many American neurosurgeons feel that the dye itself can be harmful to a brain not yet quite "dead." They argue that the arteriogram itself can cause irreversible damage. Therefore not many doctors in the United States have recommended this test.

THE CURRENT STATUS OF DEFINITIONS OF BRAIN DEATH

Today there is no consensus in the medical profession on what constitutes adequate proof of brain death. The Harvard criteria seem most widely used. However, they are very narrow. Some patients who will remain hopelessly unresponsive and may have widespread brain damage will not quite fit them. Accordingly, several other sets of criteria have been proposed. Some rely only on an examination of the patient to determine death. Some suggest arteriography. Most used mixed criteria.[4,5,6]

An important study published in 1977 examined the cases of brain death in seven different hospital centers.[7] It recommended that the following criteria be used:

1. Apnea (i.e., no spontaneous respiration).
2. Unresponsivity (i.e., no movement in response to any stimulus).
3. Absence of cephalic reflexes (i.e., no pupil response to light, no eye movements when the head is turned, no gag or cough when the throat is stimulated).
4. Electrocerebral silence on EEG (i.e., a "flat" EEG, or one showing no brain activity).
5. Until these criteria are verified, confirmatory testing indicating an absence of cerebral blood flow for thirty minutes should be added (most usually an arteriogram).

These criteria should be fulfilled for eight hours. In the study of 503 cases, 212 met these criteria, and all of them died within several months. The study's findings are liable to have substantial impact in the years to come, especially in suggesting angiography or other blood flow study as an adjunct to the diagnosis of brain death. They have not yet been widely accepted, however.

A continuing problem has been trying to correlate the findings at autopsy with the clinical state before cardiac arrest and cardiac death. Usually fulfilling these criteria means a severely damaged brain, often with fragments of it lodged in the spinal canal where they have fallen. Very rarely, however, the person without apparent brain activity on testing will not have complete brain necrosis. The correlation between clinical and pathological findings is not perfect.

Current belief is that brain swelling begins a cycle of decreased brain flow, which then causes further swelling until all circulation to the brain stops and the brain cells die. Then, with continued body oxygenation, there is a kind of disintegration of brain tissue in the otherwise living human body. The disintegrated, widely necrotic brain tissue is called the "respirator brain"; it has certain characteristics recognized by most pathologists. Presumably one way of setting the diagnosis of brain death on a firm foundation would be to be able to predict when there is a "respirator brain." [8] At present there is no perfect way to do this. Part of the trouble is that tissue destruction occurs in the brain after death and before post-mortem examination, so the changes that are seen may actually have occurred after cardiac death.

POSSIBLE FUTURE CONCEPTIONS

There is continuing work on the criteria for brain death. Although it may seem worrisome that there is a question about the precise moment when a person is to be called dead, in fact the problem is not so serious as some have suggested. There is no possibility that a person fitting the Harvard criteria will return to useful life. The question is whether for purposes of transplants or medico-legal decisions he can be called dead: whether, for example, the respirator can be turned off. Answers to this question will depend at least as much on our social needs as on our medical knowledge.

Future work is liable to proceed in at least two directions. The first is a search for better diagnostic tests. One group of radiologists in New York City has suggested a bedside test of blood flow that might make an arteriogram unnecessary.[9] Some investigators claim that cerebrospinal fluid has special enzymes released in the presence of dead cells that can be found through a lumbar puncture. Some claim that a difference in oxygen content of blood entering and leaving the brain will give the diagnosis.

Several different kinds of tests are being proposed, but none has yet been accepted. On the other hand, there is also a search for other combinations of criteria that will be more generally applicable than those of the Harvard Committee, which seem to withhold the designation of "brain dead" from a great number of patients who, according to many doctors, have no hope of recovery.

There seems to be a confusion in this area that is worth trying to clarify. The central concern in the brain-death discussion is not to decide whether a patient will ever regain consciousness. No one would at present consider calling a permanently comatose patient who can breathe independently "dead." Rather, the concern is to identify when the brain, including the brain stem, is irreversibly damaged in a way that requires respiratory support for the maintenance of cardiac activity. This is what the criteria of the Ad Hoc Committee do. If they also leave a large number of patients with irreversible severe brain damage "alive" by their guidelines, that is acceptable. In declaring death there seems a strong advantage to being conservative.

In the future, then, one is liable to find ever wider acceptance of such criteria as those of the Ad Hoc Committee or the collaborative study rather than the ready acceptance of a radically new set of guidelines. Tradition, rather than clear clinical or pathological data, will have determined our use of the term "brain dead." The carving out of categories is an ongoing part of medical work, however; and in this area, as in others, we must build on the experience of those before us. Clinical unresponsiveness to any external or internal stimuli, lack of spontaneous respiration, fixed dilated pupils, lack of brainstem reflexes, and an isoelectric electroencephalogram or absence of cerebral blood flow may one day mean "death" as clearly as an absent heartbeat does today.

Notes

1. P. Mollaret, and M. Goulon, "Le Coma depassé," *Rev. Neurol.,* 101 (1959), 3.
2. A definition of irreversible coma, "Report of the Ad Hoc Committee of the Harvard Medical School to Examine the Definition of Brain Death," *JAMA* 205 (1968), 337.
3. D. Silverman, R. Masland, S. G. Saunders, et al., "Irreversible Coma Associated with Electrocerebral Silence," *Neurology,* 20 (1970), 525.
4. P. McL. Black, "Definitions of Brain Death." Review and comparison. *Postgrad. Med.,* 57, no. 2 (1975), 69.
5. C. Kaufer, "Criteria of Cerebral Death," *Minn. Med.,* 56 (1973), 321.
6. A. Mohandas, and S. N. Chou, "Brain Death: A Clinical and Pathological Study," *J. Neurosurg.,* 35 (1971), 211.
7. "An Appraisal of the Criteria of Cerebral Death." A summary statement. A collaborative study. *JAMA,* 237, no. 10 (1977), 982.
8. A. E. Walker, et al., "The Neuropathological Findings in Irreversible Coma: A Critique of the 'Respirator Brain.' " *J. Neuropath Exp. Neurol.,* 34, no. 4 (July 1975), 295.
9. P. Braunstein, et al., "A Simple Bedside Evaluation for Cerebral Blood Flow in the Study of Cerebral Death: A Prospective Study on 34 Comatose Patients," *Am. J. Roentgenol. Radium Ther. Nucl. Med.,* 118 (1973), 757.

Dr. Black concludes that "In the future, then, one is liable to find ever wider acceptance of such criteria as those of the [Harvard] Ad Hoc Committee rather than the ready acceptance of a radically new set of guidelines." Later in our readings other writers will challenge this prediction. But first a thorough acquaintance is needed with the Harvard Criteria, as we shall call them. The original 1968 text of the "Report of the Ad Hoc Committee," as it appeared in the *Journal of the American Medical Association,* follows. The purpose of this report is to establish an exact definition of the phenomenon of "irreversible coma" to serve as a criterion of death. The report outlines three fundamental characteristics or physiological criteria of irreversible coma: (1) unreceptivity and unresponsiveness; (2) no spontaneous muscular movements or spontaneous breathing; and (3) no reflexes. A fourth listed criterion—a flat electroencephalogram—is a confirmatory criterion for determining death, rather than a criterion of death itself. And, as Dr. Black noted, certain time restrictions and excluded conditions are also mentioned.

Report of the Ad Hoc Committee of the Harvard
Medical School to Examine the Definition
of Brain Death †

A DEFINITION OF IRREVERSIBLE COMA *

Our primary purpose is to define irreversible coma as a new criterion for death. There are two reasons why there is need for a definition: (1) Improvements in resuscitative and supportive measures have led to increased efforts to save those who are desperately injured. Sometimes these efforts have only partial success, so that the result is an individual whose heart continues to beat but whose brain is irreversibly damaged. The burden is great on patients who suffer permanent loss of intellect, on their families, on the hospitals, and on those in need of hospital beds already occupied by these comatose patients. (2) Obsolete criteria for the definition of death can lead to controversy in obtaining organs for transplantation.

Irreversible coma has many causes, but *we are concerned here only with those comatose individuals who have have no discernible central nervous system activity.* If the characteristics can be defined in satisfactory terms, translatable into action—and we believe this is possible—then several problems will either disappear or will become more readily soluble.

More than medical problems are present. There are moral, ethical, religious, and legal issues. Adequate definition here will prepare the way

* From *JAMA,* 205, no. 6 (August 6, 1968) 337–40. Copyright 1968, American Medical Association.

† The Ad Hoc Committee includes Henry K. Beecher, M.D., chairman; Raymond D. Adams, M.D.; A. Clifford Barger, M.D.; William J. Curran, LL.M., S.M.Hyg.; Derek Denny-Brown, M.D.; Dana L. Farnsworth, M.D.; Jordi Folch-Pi, M.D.; Everett I. Mendelsohn, Ph.D.; John P. Merrill, M.D.; Joseph Murray, M.D.; Ralph Potter, Th.D.; Robert Schwab, M.D.; and William Sweet, M.D.

for better insight into all of these matters as well as for better law than is currently applicable.

CHARACTERISTICS OF IRREVERSIBLE COMA

An organ, brain or other, that no longer functions and has no possibility of functioning again is for all practical purposes dead. Our first problem is to determine the characteristics of a *permanently* nonfunctioning brain.

A patient in this state appears to be in deep coma. The condition can be satisfactorily diagnosed by points 1, 2, and 3 to follow. The electroencephalogram (point 4) provides confirmatory data, and when available it should be utilized. In situations where for one reason or another electroencephalographic monitoring is not available, the absence of cerebral function has to be determined by purely clinical signs, to be described, or by absence of circulation as judged by standstill of blood in the retinal vessels, or by absence of cardiac activity.

1. *Unreceptivity and Unresponsitivity.*   There is a total unawareness to externally applied stimuli and inner need and complete unresponsiveness —our definition of irreversible coma. Even the most intensely painful stimuli evoke no vocal or other response, not even a groan, withdrawal of a limb, or quickening of respiration.

2. *No Movements or Breathing.*   Observation covering a period of at least one hour by physicians is adequate to satisfy the criteria of no spontaneous muscular movements or spontaneous respiration or response to stimuli such as pain, touch, sound, or light. After the patient is on a mechanical respirator, the total absence of spontaneous breathing may be established by turning off the respirator for three minutes and observing whether there is any effort on the part of the subject to breathe spontaneously. (The respirator may be turned off for this time provided at the start of the trial period the patient's carbon dioxide tension is within the normal range, and provided also that the patient had been breathing room air for at least 10 minutes prior to the trial.)

3. *No Reflexes.*   Irreversible coma with abolition of central nervous system activity is evidenced in part by the absence of elicitable reflexes. The pupil will be fixed and dilated and will not respond to a direct source of bright light. Since the establishment of a fixed, dilated pupil is clear-cut in clinical practice, there should be no uncertainty as to its presence. Ocular movement (to head turning and to irrigation of the ears with ice water) and blinking are absent. There is no evidence of postural activity (decerebrate or other). Swallowing, yawning, vocalization are in abeyance. Corneal and pharyngeal reflexes are absent.

As a rule the stretch of tendon reflexes cannot be elicited; i.e., tapping the tendons of the biceps, triceps, and pronator muscles, quadriceps and gastrocnemius muscles with the reflex hammer elicits no contraction of the respective muscles. Plantar or noxious stimulation gives no response.

4. *Flat Electroencephalogram.* Of great confirmatory value is the flat or isoelectric EEG. We must assume that the electrodes have been properly applied, that the apparatus is functioning normally, and that the personnel in charge is competent. We consider it prudent to have one channel of the apparatus used for an electrocardiogram. This channel will monitor the ECG so that, if it appears in the electroencephalographic leads because of high resistance, it can be readily identified. It also establishes the presence of the active heart in the absence of the EEG. We recommend that another channel be used for a noncephalic lead. This will pick up space-borne or vibration-borne artifacts and identify them. The simplest form of such a monitoring noncephalic electrode has two leads over the dorsum of the hand, preferably the right hand, so the ECG will be minimal or absent. Since one of the requirements of this state is that there be no muscle activity, these two dorsal hand electrodes will not be bothered by muscle artifact. The apparatus should be run at standard gains 10 μv/ mm, 50 μv/5 mm. Also it should be isoelectric at double this standard gain, which is 5 μv/mm or 25 μv/5 mm. At least ten full minutes of recording are desirable, but twice that would be better.

It is also suggested that the gains at some point be opened to their full amplitude for a brief period (5 to 100 seconds) to see what is going on. Usually in an intensive-care unit artifacts will dominate the picture, but these are readily identifiable. There shall be no electroencephalographic response to noise or to pinch.

All of the above tests shall be repeated at least 24 hours later with no change.

The validity of such data as indications of irreversible cerebral damage depends on the exclusion of two conditions: hypothermia (temperature below 90°F [32.2°C]) or central nervous system depressants, such as barbiturates.

OTHER PROCEDURES

The patient's condition can be determined only by a physician. When the patient is hopelessly damaged as defined above, the family and all colleagues who have participated in major decisions concerning the patient, and all nurses involved, should be so informed. Death is to be declared and *then* the respirator turned off. The decision to do this and the responsibility for it are to be taken by the physician-in-charge, in consultation with one or more physicians who have been directly involved in the case. It is unsound and undesirable to force the family to make the decision.

LEGAL COMMENTARY

The legal system of the United States is greatly in need of the kind of analysis and recommendations for medical procedures in cases of irreversible brain damage as described. At present, the law of the United States, in all 50 states and in the federal courts, treats the question of human death as a question of fact to be decided in every case. When any doubt exists, the courts seek medical expert testimony concerning the time of death of the particular individual involved. However, the law makes the assumption that the medical criteria for determining death are settled and not in doubt among physicians. Furthermore, the law assumes that the traditional method among physicians for determination of death is to ascertain the absence of all vital signs. To this extent, *Black's Law Dictionary* (fourth edition, 1951) defines death as

> The cessation of life; the ceasing to exist; *defined by physicians* as a total stoppage of the circulation of the blood, and a cessation of the animal and vital functions consequent thereupon, such as respiration, pulsation, etc [italics added].

In the few modern court decisions involving a definition of death, the courts have used the concept of the total cessation of all vital signs. Two cases are worthy of examination. Both involved the issue of which one of two persons died first.

In *Thomas* v. *Anderson* (96 Cal. App. 2d 371, 211 P.2d 478), a California District Court of Appeal in 1950 said, "In the instant case the question as to which of the two men died first was a question of fact for the determination of the trial court. . . ."

The appellate court cited and quoted in full the definition of death from *Black's Law Dictionary* and concluded, ". . . death occurs precisely when life ceases and does not occur until the heart stops beating and respiration ends. Death is not a continuous event and is an event that takes place at a precise time."

The other case is *Smith* v. *Smith* (229 Ark. 579, 317 S.W.2d 275), decided in 1958 by the Supreme Court of Arkansas. In this case the two people were husband and wife involved in an auto accident. The husband was found dead at the scene of the accident. The wife was taken to the hospital unconscious. It is alleged that she "remained in coma due to brain injury" and died at the hospital 17 days later. The petitioner in court tried to argue that the two people died simultaneously. The judge writing the opinion said the petition contained a "quite unusual and unique allegation." It was quoted as follows:

> That the said Hugh Smith and his wife, Lucy Coleman Smith, were in an automobile accident on the 19th day of April, 1957, said accident being instantly fatal to each of them at the same time, although the doctors maintained a vain hope of survival and made every effort to revive and resuscitate said Lucy Coleman Smith until May 6th, 1957, when it was finally determined by the attending physicians that their hope of

resuscitation and possible restoration of human life to the said Lucy Coleman Smith was entirely vain, and

That as a matter of modern medical science, your petitioner alleges and states, and will offer the Court competent proof that the said Hugh Smith, deceased, and said Lucy Coleman Smith, deceased, lost their power to will at the same instant, and that their demise as earthly human beings occurred at the same time in said automobile accident, neither of them ever regaining any consciousness whatsoever.

The court dismissed the petition as a *matter of law.* The court quoted *Black's* definition of death and concluded,

Admittedly, this condition did not exist, and as a matter of fact, it would be too much of a strain of credulity for us to believe any evidence offered to the effect that Mrs. Smith was dead, scientifically or otherwise, unless the conditions set out in the definition existed.

Later in the opinion the court said, "Likewise, we take judicial notice that one breathing, though unconscious, is not dead."

"Judicial notice" of this definition of death means that the court did not consider that definition open to serious controversy; it considered the question as settled in responsible scientific and medical circles. The judge thus makes proof of uncontroverted facts unnecessary so as to prevent prolonging the trial with unnecessary proof and also to prevent fraud being committed upon the court by quasi-"scientists" being called into court to controvert settled scientific principles at a price. Here, the Arkansas Supreme Court considered the definition of death to be a settled, scientific, biological fact. It refused to consider the plaintiff's offer of evidence that "modern medical science" might say otherwise. In simplified form, the above is the state of the law in the United States concerning the definition of death.

In this report, however, we suggest that responsible medical opinion is ready to adopt new criteria for pronouncing death to have occurred in an individual sustaining irreversible coma as a result of permanent brain damage. If this position is adopted by the medical community, it can form the basis for change in the current legal concept of death. No statutory change in the law should be necessary, since the law treats this question essentially as one of fact to be determined by physicians. The only circumstance in which it would be necessary that legislation be offered in the various states to define "death" by law would be in the event that great controversy were engendered surrounding the subject and physicians were unable to agree on the new medical criteria.

It is recommended as a part of these procedures that judgment of the existence of these criteria is solely a medical issue. It is suggested that the physician in charge of the patient consult with one or more other physicians directly involved in the case before the patient is declared dead on the basis of these criteria. In this way, the responsibility is shared over a wider range of medical opinion, thus providing an important degree of protection against later questions which might be raised about the particular case. It is further suggested that the decision to declare the person dead, and then to turn off the respirator, be made by physicians not involved in any later effort to transplant organs or tissue from the deceased individual. This is advisable in order to avoid any appearance of self-interest by the physicians involved.

It should be emphasized that we recommend the patient be declared dead before any effort is made to take him off a respirator, if he is then on a respirator. This declaration should not be delayed until he has been taken off the respirator and all artificially stimulated signs have ceased. The reason for this recommendation is that in our judgment it will provide a greater degree of legal protection to those involved. Otherwise, the physicians would be turning off the respirator on a person who is, under the present strict, technical application of law, still alive.

COMMENT

Irreversible coma can have various causes: cardiac arrest; asphyxia with respiratory arrest; massive brain damage; intracranial lesions, neoplastic or vascular. It can be produced by other encephalopathic states such as the metabolic derangements associated, for example, with uremia. Respiratory failure and impaired circulation underlie all of these conditions. They result in hypoxia and ischemia of the brain.

From ancient times down to the recent past it was clear that, when the respiration and heart stopped, the brain would die in a few minutes; so the obvious criterion of no heart beat as synonymous with death was sufficiently accurate. In those times the heart was considered to be the central organ of the body; it is not surprising that its failure marked the onset of death. This is no longer valid when modern resuscitative and supportive measures are used. These improved activities can now restore "life" as judged by the ancient standards of persistent respiration and continuing heart beat. This can be the case even when there is not the remotest possibility of an individual recovering consciousness following massive brain damage. In other situations "life" can be maintained only by means of artificial respiration and electrical stimulation of the heart beat, or in temporarily bypassing the heart, or, in conjunction with these things, reducing with cold the body's oxygen requirement.

In an address, "The Prolongation of Life" (1957),[1] Pope Pius XII raised many questions; some conclusions stand out: (1) In a deeply unconscious individual vital functions may be maintained over a prolonged period only by extraordinary means. Verification of the moment of death can be determined, if at all, only by a physician. Some have suggested that the moment of death is the moment when irreparable and overwhelming brain damage occurs. Pius XII acknowledged that it is not "within the competence of the Church" to determine this. (2) It is incumbent on the physician to take all reasonable, ordinary means of restoring the spontaneous vital functions and consciousness, and to employ such extraordinary means as are available to him to this end. It is not obligatory, however, to continue to use extraordinary means indefinitely in hopeless cases. "But normally one is held to use only ordinary means—according to circumstances of persons, places, times, and cultures—that is to say, means that do not involve any grave burden for oneself or another." It is the church's view that a time comes when resuscitative efforts should stop and death be unopposed.

SUMMARY

The neurological impairment to which the terms "brain-death syndrome" and "irreversible coma" have become attached indicates diffuse disease. Function is abolished at cerebral, brain-stem, and often spinal levels. This should be evident in all cases from clinical examination alone. Cerebral, cortical, and thalamic involvement are indicated by a complete absence of receptivity of all forms of sensory stimulation and a lack of response to stimuli and to inner need. The term "coma" is used to designate this state of unreceptivity and unresponsivity. But there is always coincident paralysis of brain-stem and basal ganglionic mechanisms as manifested by an abolition of all postural reflexes, including induced decerebrate postures; a complete paralysis of respiration; widely dilated, fixed pupils; paralysis of ocular movements; swallowing; phonation; face and tongue muscles. Involvement of spinal cord, which is less constant, is reflected usually in loss of tendon reflex and all flexor withdrawal or nocifensive reflexes. Of the brain-stem-spinal mechanisms which are conserved for a time, the vasomotor reflexes are the most persistent, and they are responsible in part for the paradoxical state of retained cardiovascular function, which is to some extent independent of nervous control, in the face of widespread disorder of cerebrum, brain stem, and spinal cord.

Neurological assessment gains in reliability if the aforementioned neurological signs persist over a period of time, with the additional safeguards that there is no accompanying hypothermia or evidence of drug intoxication. If either of the latter two conditions exist, interpretation of the neurological state should await the return of body temperature to normal level and elimination of the intoxicating agent. Under any other circumstances, repeated examinations over a period of 24 hours or longer should be required in order to obtain evidence of the irreversibility of the condition.

Note

1. Pius XII, "The Prolongation of Life," *Pope Speaks,* 4, no. 4 (1958), 393–98.

In the following selection from his book *Death, Dying, and the Biological Revolution,* Robert M. Veatch argues that a philosophical view of man and of human values is needed in order to provide an adequate medical definition of death. Veatch first establishes a framework for his argument by distinguishing between four levels in the definition of death: the formal definition of death, the concept of death, the locus of death, and criteria for the determination of death. He then argues that the Harvard Committee "updating" of death confuses these levels and also does not go far enough in the direction of updating. While he agrees that not all the empirical evidence is in, Veatch is inclined to think that the irreversible loss of functioning in the cerebral neocortex rather than in the *whole brain* ought to be the fundamental physiological criterion for the determination of death. Indeed, he sees more conventional criteria, as well as spinal and brainstem reflexes, as largely irrelevant to the determination of death. Veatch's position is thus substantially different from that of the Harvard Report.

Robert M. Veatch

DEFINING DEATH ANEW: TECHNICAL AND ETHICAL PROBLEMS *

It seems strange to ask what death means. Throughout history men have had a good enough idea to transact the business of society—to cover the corpse, bury the dead, transmit authority. But now that technology permits us to treat the body organ by organ, cell by cell, we are forced to develop a more precise understanding of what it means to call a person dead. There is a complex interaction between the technical aspects of deciding a person is dead—all the business involving stethoscopes, electro-

* From *Death, Dying, and the Biological Revolution.* Copyright © 1976. Reprinted by permission of Yale University Press.

encephalograms, and intricately determined medical diagnoses and prognoses—and the more fundamental philosophical considerations which underlie the judgment that a person in a particular condition should be called dead.

On May 24, 1968, a black laborer named Bruce Tucker fell and suffered a massive head injury. He was rushed by ambulance to the emergency room of the Medical College of Virginia Hospital, where he was found to have a skull fracture, a subdural hematoma, and a brain-stem contusion. At eleven o'clock that evening an operation was performed (described as "a right temporoparietal craniotomy and right parietal bur hole" in a later court record of the case), opening the skull to relieve the strain on the brain. A tracheotomy was also done to help his labored breathing. By the next morning Tucker was being fed intravenously, had been given medication, and was attached to a respirator. According to the court record, he was "mechanically alive"; the treating physician noted, his "prognosis for recovery is nil and death imminent."

In cases like Tucker's, the patient has frequently stopped breathing by the time he arrives at the hospital, and his heart may have gone into fibrillation. However, the rapid application of an electrical shock can cajole the heart back into a normal rhythm, while a respirator forces the breath of life from the tube of the machine into the tube of the patient's trachea. Thus technology can arrest the process of dying.

The Medical College of Virginia, where Tucker was taken, is the hospital of David M. Hume who, until his own recent accidental death, headed one of the eminent heart transplant teams of the world. At the time Tucker was brought in, there was a patient on the ward named Joseph Klett who was an ideal recipient. Bruce Tucker, with irreversible loss of brain function from a period of oxygen starvation in the brain and an otherwise healthy body, was an ideal heart donor.

Early in the afternoon a neurologist obtained an electroencephalogram (EEG) to determine the state of Tucker's brain activity. He saw that the electrical tracing was a flat line "with occasional artifact." Assuming the artifacts were the kind normally found from extraneous causes, this meant there was no evidence of cortical activity at that time. If the flat line on the EEG is not caused by drug overdose or low body temperature and is found again in repeated tests over several hours, most neurologists would take it to mean that consciousness would never return. Nevertheless, the respirator continued pumping oxygen into Tucker's lungs and, according to the judge's later summary, "his body temperature, pulse, and blood pressure were all normal for a patient in his condition."

In August of the same year a prestigious committee from the Harvard Medical School published more rigorous criteria for irreversible coma. Drafts of the report were circulating among professionals early in the year, but there is no evidence that the physicians in Virginia had access to it. Their use of their own judgment about criteria for diagnosing irreversible coma is still the subject of controversy.

At 2:45 that afternoon Tucker was taken back into the operating room to be prepared for the removal of his heart and both kidneys. Oxygen was given to preserve the viability of these organs. According to the court record, "he maintained, for the most part, normal body temperature, normal blood pressure and normal rate of respiration," but, in spite of the presence of these vital signs, at 3:30 the respirator was cut off. Five minutes later the patient was pronounced dead and the mechanical support was resumed to preserve the organs, and his heart was removed and transplanted to Joseph Klett. According to the record, Tucker's vital signs continued to be normal until 4:30, soon before the heart was removed.

The heart was removed although it had continued functioning while the respirator continued to pump. It was removed without any attempt to get the permission of relatives, although Tucker's wallet contained his brother's business card with a phone number and an address only fifteen blocks away. The brother was in his place of business that day, and a close friend had made unsuccessful inquiries at three information desks in the hospital. The heart was removed although Virginia law, according to the interpretation of the judge in the subsequent trial, defines death as total cessation of all body functions.

William Tucker, the "donor's" brother, brought suit against the surgical team for wrongfully ending Bruce Tucker's life. During the trial, physicians testified that Tucker was "neurologically dead" several hours before the transplant and that his heart and respiratory system were being kept viable by mechanical means. To this William Tucker responded, "There's nothing they can say to make me believe they didn't kill him." [1] Commenting on the decision in favor of the surgeons, Dr. Hume said, "This simply brings the law in line with medical opinion."

The *New York Times* headline read, "Virginia Jury Rules That Death Occurs When Brain Dies." Victor Cohn's *Washington Post* story announced, " 'Brain Death' Upheld in Heart Transplant." The medical news services were equally quick to treat this unquestioningly as a brain-death case. The *Internal Medicine News* claimed, " 'Brain Death' Held Proof of Demise in Va. Jury Decision." Even a law review article considered the judgment to affirm that cesessation of brain activity can be used in determining the time of death.[2] There has been some outcry, especially in the black community, over the hasty removal of a man's heart without permission from the next of kin, but the general public seemed undisturbed by the decision. The medical community felt that one of their outstanding members had been exonerated.

Although the press, public, and some legal opinion treat this case as crucial in establishing the legitimacy of the use of brain criteria for death (thus bringing the law in line with "medical opinion"), more issues than that are at stake. The case raises basic questions about the definition of death.

The debate has become increasingly heated in the past decade, because fundamental moral and religious issues are at stake. The very meaning of the word *definition* is ambiguous. Some of the issues are indeed matters of neurobiological fact and as such are appropriate for interpretation by medical opinion. But judgments about facts made by scientists with expertise in a particular and relevant field can be called *definitions* only in an operational sense. The debate over the definition of death also takes place at philosophical, religious, and ethical levels, probing into the meaning of life and its ending. The more practical, empirical problems are an important part of the debate, but they must be separated from the philosophical issues. The philosophical question is, What is lost at the point of death that is essential to human nature? We can avoid the serious philosophical errors committed in the Virginia trial only by carefully separating the levels of the debate.

Four separate levels in the definition of death debate must be distinguished. First, there is the purely formal analysis of the term *death,* an analysis that gives the structure and specifies the framework that must be filled in with content. Second, the *concept* of death is considered, attempting to fill the content of the formal definition. At this level the question is, What is so essentially significant about life that its loss is termed *death?* Third, there is the question of the locus of death: where in the organism ought one to look to determine whether death has occurred? Fourth, one must ask the question of the criteria of death: what technical tests must be applied at the locus to determine if an individual is living or dead?

Serious mistakes have been made in slipping from one level of the debate to another and in presuming that expertise on one level necessarily implies expertise on another. For instance, the Report of the Ad Hoc Committee of the Harvard Medical School to Examine the Definition of Brain Death is titled "A Definition of Irreversible Coma." [3] The report makes clear that the committee members are simply reporting empirical measures which are criteria for predicting an irreversible coma. (I shall explore later the possibility that they made an important mistake even at this level.) Yet the name of the committee seems to point more to the question of locus, where to look for measurement of death. The committee was established to examine the death of the brain. The implication is that the empirical indications of irreversible coma are also indications of "brain death." But by the first sentence of the report the committee claims that "Our primary purpose is to define irreversible coma as a new criterion for death." They have now shifted so that they are interested in "death." They must be presuming a philosophical concept of death—that a person in irreversible coma should be considered dead—but they nowhere argue this or even state it as a presumption.

Even the composition of the Harvard committee membership signals some uncertainty of purpose. If empirical criteria were their concern, the inclusion of nonscientists on the panel was strange. If the philosophical concept of death was their concern, medically trained people were over-represented. As it happened, the committee did not deal at all with conceptual matters. The committee and its interpreters have confused the questions at different levels. The remainder of this [paper] will discuss the meaning of death at these four levels.

The Formal Definition of Death

A strictly formal definition of death might be the following:

> Death means a complete change in the status of a living entity characterized by the irreversible loss of those characteristics that are essentially significant to it.

Such a definition would apply equally well to a human being, a non-human animal, a plant, an organ, a cell, or even metaphorically to a social phenomenon like a society or to any temporally limited entity like a research project, a sports event, or a language. To define the death of a human being, we must recognize the characteristics that are essential to humanness. It is quite inadequate to limit the discussion to the death of the heart or the brain.

Henry Beecher, the distinguished physician who chaired the Harvard committee that proposed a "definition of irreversible coma," has said that "at whatever level we *choose* . . . , it is an arbitrary decision" [italics added].[4] But he goes on, "It is *best* to choose a level where although the brain is dead, usefulness of other organs is still present" [italics added]. Now, clearly he is not making an "arbitrary decision" any longer. He recognizes that there are policy payoffs. He, like the rest of us, realizes that death already has a well-established meaning. It is the task of the current debate to clarify that meaning for a few rare and difficult cases. We use the term *death* to mean the loss of what is essentially significant to an entity—in the case of man, the loss of humanness. The direct link of a word *death* to what is "essentially significant" means that the task of defining it in this sense is first and foremost a philosophical, theological, ethical task. . . .

The Concept of Death

To ask what is essentially significant to a human being is a philosophical question—a question of ethical and other values. Many elements make human beings unique—their opposing thumbs, their possession of rational souls, their ability to form cultures and manipulate symbol systems, their upright postures, their being created in the image of God, and so on. Any concept of death will depend directly upon how one evaluates these qualities. Four choices seem to me to cover the most plausible approaches.

Irreversible Loss of Flow of Vital Fluids

At first it would appear that the irreversible cessation of heart and lung activity would represent a simple and straightforward statement of the traditional understanding of the concept of death in Western culture. Yet upon reflection this proves otherwise. If patients simply lose control of their lungs and have to be permanently supported by a mechanical respirator, they are still living persons as long as they continue to get oxygen. If modern technology produces an efficient, compact heart-lung machine capable of being carried on the back or in a pocket, people using such devices would not be considered dead, even though both heart and lungs were permanently nonfunctioning. Some might consider such a technological man an affront to human dignity; some might argue that such a device should never be connected to a human; but even they would, in all likelihood, agree that such people are alive.

What the traditional concept of death centered on was not the heart and lungs as such, but the flow of vital fluids, that is, the breath and the blood. It is not without reason that these fluids are commonly referred to as "vital." The nature of man is seen as related to this vitality—or vital activity of fluid flow—which man shares with other animals. This fluidity, the movement of liquids and gases at the cellular and organismic level, is a remarkable biological fact. High school biology students are taught that the distinguishing characteristics of "living" things include respiration, circulation of fluids, movement of fluids out of the organism, and the like. According to this view the human organism, like other living organisms, dies when there is an irreversible cessation of the flow of these fluids.

Irreversible Loss of the Soul from the Body

There is a long-standing tradition, sometimes called vitalism, that holds the essence of man to be independent of the chemical reactions and electrical forces that account for the flow of the bodily fluids. Aristotle and the Greeks spoke of the soul as the animating principle of life. The human being, according to Aristotle, differs from other living creatures in possessing a rational soul as well as vegetative and animal souls. This idea later became especially pronounced in the dualistic philosophy of gnosticism, where salvation was seen as the escape of the enslaved soul from the body. Christianity in its Pauline and later Western forms shares the view that the soul is an essential element in the living man. While Paul and some later theologian-scholars including Erasmus and Luther some-times held a tripartite anthropology that included spirit as well as body and soul, a central element in all their thought seems to be animation of the body by a noncorporeal force. In Christianity, however, contrasting to the gnostic tradition, the body is a crucial element—not a prison from which the soul escapes, but a significant part of the person. This will become important later in this discussion. The soul remains a central element in the concept of man in most folk religion today.

The departure of the soul might be seen by believers as occurring at about the time that the fluids stop flowing. But it would be a mistake to equate these two concepts of death, as according to the first fluid stops from natural, if unexplained, causes, and death means nothing more than that stopping of the flow which is essential to life. According to the second view, the fluid stops flowing at the time the soul departs, and it stops because the soul is no longer present. Here the essential thing is the loss of the soul, not the loss of the fluid flow.

Irreversible Loss of the Capacity
for Bodily Integration

In the debate between those who held a traditional religious notion of the animating force of the soul and those who had the more naturalistic concept of the irreversible loss of the flow of bodily fluids, the trend to secularism and empiricism made the loss of fluid flow more and more the operative concept of death in society. But man's intervention in the dying process through cardiac pacemakers, respirators, intravenous medication and feeding, and extravenous purification of the blood has forced a sharper examination of the naturalistic concept of death. It is now possible to ma-nipulate the dying process so that some parts of the body cease to function while other parts are maintained indefinitely. This has given rise to dis-agreements within the naturalistic camp itself. In their report, published in 1968, the interdisciplinary Harvard Ad Hoc Committee to Examine the Definition of Brain Death gave two reasons for their undertaking. First, they argued that improvements in resuscitative and supportive measures had sometimes had only partial success, putting a great burden on "patients who suffer permanent loss of intellect, on their families, on the hospitals, and on those in need of hospital beds already occupied by these comatose patients." Second, they argued that "obsolete criteria for the definition of death can lead to controversy in obtaining organs for transplantation."

These points have proved more controversial than they may have seemed at the time. In the first place, the only consideration of the patient among the reasons given for changing the definition of death was the sug-gestion that a comatose patient can feel a "great burden." If the committee is right, however, in holding that the person is in fact dead despite con-tinued respiration and circulation, then all the benefits of the change in definition will come to other individuals or to society at large. For those who hold that the primary ethical consideration in the care of the patient should be the patient's own interest, this is cause for concern.

In the second place, the introduction of transplant concerns into the discussion has attracted particular criticism. Paul Ramsey, among others, has argued against making the issue of transplant a reason for updating the definition of death. . . .

At first it would appear that the irreversible loss of brain activity is the concept of death held by those no longer satisfied with the vitalistic concept of the departure of the soul or the animalistic concept of the irreversible cessation of fluid flow. This is why the name *brain death* is frequently given to the new proposals, but the term is unfortunate for two reasons.

First, as we have seen, it is not the heart and lungs as such that are essentially significant but rather the vital functions—the flow of fluids—which we believe according to the best empirical human physiology to be associated with these organs. An "artificial brain" is not a present-day possibility, but a walking, talking, thinking individual who had one would certainly be considered living. It is not the collection of physical tissues called the brain, but rather their functions—consciousness; motor control; sensory feeling; ability to reason; control over bodily functions including respiration and circulation; major integrating reflexes controlling blood pressure, ion levels, and pupil size; and so forth—which are given essential significance by those who advocate adoption of a new concept of death or clarification of the old one. In short they see the body's capacity for integrating its functions as the essentially significant indication of life.

Second, as suggested earlier, we are not interested in the death of particular cells, organs, or organ systems, but in the death of the person as a whole—the point at which the person as a whole undergoes a quantum change through the loss of characteristics held to be essentially significant, the point at which "death behavior" becomes appropriate. Terms such as *brain death* or *heart death* should be avoided, because they tend to obscure the fact that we are searching for the meaning of the death of the person as a whole. At the public policy level, this has very practical consequences. A statute adopted in Kansas specifically refers to "alternative definitions of death" and says that they are "to be used for all purposes in this state. . . ." According to this language, which has resulted from talking of brain and heart death, a person in Kansas may be simultaneously dead according to one definition and alive according to another. When a distinction must be made, it should be made directly on the basis of the philosophical significance of the functions mentioned above rather than on the importance of the tissue collection called the brain. For purposes of simplicity we shall use the phrase *the capacity for bodily integration* to refer to the total list of integrating mechanisms possessed by the body. The case for these mechanisms being the ones that are essential to humanness can indeed be made. Man is more than the flowing of fluids. He is a complex, integrated organism with capacities for internal regulation. With and only with these integrating mechanisms is homo sapiens really a human person.

There appear to be two general aspects to this concept of what is essentially significant: first, a capacity for integrating one's internal bodily environment (which is done for the most part unconsciously through highly complex homeostatic, feedback mechanisms) and, second, a capacity for integrating one's self, including one's body, with the social environment through consciousness which permits interaction with other persons. Clearly these taken together offer a more profound understanding of the nature of man than does the simple flow of bodily fluids. Whether or not it is more a profound concept of man than that which focuses simply on the presence or absence of the soul, it is clearly a very different one. The ultimate test between the two is that of meaningfulness and plausibility. For many in the modern secular society, the concept of loss of capacity for bodily integration seems much more meaningful and plausible, that is, we see it as a much more accurate description of the essential significance of man and of what is lost at the time of death. According to this view, when individuals lose all of these "truly vital" capacities we should call them dead and behave accordingly.

At this point the debate may just about have been won by the defenders of the neurologically oriented concept. For the most part the public sees the main dispute as being between partisans of the heart and the brain. Even court cases like the Tucker suit and the major articles in the scientific and philosophical journals have for the most part confined themselves to contrasting these two rather crudely defined positions. If these were the only alternatives, the discussion probably would be nearing an end. There are, however, some critical questions that are just beginning to be asked. This new round of discussion was provoked by the recognition that it may be possible in rare cases for a person to have the higher brain centers destroyed but still retain lower brain functions including spontaneous respiration.[5] This has led to the question of just what brain functions are essentially significant to man's nature. A fourth major concept of death thus emerges.

Irreversible Loss of the Capacity
for Social Interaction

The fourth major alternative for a concept of death draws on the characteristics of the third concept and has often been confused with it. Henry Beecher offers a summary of what he considers to be essential to man's nature:

the individual's personality, his conscious life, his uniqueness, his capacity for remembering, judging, reasoning, acting, enjoying, worrying, and so on. . . .[6]

Beecher goes on immediately to ask the anatomical question of locus. He concludes that these functions reside in the brain and that when the brain no longer functions, the individual is dead. We shall take up the locus question later in this chapter. What is remarkable is that Beecher's list, with the possible exception of "uniqueness," is composed entirely of functions explicitly related to consciousness and the capacity to relate to one's social environment through interaction with others. All the functions which give the capacity to integrate one's internal bodily environment through unconscious, complex, homeostatic reflex mechanisms—respiration, circulation, and major integrating reflexes—are omitted. In fact, when asked what was essentially significant to man's living, Beecher replied simply, "Consciousness."

Thus a fourth concept of death is the irreversible loss of the capacity for consciousness or social integration. This view of the nature of man places even more emphasis on social character. Even, given a hypothetical human being with the full capacity for integration of bodily function, if he had irreversibly lost the capacity for consciousness and social interaction, he would have lost the essential character of humanness and, according to this definition, the person would be dead.

Even if one moves to the so-called higher functions and away from the mere capacity to integrate bodily functions through reflex mechanisms, it is still not clear precisely what is ultimately valued. We must have a more careful specification of "consciousness or the capacity for social integration." Are these two capacities synonymous and, if not, what is the relationship between them? Before taking up that question, we must first make clear what is meant by capacity.

Holders of this concept of death and related concepts of the essence of man specifically do not say that individuals must be valued by others in order to be human. This would place life at the mercy of other human beings, who may well be cruel or insensitive. Nor does this concept imply that the essence of man is the fact of social interaction with others, as this would also place a person at the mercy of others. The infant raised in complete isolation from other human contact would still be human, provided that the child retained the mere capacity for some form of social interaction. This view of what is essentially significant to the nature of man makes no quantitative or qualitative judgments. It need not, and for me could not, lead to the view that those who have more capacity for social integration are more human. The concepts of life and death are essentially bipolar, threshold concepts. Either one has life or one does not. Either a particular type of death behavior is called for or it is not. One does not pronounce death halfway or read a will halfway or become elevated from the vice-presidency to the presidency halfway.

One of the real dangers of shifting from the third concept of death to the fourth is that the fourth, in focusing exclusively on the capacity for consciousness or social interaction, lends itself much more readily to quantitative and qualitative considerations. When the focus is on the complete capacity for bodily integration, including the ability of the body to carry out spontaneous respiratory activity and major reflexes, it is quite easy to maintain that if any such integrating function is present the person is alive. But when the question begins to be, "What kinds of integrating capacity are really significant?" one finds oneself on the slippery slope of evaluating kinds of consciousness or social interaction. If consciousness is what counts it might be asked if a long-term, catatonic schizophrenic or a patient with extreme senile dementia really has the capacity for consciousness. To position oneself for such a slide down the slope of evaluating the degree of capacity for social interaction is extremely dangerous. It seems to me morally obligatory to stay off the slopes.

Precisely what are the functions considered to be ultimately significant to human life according to this concept? There are several possibilities.

The capacity for rationality is one candidate. . . . Consciousness is a second candidate that dominates much of the medical and biological literature. . . .

Social interaction is a third candidate. . . .

The concept presents one further problem. The Western tradition which emphasizes social interaction also emphasizes, as we have seen, the importance of the body. Consider the admittedly remote possibility that the electrical impulses of the brain could be transferred by recording devices onto magnetic computer tape. Would that tape together with some kind of minimum sensory device be a living human being and would erasure of the tape be considered murder? If the body is really essential to man, then we might well decide that such a creature would not be a living human being.

Where does this leave us? The alternatives are summarized in Table 1 at the end of the paper. The earlier concepts of death—the irreversible loss of the soul and the irreversible stopping of the flow of vital body fluids—strike me as quite implausible. The soul as an independent nonphysical entity that is necessary and sufficient for a person to be considered alive is a relic from the era of dichotomized anthropologies. Animalistic fluid flow is simply too base a function to be the human essence. The capacity for bodily integration is more plausible, but I suspect it is attractive primarily because it includes those higher functions that we normally take to be central—consciousness, the ability to think and feel and relate to others. When the reflex networks that regulate such things as blood pressure and respiration are separated from the higher functions, I am led to conclude that it is the higher functions which are so essential that their loss ought to be taken as the death of the person. While consciousness is certainly important, man's social nature and embodiment seem to me to be the truly essential characteristics. I therefore believe that death is most appropriately thought of as the irreversible loss of the embodied capacity for social interaction.

The Locus of Death

Thus far I have completely avoided dealing with anatomy. Whenever the temptation arose to formulate a concept of death by referring to organs or tissues such as the heart, lungs, brain, or cerebral cortex, I have carefully resisted. Now finally I must ask, "Where does one look if one wants to know whether a person is dead or alive?" This question at last leads into the field of anatomy and physiology. Each concept of death formulated in the previous section (by asking what is of essential significance to the nature of man) raises a corresponding question of where to look to see if death has occurred. This level of the definitional problem may be called the locus of death.

The term *locus* must be used carefully. I have stressed that we are concerned about the death of the individual as a whole, not a specific part. Nevertheless, differing concepts of death will lead us to look at different body functions and structures in order to diagnose the death of the person as a whole. This task can be undertaken only after the conceptual question is resolved, if what we really want to know is where to look to determine if a person is dead rather than where to look to determine simply if the person has irreversibly lost the capacity for vital fluid flow or bodily integration or social interaction. What then are the different loci corresponding to the different concepts?

The *loci* corresponding to the irreversible loss of vital fluid flow are clearly the heart and blood vessels, the lungs and respiratory tract. At least according to our contemporary empirical knowledge of physiology and anatomy, in which we have good reason to have confidence, these are the vital organs and organ systems to which the tests should have applied to determine if a person has died. Should a new Harvey reveal evidence to the contrary, those who hold to the concept of the irreversible loss of vital fluid flow would probably be willing to change the site of their observations in diagnosing death.

The locus, or the "seat," of the soul has not been dealt with definitely since the day of Descartes. In his essay, "The Passions of the Soul," Descartes pursues the question of the soul's dwelling place in the body. He argues that the soul is united to all the portions of the body conjointly, but, nevertheless, he concludes:

> There is yet . . . a certain part in which it exercises its functions more particularly than in all the others; and it is usually believed that this part is

the brain, or possibly the heart: the brain, because it is with it that the organs of sense are connected, and the heart because it is apparently in it that we experience the passions. But in examining the matter with care, it seems as though I had clearly ascertained that the part of the body in which the soul exercises its functions immediately is in no wise the heart, not the whole of the brain, but merely the most inward of all its parts, to wit, a certain very small gland which is situated in the middle of its substance. . . .[7]

Descartes is clearly asking the questions of locus. His anatomical knowledge is apparently sound, but his conclusion that the soul resides primarily and directly in the pineal body raises physiological and theological problems which most of us are unable to comprehend today. What is significant is that he seemed to hold that the irreversible loss of the soul is the critical factor in determining death, and he was asking the right kind of question about where to look to determine whether a man is dead.

The fact that the Greek term *pneuma* has the dual meaning of both breath and soul or spirit could be interpreted to imply that the presence of this animating force is closely related to (perhaps synonymous with) breath. This gives us another clue about where holders of the irreversible-loss-of-the-soul concept of death might look to determine the presence or absence of life.

The locus for loss of capacity for bodily integration is a more familiar concept today. The anatomist and physiologist would be sure that the locus of the integrating capacity is the central nervous system, as Sherrington has ingrained into the biomedical tradition. Neurophysiologists asked to find this locus might reasonably request a more specific concept, however. They are aware that the automatic nervous system and spinal cord play a role in the integrating capacity, both as transmitters of nervous impulses and as the central analyzers for certain simple acts of integration (for example, a withdrawal reflex mediated through the spinal cord); they would have to know whether one was interested in such simple reflexes.

Beecher gives us the answer quite specifically for his personal concept of death: he says spinal reflexes are to be omitted.[8] This leaves the brain as essentially the place to look to determine whether a man is dead according to the third concept of death. The brain's highly complex circuitry provides the minimal essentials for the body's real integrating capacity. This third concept quite specifically includes unconscious homeostatic and higher reflex mechanisms such as spontaneous respiration and pupil reflexes. Thus, anatomically, according to our reading of neurophysiology, we are dealing with the whole brain, including the cerebellum, medulla, and brain stem. This is the basis for calling the third concept of death *brain death,* and we already discussed objections to this term.

Where to seek the locus for irreversible loss of the capacity for social interaction, the fourth conception of death, is quite another matter. We have eliminated unconscious reflex mechanisms. The answer is clearly not the whole brain—it is much too massive. Determining the locus of consciousness and social interaction certainly requires greater scientific understanding, but evidence points strongly to the neocortex or outer surface of the brain as the site.[9] Indeed, if this is the locus of consciousness, the presence or absence of activity in the rest of the brain will be immaterial to the holder of this view.

THE CRITERIA OF DEATH

Having determined a concept of death, which is rooted in a philosophical analysis of the nature of man, and a locus of death, which links this philosophical understanding to the anatomy and physiology of the human body, we are finally ready to ask the operational question, What tests or measurements should be applied to determine if an individual is living or dead? At this point we have moved into a more technical realm in which the answer will depend primarily on the data gathered from the biomedical sciences.

Beginning with the first concept of death, irreversible loss of vital fluid flow, what criteria can be used to measure the activty of the heart and lungs, the blood vessels and respiratory tract? The methods are simple: visual observation of respiration, perhaps by the use of the classic mirror held at the nostrils; feeling the pulse; and listening for the heartbeat. More technical measures are also now available to the trained clinician: the electrocardiogram and direct measures of oxygen and carbon dioxide levels in the blood.

If Descartes' conclusion is correct that the locus of the soul is in the pineal body, the logical question would be, "How does one know when the pineal body has irreversibly ceased to function?" or more precisely "How does one know when the soul has irreversibly departed from the gland?" This matter remains baffling for the modern neurophysiologist. If, however, holders of the soul-departing concept of death associate the soul with the breath, as suggested by the word *pneuma,* this might give us another clue. If respiration and specifically breath are the locus of the soul, then the techniques discussed above as applying to respiration might also be the appropriate criteria for determining the loss of the soul.

We have identified the (whole) brain as the locus associated with the third concept of death, the irreversible loss of the capacity for bodily integration. The empirical task of identifying criteria in this case is to develop accurate predictions of the complete and irreversible loss of brain activity. This search for criteria was the real task carried out by the Ad Hoc Committee to Examine the Definition of Brain Death of Harvard Medical School;

the simple criteria they proposed have become the most widely recognized in the United States:

1. Unreceptivity and unresponsitivity.
2. No movements or breathing.
3. No reflexes.
4. Flat electroencephalogram.

The report states that the fourth criterion is "of great confirmatory value." It also calls for the repetition of these tests twenty-four hours later. Two types of cases are specifically excluded: hypothermia (body temperature below 90°F) and the presence of central nervous system depressants such as barbiturates.[10]

Other criteria have been proposed to diagnose the condition of irreversible loss of brain function. James Toole, a neurologist at the Bowman Gray School of Medicine, has suggested that metabolic criteria such as oxygen consumption of the brain or the measure of metabolic products in the blood or cerebrospinal fluid could possibly be developed as well.[11]

European observers seem to place more emphasis on demonstrating the absence of circulation in the brain. This is measured by angiography, radioisotopes, or sonic techniques. In Europe sets of criteria analogous to the Harvard criteria have been proposed. G. P. J. Alexandre, a surgeon who heads a Belgian renal transplant department, reports that in addition to absence of reflexes as criteria of irreversible destruction of the brain, he uses lack of spontaneous respiration, a flat EEG, complete bilateral mydriasis, and falling blood pressure necessitating increasing amounts of vasopressive drugs.[12] J. P. Revillard, a Frenchman, reportedly uses these plus angiography and absence of reaction to atropine.[13] Even among those who agree on the types of measures, there may still be disagreement on the levels of measurement. This is especially true for the electroencephalogram, which can be recorded at varying sensitivities and for different time periods. The Harvard-proposed twenty-four-hour period is now being questioned as too conservative.

While these alternate sets of criteria are normally described as applicable to measuring loss of brain function (or "brain death," as in the name of the Harvard committee), it appears that many of these authors, especially the earlier ones, have not necessarily meant to distinguish them from criteria for measuring the narrower loss of cerebral function.

The criteria for irreversible loss of the capacity for social interaction are far more selective. It should be clear from the above criteria that they measure loss of all brain activity, including spontaneous respiration and higher reflexes and not simply loss of consciousness. This raises a serious problem about whether the Harvard criteria really measure "irreversible coma" as the report title indicates. Exactly what is measured is an entirely empirical matter. In any case, convincing evidence has been cited by the committee and more recently by a committee of the Institute of Society,

Ethics and the Life Sciences that no one will falsely be pronounced in irreversible coma. In 128 patients who underwent autopsy, the brain was found to be "obviously destroyed" in each case.[14] Of 2650 patients with isoelectric EEGs of twenty-four hours' duration, not one patient recovered ("excepting three who had received anesthetic doses of CNS depressants, and who were, therefore, outside the class of patients covered by the report").[15]

What then is the relationship between the more inclusive Harvard criteria and the simple use of electrocerebral silence as measured by an isoelectric or flat electroencephalogram? The former might be appropriate for those who associate death with the disappearance of any neurological function of the brain. For those who hold the narrower concept based simply on consciousness or capacity for social interaction, however, the Harvard criteria may suffer from exactly the same problem as the old heart- and lung-oriented criteria. With those criteria, every patient whose circulatory and respiratory function had ceased was indeed dead, but the criteria might be too conservative, in that some patients dead according to the "loss of bodily integrating capacity" concept of death (for which the brain is the corresponding locus) would be found alive according to heart- and lung-oriented criteria. It might also happen that some patients who should be declared dead according to the irreversible loss of consciousness and social interaction concept would be found to be alive according to the Harvard criteria.[16] All discussions of the neurological criteria fail to consider that the criteria might be too inclusive, too conservative. The criteria might, therefore, give rise to classifying patients as dead according to the consciousness or social-interaction conception, but as alive according to the full Harvard criteria.

A report in *Lancet* by the British physician J. B. Brierley and his colleagues implies this may indeed be the case.[17] In two cases in which patients had undergone cardiac arrest resulting in brain damage, they report, "the electroencephalogram (strictly defined) was isoelectric throughout. Spontaneous respiration was resumed almost at once in case 2, but not until day 21 in case 1." [18] They report that the first patient did not "die" until five months later. For the second patient they report, "The Patient died on day 153." Presumably in both cases they were using the traditional heart and lung locus and correlated criteria for death as they pronounced it. They report that subsequent detailed neuropathological analysis confirmed that the "neocortex was dead while certain brainstem and spinal centers remained intact." These intact centers specifically involved the functions of spontaneous breathing and reflexes: eye-opening, yawning, and "certain reflex activities at brain-stem and spinal cord levels." As evidence that lower brain activity remained, they report that an electroretinogram (measuring electrical activity of the eye) in patient 1 was normal on day 13. After day 49 there still remained reactivity of the pupils to light in addition to spontaneous respiration.

If this evidence is sound, it strongly suggests that it is empirically as well as theoretically possible to have irreversible loss of cortical function (and therefore loss of consciousness) while lower brain functions remain intact.

This leaves us with the empirical question of the proper criteria for the irreversible loss of consciousness which is thought to have its locus in the neocortex of the cerebrum. Brierley and his colleagues suggest that the EEG alone (excluding the other three criteria of the Harvard report) measures the activity of the neocortex.[19] Presumably this test must also meet the carefully specified conditions of amplifier gain, repeat of the test after a given time period, and exclusion of the exceptional cases, if it is to be used as the criterion for death according to our fourth concept, irreversible loss of capacity for social interaction. The empirical evidence is not all in, but it would seem that the 2650 cases of flat EEG without recovery which are cited to support the Harvard criteria would also be persuasive preliminary empirical evidence for the use of the EEG alone as empirical evidence for the irreversible loss of consciousness and social interaction which (presumably) have their locus in the neocortex. What these 2650 cases would have to include for the data to be definitive would be a significant number of Brierley-type patients where the EEG criteria were met without the other Harvard criteria being met. This is a question for the neurophysiologists to resolve.

There is another problem with the use of electroencephalogram, angiography, or other techniques for measuring cerebral function as a criterion for the irreversible loss of consciousness. Once again we must face the problem of a false positive diagnosis of life. The old heart and lung criteria may provide a false positive diagnosis for a holder of the bodily integrating capacity concept, and the Harvard criteria may give false positive indications for a holder of the consciousness or social interaction concept. Could a person have electroencephalographic activity but still have no capacity for consciousness or social interaction? Whether this is possible empirically is difficult to say, but at least theoretically there are certainly portions of the neocortex which could be functioning and presumably be recorded on an electroencephalogram without the individual having any capacity for consciousness. For instance, what if through an accident or vascular occlusion the motor cortex remained viable but the sensory cortex did not? Even the most narrow criterion of the electroencephalogram alone may still give false positive diagnoses of living for holders of the social interaction concept.

COMPLEXITIES IN MATCHING CONCEPTS WITH LOCI AND CRITERIA

It has been our method throughout this paper to identify four major concepts of death and then to determine, primarily by examining the empirical evidence, what the corresponding loci and criteria might be. But there are good reasons why the holders of a particular concept of death might not want to adopt the corresponding criteria as the means of determining the status of a given patient. These considerations are primarily pragmatic and empirical. In the first place, as a matter of policy we would not want to have to apply the Harvard criteria before pronouncing death while standing before every clearly dead body. It is not usually necessary to use such technical measures as an EEG, whether one holds the fluid-flow concept, the loss of bodily integration concept, or the loss of social interaction concept.

Reliance on the old circulatory and respiratory criteria in cases where the individual is obviously dead may be justified in either of two ways. First, there is the option implied in the new Kansas statute . . . of maintaining two operating concepts of death, either of which will be satisfactory. This appears, however, to be philosophically unsound, since it means that a patient could be simultaneously dead and alive. If the philosophical arguments for either of the neurological concepts are convincing, and I think they are, we should not have to fall back on the fluid-flow concept for pronouncing death in the ordinary case.

A second way to account for the use of the heart- and lung-oriented criteria is that they do indeed correlate empirically with the neurological concepts. When there is no circulatory or respiratory activity for a sufficient time, there is invariably a loss of capacity for bodily integration or capacity for consciousness or social interaction. Using circulatory and respiratory activity as tests is crude, and in some cases the presence of such activity will lead to a false positive diagnosis of life; but the prolonged absence of circulation and respiration is a definitive diagnosis of death even according to the neurologically oriented concepts. Their use is thus an initial shortcut; if these criteria are met, one need not go on to the other criteria for the purpose of pronouncing death. This would appear to be a sound rationale for continuing the use of the old criteria of respiratory and circulatory activity.

A second practical difficulty is inherent in correlating concept and criteria. Let us examine this by asking why one might not wish at this time to adopt the EEG alone as a definitive criterion for pronouncing death. There are two possible reasons. First, quite obviously, there will be those who do not accept the correlated concept of death. They reject the irreversible loss of the capacity for consciousness or social interaction in favor of the irreversible loss of capacity for bodily integration or for fluid flow. Second, there are those who accept the concept of irreversible loss of consciousness or social interaction, but still are not convinced that the EEG unfailingly predicts this. If and when they can be convinced that the EEG alone accurately predicts irreversible loss of consciousness or social interaction without any false diagnosis of death, they will adopt it as the criterion. In the meantime they would logically continue to advocate the concept

TABLE 1   LEVELS OF THE DEFINITION OF DEATH

Formal Definition: Death means a complete change in the status of a living entity characterized by the irreversible loss of those characteristics that are essentially significant to it.

Concept of death: philosophical or theological judgment of the essentially significant change at death	*Locus of death:* place to look to determine if a person has died	*Criteria of death:* measurements physicians or other officials use to determine whether a person is dead—to be determined by scientific empirical study
1. The irreversible stopping of the flow of "vital" body fluids, i.e., the blood and breath	Heart and lungs	1. Visual observation of respiration, perhaps with the use of a mirror 2. Feeling of the pulse, possibly supported by electrocardiogram
2. The irreversible loss of the soul from the body	The pineal body? (according to Descartes) The respiratory tract?	Observation of breath?
3. The irreversible loss of the capacity for bodily integration and social interaction	The brain	1. Unreceptivity and unresponsivity 2. No movements or breathing 3. No reflexes (except spinal reflexes) 4. Flat electroencephalogram (to be used as confirmatory evidence) —All tests to be repeated 24 hours later (excluded conditions: hypothermia and central nervous system drug depression)
4. Irreversible loss of consciousness or the capacity for social interaction	Probably the neocortex	Electroencephalogram

Note: The possible concepts, loci, and criteria of death are much more complex than the ones given here. These are meant to be simplified models of types of positions being taken in the current debate. It is obvious that those who believe that death means the irreversible loss of the capacity for bodily integration (3) or the irreversible loss of consciousness (4) have no reservations about pronouncing death when the heart and lungs have ceased to function. This is because they are willing to use loss of heart and lung activity as shortcut criteria for death, believing that once heart and lungs have stopped, the brain or neocortex will necessarily stop as well.

while adhering to the more conservative Harvard criteria, which appear to measure the loss of whole brain function. Since the distinction is a new one and the empirical evidence may not yet be convincing, it is to be expected that many holders of this concept will, for the time being and as a matter of policy, prefer the Harvard Committee's older and more conservative criteria for determining death. The entire analysis of the four levels of definition presented thus far is summarized in Table 1.

Notes

1. "Clear MD's in 'Living' Donor Case," *New York Post,* May 26, 1972, p. 2.

2. Richmond Stanfield Frederick, "Medical Jurisprudence—Determining the Time of Death of the Heart Transplant Donor," 51 *North Carolina Law Review* 172–84 (1972). For another review of the case see Ronald Converse, "But *When* Did He Die?: *Tucker* v. *Lower* and the Brain-Death Concept," 12 *San Diego Law Review* 424–35 (1975).

3. Ad Hoc Committee of the Harvard Medical School to Examine the Definition of Brain Death, "A Definition of Irreversible Coma," *Journal of the American Medical Association,* 205 (1968), 337–40.

4. Henry K. Beecher, "The New Definition of Death, Some Opposing Views," unpublished paper presented at the meeting of the American Association for the Advancement of Science, December 1970, p. 2.

5. J. B. Brierley, J. A. H. Adams, D. I. Graham, and J. A. Simpson, "Neocortical Death after Cardiac Arrest," *Lancet* (September 11, 1971), pp. 560–65.

6. Beecher, "The New Definition of Death," p. 4.

7. René Descartes, "The Passions of the Soul," in *The Philosophical Works of Descartes,* vol. 1 (Cambridge: Cambridge University Press, 1911), p. 345.

8. Beecher, "The New Definition of Death," p. 2.

9. Brierley et al., "Neocortical Death."

10. Ad Hoc Committee of the Harvard Medical School, "A Definition of Irreversible Coma," pp. 337–38.

11. James F. Toole, "The Neurologist and the Concept of Brain Death," *Perspectives in Biology and Medicine,* Summer 1971, p. 602.

12. G. E. W. Wolstenholme and Maeve O'Connor, eds., *Ethics in Medical Progress: With Special Reference to Transplantation* (Boston: Little, Brown, 1966), p. 69.

13. *Ibid.,* p. 71.

14. Task Force on Death and Dying of the Institute of Society, Ethics, and the Life Sciences, "Refinements in Criteria for the Determination of Death: An Appraisal," *Journal of the American Medical Association,* 221 (1972), 50–51.

15. Daniel Silverman, Richard L. Masland, Michael G. Saunders, and Robert S. Schwab, "Irreversible Coma Associated with Electrocerebral Silence," *Neurology,* 20 (1970), 525–33.

16. The inclusion of absence of breathing and reflexes in the criteria suggests

this, but does not necessarily lead to this. It might be that, empirically, it is necessary for lower brain reflexes and breathing to be absent for twenty-four hours in order to be sure that the patient not only will never regain these functions but will never regain consciousness.

17. Brierley et al., "Neocortical Death." See also Ricardo Ceballos and Samuel C. Little, "Progressive Electroencephalographic Changes in Laminar Necrosis of the Brain," *Southern Medical Journal,* 64 (1971), 1370–76.
18. *Ibid.,* p. 560.
19. Brierley et al., "Neocortical Death."

In the following selection Robert Schwager considers the views of both Paul Ramsey and Veatch—Ramsey sympathetically and Veatch critically. Like the Harvard Committee, Schwager concentrates on the irreversibly comatose, where removal from an artificial respirator results in death. He is interested not only in the definition of death but equally in the related question of whether turning off respirators is killing patients, allowing them to die, or merely disconnecting a machine from a dead body. Schwager argues: (1) that when cerebral activity has been totally destroyed the patient is dead, so that disconnecting a respirator is *not* allowing the patient to die, but (2) that when there remains some cerebral capacity (even in irreversibly comatose patients), the patient is alive, so that to disconnect the respirator is to allow those individuals to die. Schwager then considers Veatch's view that even when there is some cerebral activity, the person is dead if there is neocortex death. He criticizes Veatch's view as both too conservative and too radical. It is too conservative because there are justifying reasons for discontinuing treatment other than the death of a person; and it is too radical in permitting the burial of individuals who have independently functioning heartbeat and respiration.

Robert L. Schwager

LIFE, DEATH, AND THE IRREVERSIBLY COMATOSE *

Medical science has truly awesome power to do battle with death and disease. From prenatal diagnosis to the latest improvements in resuscitative technique, from the development of vaccines to the therapeutic use of organ transplantation, medicine has worked miracles in saving human beings from crippling disease and early death. Unfortunately, every silver lining is attached to a cloud. In the case of medical science, the same techniques that prevent death and allow recovery from hithertofore fatal conditions are often used to maintain life in those who can never recover from their diseases, illnesses, or injuries. Cardiac resuscitative techniques can be used to save patients suffering the agonies of terminal cancer[1] as well as those who have gone on to lead long and satisfying lives. Antibiotics can be used to ward off infection in the permanently moribund as well as to fight strep throat in the otherwise healthy child. And respirators can maintain pulmonary function in the irreversibly comatose as well as the victim of a temporary inability to breathe spontaneously. Thus the very success of modern medical science raises both ethical and legal questions where previously none existed. For in the past the ability to save life was so limited that doing so rarely became problematical. Now, however, our abilities in this area are so prodigious that questions about their appropriate use arise daily.

In this paper I shall discuss some issues that arise in the treatment of the irreversibly comatose. Consider a person who is permanently comatose and for whom removal from an artificial respirator means death. In connection with this example, suppose societal agreement has been reached on three related issues. First, it is neither morally nor legally permissible to kill a patient. Second, removing a patient from life-support systems is not in all cases to kill that patient.[2] Third, it is morally and legally permissible to allow the irreversibly comatose patient to be removed from a respirator. I do not claim that such societal agreement is to be found, though the decision of the New Jersey Supreme Court in the case of Karen Ann Quinlan, together with the refusal of the United States Supreme Court to review that decision, reflects some degree of support for this claim.[3] Nor do I intend to argue that society ought to agree with these contentions. Rather, my purpose is to examine the implications of these claims for the problem of how to conceptualize turning off the respirator on an irreversibly comatose patient unable to maintain spontaneous respiration. A second purpose is to examine the distinction between ordinary and extraordinary means. Specifically, I am concerned to see if that distinction can serve as a basis for deciding which treatments may be omitted in the case of the irreversibly comatose. I shall argue that it cannot, and that its use is more likely to obscure, rather than illuminate, the true nature of the questions we need to ask about some of the situations in which it is customarily invoked.

I

How ought we to conceptualize turning off the respirator in the case of an irreversibly comatose patient who is unable to maintain spontaneous respiration? The assumptions above jointly entail that this is not a case of killing the patient. Since it is both morally and legally permissible to disconnect the respirator in this case, but neither morally nor legally permissible to kill a patient, disconnecting the respirator from a permanently unconscious patient cannot be to kill that patient. This leaves two possibilities. To turn off the respirator may be to allow the patient to die. If so, the patient is alive prior to the disconnection. Since the disconnection will lead to a cessation of breathing, which in turn will lead to the irreversible loss of cardiac and cerebral function, turning off the respirator is, according to this view, allowing death in the traditional sense [4] to occur. The second alternative is to treat disconnecting the respirator as terminating the application of a useless mechanical contrivance to a dead body. In this case we do not cease to treat the patient, since the patient has died prior to the disconnection. Since both respiration and cardiac activity continue after the patient is said to have died, it seems necessary to deny that this death is death in the traditional sense. How, then, can we say that such a patient has died?

To handle this question a distinction must be drawn between two kinds of irreversible coma: that in which the capacity for cerebral activity has been totally destroyed and that in which there remains some such capacity. To simplify matters, I shall refer to individuals irreversibly comatose in the first way as *decerebrate*. Those who are irreversibly comatose without being decerebrate will be referred to as *irreversibly comatose simpliciter (ICS)*. The claims to be defended can be stated as follows: (a) there are good reasons for counting a decerebrate individual as dead, so that disconnecting a respirator is not allowing that patient to die; and (b) those individuals who are ICS are still alive, so that to disconnect the respirator is to allow those individuals to die. (Of course, given the assumptions of this discussion, such a course of action is both morally and legally permissible.)

(a) In 1968 the report of the Ad Hoc Committee of the Harvard Medical School to Examine the Definition of Brain Death appeared under the rather misleading title "A Definition of Irreversible Coma." [5] The report indicates that its "primary purpose is to define irreversible coma as a new criterion of death." [6] In the second paragraph, however, the report makes it clear that it is concerned only with decerebrate individuals.[7] After setting out "the characteristics of a *permanently* nonfunctioning brain," [8] the report recommends that decerebrate individuals be declared dead prior to removing the respirator. Though recognizing that both respiration and circulation, the usual signs of life, can be present in a decerebrate patient maintained on a respirator, the report states that if its recommendation "is adopted by the medical community, it can form the basis for a change in the current legal concept of death. No statutory change in the law should be necessary, since the law treats this question essentially as one of fact to be determined by physicians." [9]

Since 1968 a number of states have enacted statutes giving legislative sanction to the idea that a decerebrate individual is dead.[10] In California, a court refused to agree with an accused murderer that it was the act of transplanting to another the heart of the decerebrate victim which had caused the victim's death. The court ruled that the decerebrate victim was dead when the surgeon removed his heart.[11] Thus the last decade has seen a substantial trend toward counting the decerebrate as dead.

The Harvard report recommended that a declaration of death be made prior to disconnecting the respirator. One reason for this was to emphasize that the report deals with determining that one has died as opposed to when it is legitimate to allow death to occur. An example of the confusion that results when these two different matters are run together is the following recommendation by Dr. Martin Halley and Professor William Harvey:

> We propose this general definition of human death: Death is irreversible cessation of *all* of the following: (1) total cerebral function, (2) spontaneous function of the respiratory system, and (3) spontaneous function of the circulatory system.
>
> Special circumstances may, however, justify the pronouncement of death when consultations consistent with established professional standards have been obtained and when valid consent to withhold or stop resuscitative measures has been given by the appropriate relative or legal guardian.[12]

The special circumstances referred to are essentially those of a decerebrate patient maintained on a respirator. There the authors would countenance a declaration of death. This is permissible, however, only if valid consent to turn off the respirator has been given. But if the patient is *dead,* then why should any consent be necessary? On the other hand, if such consent is really necessary, how can it be that the patient is dead? Where it is necessary to seek "consent to withhold or stop resuscitative measures," withholding or stopping such measures is allowing the patient to die, not giving up because the patient is already dead.

More important, however, is that the authors believe it necessary to treat this case as special. Since a decerebrate individual has undergone irreversible cessation of both total cerebral function and spontaneous function of the respiratory system ("Actual or recoverable respiratory function is always a test for a still-functioning brain"),[13] what makes this a special case, presumably, is the presence of spontaneous activity of the circulatory system. In placing such emphasis on the circulatory system, the authors' position is consistent with Paul Ramsey's view (with which I concur) that "the presence or absence of truly spontaneous cardiac activity . . . ought not hastily to be removed from our tests of whether a man is still alive or has died." [14] In treating this as a special case of *death,* however, the authors muddy the waters by neglecting Ramsey's warning that "it would be far more reasonable to open decisively the question under what conditions and by what means we should continue 'heroic' efforts to save life than by an intellectual tour de force to pronounce a man dead whose heart still beats spontaneously." [15]

Having cited with approval Ramsey's claim that spontaneous heart function is a sign of life, and having criticized Halley and Harvey for their failure to separate questions of when death has occurred from questions concerning allowing patients to die, I would appear to be backing away from the claim that the decerebrate patient is dead. Appearances, however, are deceptive, the more so because I am also willing to accept the general definition of death proposed by Halley and Harvey. The reason why accepting their definition of death, together with Ramsey's point about spontaneous heart function as a sign of life, does not involve withdrawing the claim that a decerebrate individual is dead, is that (like Ramsey) I do not believe that the decerebrate individual has truly spontaneous circulatory function.

For consider the following extreme case. It has proved possible to maintain both respiration and circulation in the body of an individual who had been decapitated.[16] Now suppose respiration was maintained by the use of an artificial respirator while no further contrivances were necessary to stimulate cardiovascular function. If such circulatory activity were to count as spontaneous, and thus as a sign of life, we should be forced to say that death had not yet taken place and that the individual, *sans* head, was still alive. But this is absurd. Where there has been an irreversible cessation of natural, spontaneous cerebral and pulmonary function, so that circulatory activity continues only because artificial respiration continues to oxygenate the blood, such circulatory activity is neither truly spontaneous nor a sign of life. Where irreversible cessation of total brain activity has occurred, the absence of "recoverable capacity to breathe by . . . [oneself precludes the existence of] recoverable permanent capacity to circulate [oneself]." [17] Thus circulation is no more spontaneous here than is respiration. This is obscured by our failure to realize that the absence of a direct mechanical aid to circulation, such as a heart-lung machine, does not guarantee the spontaneity of that circulation. And once this is understood, we see that the real upshot of the Harvard Committee's recommendation is not really a new definition of death, but rather "a return to a rather traditionalistic understanding of the procedure for stating that a man has died." [18]

(b) Now consider the individual who is irreversibly comatose simpliciter (ICS). ICS individuals fall into two classes: those in whom irreversible neocortical destruction (neocortical death) has been established (perhaps by use of an EEG together with "a biopsy specimen . . . taken from the posterior half of a cerebral hemisphere") [19] and those in whom the neocortex retains some functional capacity. In what follows, I should be understood as referring to those ICS individuals who have undergone neocortical death. By "neocortical death" I mean a state in which, though brain-stem activity remains, the neocortex is irreversibly and totally non-functional.

In recent years, a number of suggestions have been made to extend the definition of death to include those who have undergone neocortical death but are not decerebrate.[20] Since ICS individuals might maintain both spontaneous respiration and circulation, critics of this further updating have appealed to our basic intuitions concerning the presence of spontaneous respiration. Henry Beecher, chairman of the Harvard Committee, said: "Although some have attempted to make a case for the concept of a corpse as one who is unconscious and suffering from incurable brain damage, one can nevertheless orient the situation swiftly by a simple wry question: 'Would you bury such a man whose heart was beating?' "[21] Since burying a person attached to a respirator is too bizarre to contemplate, we must assume that Beecher was not referring to patients whose hearts continue to beat only because they are supplied with oxygen by a respirator.

Our reluctance to bury the spontaneously breathing is important in considering whether to count the ICS as dead. This point is ignored by Robert M. Veatch when he recommends that we adopt a concept of death which includes the ICS. After suggesting a *formal* definition of death as "the irreversible loss of that which is essentially significant to the nature of man," [22] he reminds us that a finding of human death is much more than a statement of biological fact.[23] Veatch treats a pronouncement of death as a justification for stopping treatments that until then remained obligatory and the initiation of steps leading to burial, cremation, etc. When combined with his contention that the ICS can be considered dead, this set of claims is at once too conservative and too radical. It is too conservative in asserting that *only* the death of the patient justifies discontinuing certain medical treatments; it is too radical in permitting the burial of individuals who respirate and circulate themselves. I shall return to this point.

After giving his formal definition of death, Veatch examines different material concepts. The earliest was the separation of the soul from the body. This was replaced by one equating death with "the irreversible loss of the ability of the body to maintain the flowing of vital fluids, i.e., the blood and the breath." [24] More recently, he claims, our idea of death has shifted to neurological criteria supported by the concept of "the capacity to integrate bodily functioning through the neurological system" [25] as what is essentially significant to man's nature. Veatch traces this shift to the false positives produced by the heart-lung criteria. For similar reasons he advocates adopting "irreversible loss of the capacity for experience or social interaction" [26] as our concept of death. This would eliminate what false positives remain under the neurologically based whole-brain criteria by allowing death to be declared whenever an individual is ICS. Veatch argues that once you elect to move away from the heart-lung concept of death to a brain-oriented one, there can be no good reason for requiring *total* cessation of brain activity as opposed to total cessation of the kind of brain activity that controls consciousness.

There may be good reasons for agreeing with Veatch that *if* we ought to move away from the earlier understanding of death to one that is brain-oriented, there is little sense in requiring total loss of cerebral function. What ought not to be agreed with, however, is his claim that this is the correct way to characterize the recent updating of death. As was argued above, using total cessation of cerebral function to determine death in the presence of artificially maintained respiration and superficially natural circulation is a way of applying the older concept of death that treated spontaneous respiration and spontaneous circulation as signs of life. Thus the underlying concept of death remains unchanged. What changes are the criteria for deciding that death has taken place. Rather than turning off the respirator and waiting for the heart to stop beating, death can be pronounced while heartbeat continues, since, given the total and irreversible loss of cerebral function, *that* heartbeat is no sign of life. But where cerebral function has not irreversibly ceased, a patient removed from a respirator will attempt to breathe. Where efforts at breathing continue, heartbeat is a sign of life and using the respirator is not maintaining the illusion of life in a corpse. Thus removing the respirator from ICS patients who cannot maintain spontaneous respiration is allowing them to die and not removing useless mechanical contrivances from dead bodies. Furthermore, since death will not be pronounced in the presence of truly spontaneous heartbeat, there can be no problem of initiating death behavior toward ICS individuals who maintain respiration and heartbeat without the help of a respirator.

But ought we to change our concept of death as Veatch recommends? I think not. First, because to do so would on certain occasions lead to declaring dead individuals maintaining spontaneous respiration and heartbeat, with all the problems attendant thereunto. Second, and more significant, to do so would be to underplay the importance of the human body in our idea of ourselves. Indeed, one problem with the concept of death as the departure of the soul from the body is that it gives too short shrift to bodily functioning. While I would agree that what gives human life its *value* is the capacity for experience and/or social interaction, the loss of what gives life its value is not identical with the loss of life. It may, however, be identical with the loss of any good reason for striving to preserve that life, which brings us back to what I have called the overly conservative, yet too radical, nature of Veatch's position.

One possible response to my claim is this. Consider those ICS individuals with spontaneous respiration and heartbeat. On the heart-lung concept they are alive. Since consciousness has been irreversibly lost, it is not obligatory to continue extraordinary treatments, e.g., a respirator. However, since they are still alive, ordinary treatments, e.g., intravenous feeding and antibiotics, must be continued, for to discontinue them would be to kill the patient, which is forbidden. But if they are counted as dead, heartbeat and respiration can be stopped, which in turn will lead to the irreversible loss of remaining cerebral function. Once these have all ended, the corpse can be prepared for burial. So, this argument concludes, the existence of ICS individuals with spontaneous respiration and heartbeat is really a reason in favor of an experience-oriented concept of death.

This argument presupposes that some treatments may only be stopped when the patient has died, which is just the overly conservative element of Veatch's position. It also uses the distinction between ordinary and extraordinary means to determine which treatments may be omitted and which may not. In this respect it is not unlike many other arguments in the philosophical and medical literature on the treatment of the terminally ill, which makes it of interest in its own right. What I shall argue is that the ordinary-extraordinary distinction cannot serve as the basis for this decision, and that any and all treatments may be omitted in the case of the ICS.

II

If the ordinary-extraordinary distinction is to determine what treatments may be omitted, then some way of deciding which treatments are which must be found. Furthermore, if that distinction is to be used to show that some treatments may not be dispensed with until death has occurred, there must be some procedures whose use is ordinary for any patient for whom they are medically indicated. For if there were no such treatments, then either all treatments would be dispensable or the ordinary-extraordinary distinction would not serve to distinguish indispensable treatments from dispensable ones.

One way to understand the ordinary-extraordinary distinction is by reference to customary medical practice.[27] On this view it might seem that there would be little difficulty in determining which treatments are and which are not extraordinary. Yet this was one of the problems facing the medical community in the Karen Quinlan case. When it was generally believed that Ms. Quinlan could not live without continued use of a respirator, there was no medical consensus about its status in her situation. When the respirator proved dispensable, the lack of consensus "shifted" to the use of antibiotics and forced feedings. Thus, if the ordinary-extraordinary distinction is identical with the distinction between customary and unusual medical practice, there seems to be no real agreement as to what constitutes customary practice. Alternatively, the lack of agreement as to what is to count as ordinary or extraordinary may indicate that more is at issue than customary medical practice.

The main problem with basing the ordinary-extraordinary distinction on customary medical practice is that as such it is singularly ill-suited to the role it is supposed to play. For suppose all physicians agreed that a respirator for an ICS patient is extraordinary, but antibiotics and intravenous feedings are ordinary. If all this means is that physicians customarily discontinue the one but not the others, then what moral and/or legal import does that have? To conclude from the actual behavior of physicians that such behavior is morally justified, or required, is to confer upon them a degree of authority far exceeding that which can be founded on their *medical* expertise. Moreover, physicians' attitudes toward death are such that, as a class, they may be among the least well-equipped members of society to decide when, and in what ways, death should be left unopposed.[28] Thus, if the ordinary-extraordinary distinction rests on customary medical practice, there is little reason to use it to determine which treatments may be omitted in the case of the ICS.

The legal import of this account of the distinction is much more obscure. It has been argued that what counts as an omission, as opposed to an action, and thus as a letting die rather than a killing, depends upon the relationship of physician to patient, which depends upon the patient's expectations. "Those expectations, in turn, are a function of the practices prevailing in the community at the time, and practices in the use of respirators to prolong life are no more and no less than what doctors do in the time and place."[29] Assuming that it is both morally and legally wrong to kill a patient, on this view of the legal situation, what physicians customarily do will serve as the basis in law for deciding which treatments may be omitted.

On the other hand, in the decade since this argument was advanced, the law has moved away from allowing what is customary to settle the legal status of medical practices.[30] Coupled with society's increased willingness to face up to death and dying, this makes it unlikely that pointing to customary medical practice will settle legal issues that arise concerning the duty to continue treatments for the ICS patient. As society confronts death in relation to modern medicine, customary medical practice must adjust to society's values. So it will be the values of society, and not customary medical practice *per se,* that will resolve the legal questions arising from treatment of the terminally ill, including the ICS.

The second way in which the ordinary-extraordinary distinction has been understood equates ordinary means with morally required means and extraordinary means with those that need not be initiated or continued.[31] Understood in this way, it cannot serve as the basis for deciding which treatments may and which may not be omitted. For on this view, to say that a treatment is extraordinary is just to say that it may be omitted. To offer its extraordinary nature as a *reason* for omitting it would be to say that it may be omitted because it may be omitted.

To avoid this circularity we must find some set of features reference to which will decide which treatments are ordinary and which extraordinary. But what will this accomplish? These features must be the same ones that justify omitting procedures deemed extraordinary and mandate using those deemed ordinary. But if this is so, why not simply ask what factors need to be considered in deciding when, if ever, life-preserving procedures may be omitted? Having answered *this* question, we will know what to look for when deciding to continue or initiate some procedure that has been called into question on moral grounds. Going on to characterize the procedure as extraordinary does not advance our understanding of the situation one bit.

More important, however, is the likelihood that such a characterization will obscure the real nature of the problem. Where we think of its extraordinary character when deciding not to use a treatment, there is a danger of thinking that just referring to it as extraordinary explains why it need not be used. This can lead to a failure to appreciate the real basis of the decision, which can cause trouble in a rapidly changing environment. And this problem is compounded by the fact that, as ordinarily used, the word "extraordinary" just *means* "unusual or out of the ordinary" while the word "ordinary" means "customary, normal, regular, or usual." For this means that the temptation to identify ordinary as opposed to extraordinary in terms of the usual rather than the unusual is ever present. Indeed, when a writer as careful as Paul Ramsey can, without warning, use the terms in different ways in successive paragraphs,[32] one can sympathize with the careful reader if by the end of a typical discussion of the subject he is inclined to think that deciding how many angels can fit on the head of a pin is probably simpler.

To recapitulate. If the ordinary-extraordinary distinction is relative to customary medical practice, it cannot establish that some procedures must be used until the patient dies. If it is the distinction between obligatory and elective means, then it cannot *justify* the use or omission of certain procedures. So whichever alternative one chooses, Veatch's claim that there are certain treatments which may not be stopped prior to the patient's death cannot be supported by appeal to this distinction. What is needed to assess his claim on its own merits is a complete discussion of the conditions, if any, under which patients may be allowed to die and how this may be accomplished. This is neither the time nor the place to enter into such a discussion.

One thing, however, can be said, and it should suffice for our limited purposes. Since Veatch claims that the ICS have lost what is essentially significant to the nature of man, it is difficult to see how *he* could disagree with the judgment that such persons, if not yet dead, are leading lives devoid of any of the features that give life its value. For if there were anything of value left to such persons, how could they be dead? Only if life itself is so sacred that everything must be done to preserve it, can such a life retain value to the individual. So once it is assumed that any patients may be allowed to die in some ways (e.g., by disconnecting the respirator), it becomes impossible to defend adequately the claim that certain means of preserving life must be employed to the end on ICS patients. But this means that for the ICS patient with both spontaneous respiration and circulation, it is permissible to discontinue the feedings and antibiotics that sustain his life. Once this occurs, he will soon die and appropriate death behavior can commence. Thus the plight of ICS patients with spontaneous respiration and heartbeat is no reason for adopting the experience-oriented concept of death under which they would be considered dead. I conclude, therefore, that our concept of death is such that to disconnect the respirator from an ICS patient who cannot maintain spontaneous respiration is to allow that patient to die and not to discontinue the application of a useless mechanical contrivance to a corpse.

I have argued that if we assume that killing patients is forbidden, that not all cases of removing patients from life-support systems are cases of killing, and that the irreversibly comatose may be removed from the respirator, then (a) to remove the decerebrate patient from the respirator is to discontinue the application of a useless mechanical contrivance to a dead body, and (b) to remove the ICS patient who cannot maintain spontaneous respiration from the respirator is to allow him to die. In response to an objection to the second claim, I argued that the ordinary-extraordinary distinction cannot serve as the basis for deciding which treatments may be omitted and that in the case of the ICS all treatments are dispensable. Some might wish to go further and argue that it is morally permissible not only to discontinue treatments of the ICS, but also actively to intervene to bring about death. This further claim is beyond the scope of the present discussion.

Notes

1. A. W. Campbell, *Moral Dilemmas in Medicine* (London, 1972), pp. 90–91.
2. See George P. Fletcher, "Prolonging Life," 42 *Washington Law Review*

999–1016 (1967), and "Legal Aspects of the Decision Not to Prolong Life," *Journal of the American Medical Association*, 203, no. 1 (1968), 65–68.

3. See *In The Matter of Karen Quinlan*, Vol. II (Arlington, Va., 1976).

4. "Death is the cessation of life; the ceasing to exist; defined by physicians as a total stoppage of the circulation of the blood, and a cessation of the animal and vital functions consequent thereon, such as respiration, pulsation, etc." (*Black's Law Dictionary*, 4th ed., 1951). *Smith* v. *Smith*, 229 Ark. 579, 317 S.W.2d 275, 279 (1958); *Thomas* v. *Anderson*, Cal. App. 2d 371, 215 P.2d 478, 481 (1950).

   For a discussion of the traditional definition of death, see M. Martin Halley and William F. Harvey, "Medical v. Legal Definitions of Death," *JAMA*, 204, no. 6 (1968), 423–25.

5. *JAMA*, 205, no. 6 (1968), 337–40.

6. *Ibid.*, p. 337.

7. "Irreversible coma has many causes, but *we are concerned here only with those comatose individuals who have no discernible central nervous system activity." Ibid.*, p. 337.

8. *Ibid.*

9. *Ibid.*, p. 339.

10. Since 1968 at least eleven states have passed definition-of-death statutes. They are Alaska, California, Illinois, Indiana, Kansas, Maryland, New Mexico, Oklahoma, Tennessee, Virginia, and West Virginia.

11. *People* v. *Lyons*, 15 Crim. L. Ref. 2240 (Cal. Sup. Ct., May 21, 1974). A similar decision was reached in *State* v. *Brown*, 8 Or. App., 491 P.2d 1193 (Ct. App. 1971).

12. Halley and Harvey, *op. cit.*, p. 425.

13. Paul Ramsey, *The Patient as Person* (New Haven, 1970), p. 97.

14. *Ibid.*, pp. 76–77.

15. *Ibid.*, p. 77.

16. Gordon Wolstenholme and Maeve O'Connor, eds., *Law and Ethics of Transplantation* (London, 1966), p. 100.

17. Ramsey, *op. cit.*, p. 67.

18. *Ibid.*, p. 68. It should be noted that I do not claim that the Harvard Committee would agree with this interpretation of its report. This does not, however, seem to be a serious obstacle to accepting the interpretation offered by Ramsey.

19. J. B. Brierly, et al., "Neocortical Death after Cardiac Arrest," *The Lancet* (September 11, 1971), p. 565.

20. See Brierly, *op. cit.*, p. 564; Joseph Fletcher, "Indicators of Humanhood: A Tentative Profile of Man," *Hastings Center Report*, 2 (November 1972), 1–4; and Robert M. Veatch, "The Whole Brain-Oriented Concept of Death: An Outmoded Philosophical Formulation," *Journal of Thanatology*, 3 (1975), 13–30.

21. Henry K. Beecher, "Ethical Problems Created by the Hopelessly Unconscious Patient," *New England Journal of Medicine*, 278 (1968), 1426.

22. Veatch, *op. cit.*, p. 14.

23. "When we speak of human death . . . we are making a practical statement with policy implications. We are saying that it is now appropriate to behave toward the individual in a different way. It is now appropriate to stop certain medical treatments which could not justifiably have been stopped previously. It is appropriate to begin burial ritual and for the deceased's friends and family to begin the mourning process." *Ibid.*, p. 14.

24. *Ibid.*, p. 19.

25. *Ibid.*

26. *Ibid.*, p. 23.

27. For example, "In the past, these decisions were not so difficult because there were few effective extraordinary means of preserving life. They do exist now. Transfusions were extraordinary years ago. Respirators and pacemakers, extraordinary a short time ago, now are widely applied. The wise pronouncement of Pope Pius XII in 1957, which indicated that physicians were obligated to use all ordinary means of preserving life, but not necessarily those that were extraordinary, should offer helpful clarification of these difficulties. Yet, what is extraordinary today? And, if it is, will it be commonplace tomorrow?" Howard P. Lewis, "Machine Medicine and Its Relation to the Fatally Ill," *JAMA*, 206, no. 2 (1968), 308.

28. See Herman Feifel et al., "Physicians Consider Death," *Proceedings*, American Psychological Association Convention, 1967, pp. 201–2.

29. Fletcher, "Prolonging Life," p. 1015.

30. See Charles H. Montange, "Informed Consent and the Dying Patient," 83 *Yale Law Journal* 1632–64 (1974).

31. For example, "Past moralists, in bringing principles to cases like this one, used the term 'ordinary means' to save life as an ethical category; it *meant* imperative means. They used the term 'extraordinary means' as a term of moral permission; it *meant* electable or morally dispensable means." Ramsey, "Prolonged Dying: Not Medically Indicated," *Hastings Center Report*, 6 (February 1976), 14.

32. " 'Ordinary' or imperative, and 'extraordinary' or only elective treatments are, as we have seen, not fixed categories," and, "If in the case of terminal patients the quality of life they can expect enters into the determination of whether even ordinary or customary measures would be beneficial and should or should not be used. . . ." Ramsey, *The Patient as Person*, pp. 131, 132.

We have seen several attempts either to revise the definition of death or at least to show serious problems in the more traditional formulations. In the following article, Hans Jonas stands against these revisionary tendencies. His title, "Against the Stream," reflects his belief that there is a tide in the direction of revising the definition—a tide that ought to be resisted. On the other hand, Jonas is also critical of the Harvard Committee list of criteria, which he believes to be criteria for permitting death to take place unopposed, rather than criteria of death itself. Jonas sees no sharp borderline (medical or otherwise) between life and death, doubts that the requirement of *spontaneous* functioning is useful, and sees much of the "definition" debate as covertly asking what should be done with the patient rather than whether the patient is dead. Also, unlike Veatch and others, Jonas does not see reference either to central nervous system functioning or brain functioning as directly relevant to the problem of a *definition* of death. He sees in modern technology only new capacities for sustaining life, not new ways of determining death. Indeed, he thinks such capacities might easily lead to premature declarations of death, especially where there is need for transplant organs. Consequently, he tends toward acceptance of the conservative or traditional list of medical criteria for the *determination* that death has occurred. He even concludes that "no redefinition of death is needed." Rather, more careful *moral reasoning* about what to do with such patients is needed—not a new *definition*.

Hans Jonas

AGAINST THE STREAM:
COMMENTS ON THE DEFINITION
AND REDEFINITION OF DEATH *

The by now famous "Report of the Ad Hoc Committee of the Harvard Medical School to Examine the Definition of Brain Death" advocates the adoption of "irreversible coma as a new definition of death." The report leaves no doubt of the practical reasons "why there is need for a definition," naming these two: relief of patient, kin, and medical resources from the burdens of indefinitely prolonged coma; and removal of controversy on obtaining organs for transplantation. On both counts, the new definition is designed to give the physician the right to terminate the treatment of a condition which not only cannot be improved by such treatment, but whose mere prolongation by it is utterly meaningless to the patient himself. The last consideration, of course, is ultimately the only valid rationale for termination (and for termination only!) and must support all the others. It does so with regard to the reasons mentioned under the first head, for the relief of the patient means automatically also that of his family, doctor, nurses, apparatus, hospital space, and so on. But the other reason—freedom for organ use—has possible implications that are not equally covered by the primary rationale, which is the patient himself. For with this primary rationale (the senselessness of mere vegetative function) the Report has strictly speaking defined not death, the ultimate state, itself, but a criterion

---

* From *Philosophical Essays: From Ancient Creed to Technological Man.* Copyright © 1974 by Hans Jonas. Reprinted by permission of the author.

for permitting it to take place unopposed—e.g., by turning off the respirator. The Report, however, purports by that criterion to have defined death itself, declaring it on its evidence as already given, not merely no longer to be opposed. But if "the patient is declared dead on the basis of these criteria," i.e., if the comatose individual is not a patient at all but a corpse, then the road to other uses of the definition, urged by the second reason, has been opened in principle and will be taken in practice, unless it is blocked in good time by a special barrier. What follows is meant to reinforce what I called "my feeble attempt" to help erect such a barrier on theoretical grounds.

My original comments of 1968 on the then newly proposed "redefinition of death" . . . were marginal to the discussion of "experimentation on human subjects," which has to do with the living and not the dead. They have since, however, drawn fire from within the medical profession, and precisely in connection with the second of the reasons given by the Harvard Committee why a new definition is wanted, namely, the *transplant* interest, which my kind critics felt threatened by my layman's qualms and lack of understanding. Can I take this as corroborating my initial suspicion that this *interest,* in spite of its notably muted expression in the Committee Report, was and is the major motivation behind the definitional effort? I am confirmed in this suspicion when I hear Dr. Henry K. Beecher, author of the Committee's Report (and its Chairman), ask elsewhere: "Can society afford to discard the tissues and organs of the hopelessly unconscious patient when they could be used to restore the otherwise hopelessly ill, but still salvageable individual?" In any case, the tenor and passion of the discussion which my initial polemic provoked from my medical friends left no doubt where the surgeon's interest in the definition lies. I contend that, pure as this interest, viz., to save other lives, is in itself, its intrusion into the *theoretical* attempt to define death makes the attempt impure; and the Harvard Committee should never have allowed itself to adulterate the purity of its scientific case by baiting it with the prospect of this *extraneous* —though extremely appealing—gain. But purity of theory is not my concern here. My concern is with certain practical consequences which under the urgings of that extraneous interest can be drawn from the definition and would enjoy its full sanction, once it has been officially accepted. Doctors would be less than human if certain formidable advantages of such possible consequences would not influence their judgment as to the theoretical adequacy of a definition that yields them—just as I freely admit that my shudder at one aspect of those consequences, and at the danger of others equally sanctioned by that definition, keeps my theoretical skepticism in a state of extreme alertness.

Since the private exchanges referred to (which were conducted in the most amicable spirit of shared concern) somewhat sharpened my theoretical case and in addition brought out some of the apprehensions that haunt me in this matter—and which, I think, should be in everyone's mind before final approval of the new definition takes matters out of our hands— I base the remainder of this paper on a statement titled "Against the Stream" which I circulated among the members of the informal group in question.[1]

I had to answer three charges made à propos of the pertinent part of my *Daedalus* essay: that my reasoning regarding "cadaver donors" counteracts sincere life-saving efforts of physicians; that I counter precise scientific facts with vague philosophical considerations; and that I overlook the difference between death of "the organism as a whole" and death of "the whole organism," with the related difference between spontaneous and externally induced respiratory and other movements.

I plead, of course, guilty to the first charge for the case where the cadaver status of the donor is in question, which is precisely what my argument is about. The use of the term "cadaver donor" here simply begs the question, to which only the third charge (see below) addresses itself.

As to the charge of vagueness, it might just be possible that it vaguely reflects the fact that mine is an argument—a precise argument, I believe— *about* vagueness, viz., the vagueness of a condition. Giving intrinsic vagueness its due is not being vague. Aristotle observed that it is the mark of a well-educated man not to insist on greater precision in knowledge than the subject admits, e.g., the same in politics as in mathematics. Reality of certain kinds—of which the life-death spectrum is perhaps one—may be imprecise in itself, or the knowledge obtainable of it may be. To acknowledge such a state of affairs is more adequate to it than a precise definition, which does violence to it. I am challenging the undue precision of a definition and of its practical application to an imprecise field.

The third point—which was made by Dr. Otto Guttentag—is highly relevant and I will deal with it step by step.

a. The difference between "organism as a whole" and "whole organism" which he has in mind is perhaps brought out more clearly if for "whole organism" we write "every and all parts of the organism." If this is the meaning, then I have been speaking throughout of "death of the organism as a whole," not of "death of the whole organism"; and any ambiguity in my formulations can be easily removed. Local subsystems—single cells or tissues—may well continue to function locally, i.e., to display biochemical activity for themselves (e.g., growth of hair and nails) for some time after death, without this affecting the definition of death by the larger criteria of the whole. But respiration and circulation do not fall into this class, since the effect of their functioning, though performed by subsystems, extends through the total system and insures the functional preservation of its other parts. Why else prolong them artificially in prospective "cadaveric" organ donors (e.g., "maintain renal circulation of cadaver kidneys in situ") except to keep those other parts "in good shape"—viz., alive—for eventual transplantation? The comprehensive system thus sustained is even capable of continued overall metabolism when intravenously fed, and then, presumably, of diverse other (e.g., glandular) functions as well—in fact, I suppose, of pretty much everything not involving neural control. There are stories of comatose patients lingering on for months with those aids; the metaphor of the "human vegetable" recurring in the debate (strangely enough, sometimes in support of redefining death—as if "vegetable" were not an instance of life!) says as much. In short, what is here kept going by various artifices must—with the caution due in this twilight zone—be equated with "the organism as a whole" named in the classical definition of death—much more so, at least, than with any mere, separable part of it.

b. Nor, to my knowledge, does that older definition specify that the functioning whose "irreversible cessation" constitutes death must be spontaneous and does not count for life when artificially induced and sustained (the implications for therapy would be devastating). Indeed, "irreversible" cessation can have a twofold reference: to the function itself or only to the spontaneity of it. A cessation can be irreversible with respect to spontaneity but still reversible with respect to the activity as such—in which case the reversing external agency must continuously substitute for the lost spontaneity. This is the case of the respiratory movements and heart contractions in the comatose. The distinction is not irrelevant, because if we could do for the disabled brain—let's say, the lower nerve centers only—what we can do for the heart and lungs, viz., *make* it work by the continuous input of some external agency (electrical, chemical, or whatever), we would surely do so and not be finicky about the resulting function's lacking spontaneity: the functioning as such would matter. Respirator and stimulator could then be turned off, because the nerve center presiding over heart contractions (etc.) has again taken over and returned *them* to being "spontaneous"—just as systems presided over by circulation had enjoyed spontaneity of function when the circulation was only nonspontaneously active. The case is wholly hypothetical, but I doubt that a doctor would feel at liberty to pronounce the patient dead on the ground of the nonspontaneity at the cerebral source, when it can be *made* to function by an auxiliary device.

The purpose of the foregoing thought-experiment was to cast some doubt (a layman's, to be sure) on the seeming simplicity of the spontaneity criterion. With the stratification and interlocking of functions, it seems to me, organic spontaneity is distributed over many levels and loci—any superordinated level enabling its subordinates to be naturally spontaneous, be its own action natural or artificial.

c. The point with irreversible coma as defined by the Harvard group, of course, is precisely that it is a condition which precludes reactivation of any part of the brain in *every* sense. We then have an "organism as a whole" minus the brain, maintained in some partial state of life so long as the respirator and other artifices are at work. And here the question is not: has the patient died? but: how should he—still a patient—be dealt with? Now *this* question must be settled, surely not by a definition of death, but by a definition of man and of what life is human. That is to say, the question cannot be answered by decreeing that death has already occurred and the body is therefore in the domain of things; rather it is answered by holding, e.g., that it is humanly not justified—let alone, demanded—to artificially prolong the life of a brainless body. This is the answer I myself would advocate. On that philosophical ground, which few will contest, the physician can, indeed should, turn off the respirator and let the "definition of death" take care of itself by what then inevitably happens. (The later utilization of the corpse is a different matter I am not dealing with here, though it too resists the comfortable patness of merely utilitarian answers.) The decision to be made, I repeat, is an axiological one and not already made by clinical fact. It begins when the diagnosis of the condition has spoken: it is not diagnostic itself. Thus, as I have pointed out before, no redefinition of death is needed; only, perhaps, a redefinition of the physician's presumed duty to prolong life under all circumstances.

d. But, it might be asked, is not a definition of death made into law the simpler and more precise way than a definition of medical ethics (which is difficult to legislate) for sanctioning the same practical conclusion, while avoiding the twilight of value judgment and possible legal ambiguity? It would be, if it really sanctioned the same conclusion, and no more. But it sanctions indefinitely more: it opens the gate to a whole range of other possible conclusions, the extent of which cannot even be foreseen, but some of which are disquietingly close at hand. The point is, if the comatose patient is by definition dead, he is a patient no more but a corpse, with which can be done whatever law or custom or the deceased's will or next of kin permit and sundry interests urge doing with a corpse. This includes— why not?—the protracting of the in-between state, for which we must find a new name ("simulated life"?), since that of "life" has been preempted by the new definition of death, and extracting from it all the profit we can. There are many. So far the "redefiners" speak of no more than keeping the respirator going until the transplant organ is to be removed, then turning it off,[2] then beginning to cut into the "cadaver," this being the end of it—which sounds innocent enough. But why must it be the end? Why turn the respirator off? Once we are assured that we are dealing with a cadaver, there are no logical reasons against (and strong pragmatic reasons for) going on with the artificial "animation" and keeping the "deceased's" body on call, as a bank for life-fresh organs, possibly also as a plant for manufacturing hormones or other biochemical compounds in demand. I have no doubts that methods exist or can be perfected which allow the natural powers for the healing of surgical wounds by new tissue growth to stay "alive" in such a body. Tempting also is the idea of a self-replenishing blood bank. And that is not all. Let us not forget research. Why shouldn't the most wonderful surgical and grafting experiments be conducted on the complaisant subject-nonsubject, with no limits set to daring? Why not immunological explorations, infection with diseases old and new, trying out of drugs? We have the active cooperation of a functional organism declared to be dead: we have, that is, the advantages of the living donor without the disadvantages imposed by his rights and interests (for a corpse has none). What a boon for medical instruction, for anatomical and physiological demonstration and practicing on so much better material than the inert cadavers otherwise serving in the dissection room! What a chance for the apprentice to learn *in vivo,* as it were, how to amputate a leg, without his mistakes mattering! And so on, into the wide open field. After all, what is advocated is "the full utilization of modern means to maximize the value of cadaver organs." Well, this is it.

Come, come, the members of the profession will say, nobody is thinking of this kind of thing. Perhaps not; but I have just shown that one *can* think of them. And the point is that the proposed definition of death has removed any reasons not to think of them and, once thought of, not to do them when found desirable (and the next of kin are agreeable). We must remember that what the Harvard group offered was not a definition of irreversible coma as a rationale for breaking off sustaining action, but a definition of death by the criterion of irreversible coma as a rationale for conceptually transposing the patient's body to the class of dead things, *regardless* of whether sustaining action is kept up or broken off. It would be hypocritical to deny that the redefinition amounts to an antedating of the accomplished fact of death (compared to conventional signs that may outlast it); that it was motivated not by exclusive concern with the patient but with certain extraneous interests in mind (organ donorship mostly named so far); and that the actual use of the general license it grants is implicitly anticipated. But no matter what particular use is or is not anticipated at the moment, or even anathematized—it would be naive to think that a line can be drawn anywhere for such uses when strong enough interests urge them, seeing that the definition (which is absolute, not graded) negates the very principle for drawing a line. (Given the ingenuity of medical science, in which I have great faith, I am convinced that the "simulated life" can eventually be made to comprise practically every extra-neural activity of the human body; and I would not even bet on its never comprising *some* artificially activated neural functions as well: which would be awkward for the argument of nonsensitivity, but still under the roof of that of nonspontaneity.)

e. Now my point is a very simple one. It is this. We do not know with certainty the borderline between life and death, and a definition cannot substitute for knowledge. Moreover, we have sufficient grounds for suspecting that the artificially supported condition of the comatose patient may still be one of life, however reduced—i.e., for doubting that, even with the brain function gone, he is completely dead. In this state of marginal ignorance and doubt the only course to take is to lean over backward toward the side of possible life. It follows that interventions as I described should be regarded on a par with vivisection and on no account be performed on a human body in that equivocal or threshold condition. And the definition that allows them, by stamping as unequivocal what at best is equivocal, must be rejected. But mere rejection in discourse is not enough. Given the pressure of the—very real and very worthy—medical interests, it can be predicted that the permission it implies in theory will be irresistible in practice, once the definition is installed in official authority. Its becoming so installed must therefore be resisted at all cost. It is the only thing that still can be resisted; by the time the practical conclusions beckon, it will be too late. It is a clear case of *principiis obsta*.

The foregoing argumentation was strictly on the plane of common sense and ordinary logic. Let me add, somewhat conjecturally, two philosophical observations.

I see lurking behind the proposed definition of death, apart from its obvious pragmatic motivation, a curious revenant of the old soul-body dualism. Its new apparition is the dualism of brain and body. In a certain analogy to the former it holds that the true human person rests in (or is represented by) the brain, of which the rest of the body is a mere subservient tool. Thus, when the brain dies, it is as when the soul departed: what is left are "mortal remains." Now nobody will deny that the cerebral aspect is decisive for the human quality of the life of the organism that is man's. The position I advanced acknowledges just this by recommending that with the irrecoverable total loss of brain function one should not hold up the naturally ensuing death of the rest of the organism. But it is no less an exaggeration of the cerebral aspect as it was of the conscious soul, to deny the extracerebral body its essential share in the identity of the person. The body is as uniquely the body of this brain and no other, as the brain is uniquely the brain of this body and no other. What is under the brain's central control, the bodily total, is as individual, as much "myself," as singular to my identity (fingerprints!), as noninterchangeable, as the controlling (and reciprocally controlled) brain itself. My identity is the identity of the whole organism, even if the higher functions of personhood are seated in the brain. How else could a man love a woman and not merely her brains? How else could we lose ourselves in the aspect of a face? Be touched by the delicacy of a frame? It's this person's, and no one else's. Therefore, the body of the comatose, so long as—even with the help of art —it still breathes, pulses, and functions otherwise, must still be considered a residual continuance of the subject that loved and was loved, and as such is still entitled to some of the sacrosanctity accorded to such a subject by the laws of God and men. That sacrosanctity decrees that it must not be used as a mere means.

My second observation concerns the morality of our time, to which our "redefiners" pay homage with the best of intentions, which have their own subtle sophistry. I mean the prevailing attitude toward death, whose faintheartedness they indulge in a curious blend with the toughmindedness of the scientist. The Catholic Church had the guts to say: under these circumstances let the patient die—speaking of the patient alone and not of outside interests (society's, medicine's, etc.). The cowardice of modern secular society which shrinks from death as an unmitigated evil needs the assurance (or fiction) that he is already dead when the decision is to be made. The responsibility of a value-laden decision replaced by the mechanics of a value-free routine. Insofar as the redefiners of death—by saying "he is already dead"—seek to allay the scruples about turning the respirator off, they cater to this modern cowardice which has forgotten that death has its own fitness and dignity, and that a man has a right to be let die. Insofar as by saying so they seek to provide an even better conscience about keeping the respirator on and freely utilizing the body thus arrested on the threshold of life and death, they serve the ruling pragmatism of our time which will let no ancient fear and trembling interfere with the relentless expanding of the realm of sheer thinghood and unrestricted utility. The "splendor and misery" of our age dwells in that irresistible tide.

POSTSCRIPT OF DECEMBER 1976

The predictions or premonitions voiced in this essay of 1970 by way of warning have meanwhile begun to come true in the glaring light of the operating theatre. On December 5, 1976, *The New York Times* brought a news report by Robert E. Tomasson under the headline "Girl is ruled dead while respirated," from which I quote the opening paragraph and the crucial statement of the act performed.

> A 17-year-old Islip, L.I., schoolgirl who suffered extensive brain damage in an apparent mugging, was pronounced dead on Thursday while she was being sustained with the aid of a respirator. The death certificate was

signed, with the consent of her parents, by the family doctor and by the head of the Suffolk County Medical Society. . . .

Within an hour, the girl's eyes and kidneys were removed for transplants. The respirator, which the doctors said was kept going to maintain the viability of the organs, was then disconnected and the forced respiration stopped.

It is to be noted that here the *new definition of death* was actually used for allowing to perform the organ excision *while the "donor" was still,* thanks to the respirator, *in the "equivocal or threshhold condition"* (as I have called it) of the comatose. The respirator was disconnected after, not before, the removal of eyes and kidneys, and then only because no further utilization of her body, now or later, happened to be contemplated (or could be because of its non-"viability" without kidneys). But to keep it going beyond the first two surgeries would have required no further legitimation and no new decision of principle. Thus by at least one precedent the door I tried to keep shut has already been opened—and with it the road to the indefinite line of practical possibilities which my lurid imagination descried and whose election no law or qualm or principle any longer blocks. The beginning has been made; fiction cedes to enterprise, and the end is nowhere in sight. All that my essay now can still do—with little hope that it or its like will—is to help ensure that "society," this blurriest of entities, goes through that door with its eyes open and not shut. Inconsistent as man blessedly is, he may still draw the line somewhere without benefit of a consistent rule.

Notes

1. Of its members I name the renal surgeon Dr. Samuel Kountz, specializing in kidney transplantation, and Drs. Harrison Sadler and Otto Guttentag, all of the Medical Center of the University of California in San Francisco.
2. This has turned out to be too charitable an assumption—see *Postscript.*

Alexander M. Capron and Leon Kass now turn to legal and public policy problems in defining death. They reject the notion that court responses to specific cases provide an effective legal remedy (as the "Tucker case" seems to demonstrate). Instead they suggest the approach of public policy formulation and legislative enactment. They argue that the matter of formally *defining* death is less important than the development of adequate standards for the *determination* that death has occurred. They are highly critical of the two-definition strategy used in the Kansas statute. Capron and Kass, furthermore, provide two useful analytical frameworks. First, they propose a fourfold division of levels in the "definition of death." Their contention is that the term "definition of death" has multiple meanings. Second, they provide a model "statutory proposal" for legislative purposes that (like the Kansas statute) contains two different physiological criteria of death but that (unlike the Kansas statute) does not allow one to infer death from just one of the criteria.

Alexander Morgan Capron

Leon R. Kass

A STATUTORY DEFINITION OF THE STANDARDS FOR DETERMINING HUMAN DEATH: AN APPRAISAL AND A PROPOSAL *

In recent years, there has been much discussion of the need to refine and update the criteria for determining that a human being has died. In light of medicine's increasing ability to maintain certain signs of life artificially and to make good use of organs from newly dead bodies, new criteria of death have been proposed by medical authorities. Several states have enacted or are considering legislation to establish a statutory "definition of death," at the prompting of some members of the medical profession who apparently feel that existing, judicially framed standards might expose physicians, particularly transplant surgeons, to civil or criminal liability. Although the leading statute in this area [1] appears to create more problems than it resolves, some legislation may be needed for the protection of the public as well as the medical profession, and, in any event, many more states will probably be enacting such statutes in the near future. . . .

PUBLIC INVOLVEMENT OR PROFESSIONAL PREROGATIVE?

In considering the possible need for and the desirability of public involvement, the central question appears to be to what extent, if at all, the "defining" of death is a medical matter, properly left to physicians because it lies within their particular sphere of competence. The belief that the matter of "defining death" is wholly medical is frequently expressed, and not only by physicians. Indeed, when a question concerning the moment at which a person died has arisen in litigation, common law courts have generally regarded this as "a question of fact" for determination at trial on the

* From *The University of Pennsylvania Law Review*, 121 (November 1972), 87–88, 92–98, 102–18. Reprinted by permission of Fred B. Rothman & Co.

basis (partially but not exclusively) of expert medical testimony.[2] Yet the standards which are applied in arriving at a conclusion, although based on medical knowledge, are established by the courts "as a matter of law." [3]

Thus while it is true that the application of particular criteria or tests to determine the death of an individual may call for the expertise of a physician, there are other aspects of formulating a "definition" of death that are not particularly within medical competence. To be sure, in practice, so long as the standards being employed are stable and congruent with community opinion about the phenomenon of death, most people are content to leave the matter in medical hands. But the underlying extramedical aspects of the "definition" become visible, as they have recently, when medicine departs (or appears to depart) from the common or traditional understanding of the concept of death. The formulation of a concept of death is neither simply a technical matter nor one susceptible of empirical verification. The idea of death is at least partly a philosophical question, related to such ideas as "organism," "human," and "living." Physicians *qua* physicians are not expert on these philosophical questions, nor are they expert on the question of which physiological functions decisively identify a "living, human organism." They, like other scientists, can suggest which "vital signs" have what significance for which human functions. They may, for example, show that a person in an irreversible coma exhibits "total unawareness to externally applied stimuli and inner need and complete unresponsiveness," [4] and they may predict that when tests for this condition yield the same results over a twenty-four-hour period there is only a very minute chance that the coma will ever be "reversed." Yet the judgment that "total unawareness . . . and complete unresponsiveness" are the salient characteristics of death, or that a certain level of risk of error is acceptable, requires more than technical expertise and goes beyond medical authority, properly understood.

The proposed departure from the traditional standards for determining death not only calls attention to the extra-medical issues involved, but is itself a source of public confusion and concern. The confusion can perhaps be traced to the fact that the traditional signs of life (the beating heart and the expanding chest) are manifestly accessible to the senses of the layman, whereas some of the new criteria require sophisticated intervention to elicit latent signs of life such as brain reflexes. Furthermore, the new criteria may disturb the layman by suggesting that these visible and palpable traditional signs, still useful in most cases, may be deceiving him in cases where supportive machinery is being used. The anxiety may also be attributable to the apparent intention behind the "new definition," which is, at least in part, to facilitate other developments such as the transplantation of cadaver organs. Such confusion and anxiety about the standards for determining death can have far-reaching and distressing consequences for the patient's family, for the physician, for other patients, and for the community at large. If the uncertainties surrounding the question of determining death are to be laid to rest, a clear and acceptable standard is needed. And if the formulation and adoption of this standard are not to be abdicated to the medical fraternity under an expanded view of its competence and authority, then the public and its representatives ought to be involved. Even if the medical profession takes the lead—as indeed it has—in promoting new criteria of death, members of the public should at least have the opportunity to review, and either to affirm or reject the standards by which they are to be pronounced dead.

WHAT MANNER OF PUBLIC INVOLVEMENT?

There are a number of potential means for involving the public in this process of formulation and review, none of them perfect. The least ambitious or comprehensive is simply to encourage discussion of the issues by the lay press, civic groups, and the community at large. This public consideration might be directed or supported through the efforts of national organizations such as the American Medical Association, the National Institutes of Health, or the National Academy of Sciences. A resolution calling for the establishment of an ad hoc body to evaluate public attitudes toward the changes wrought by biomedical advances has been sponsored by Senator Mondale since 1967 and was adopted by the Senate in December 1971. Mondale's proposed National Advisory Commission on Health Science and Society, under the direction of a board of fifteen members of the general public and professionals from "medicine, law, theology, biological science, physical science, social science, philosophy, humanities, health administration, government, and public affairs," would conduct "seminars and public hearings" as part of its two-year study.[5] As important as it is to ventilate the issues, studies and public discussions alone may not be adequate to the task. They cannot by themselves dispel the ambiguities which will continue to trouble decision makers and the public in determining whether an artificially maintained, comatose "patient" is still alive.

A second alternative, reliance upon the judicial system, goes beyond ascertaining popular attitudes and could provide an authoritative opinion that might offer some guidance for decision makers. Reliance on judge-made law would, however, neither actively involve the public in the decision-making process nor lead to a prompt, clear, and general "definition." The courts, of course, cannot speak in the abstract prospectively, but must await litigation, which can involve considerable delay and expense, to the detriment of both the parties and society. A need to rely on the courts reflects an uncertainty in the law which is unfortunate in an area where private decision makers (physicians) must act quickly and irrevocably. An ambiguous legal standard endangers the rights—and in some cases the lives —of the participants. In such circumstances, a person's choice of one course over another may depend more on his willingness to test his views in court than on the relative merits of the courses of action.

Once called upon to "redefine" death—for example, in a suit brought by a patient's relatives or, perhaps, by a revived "corpse" against the physician declaring death—the judiciary may be as well qualified to perform the task as any governmental body. If the issue could be resolved solely by a process of reasoning and of taking "judicial notice" of widely known and uncontroverted facts, a court could handle it without difficulty. If, on the other hand, technical expertise is required, problems may arise. Courts operate within a limited compass—the facts and contentions of a particular case—and with limited expertise; they have neither the staff nor the authority to investigate or to conduct hearings in order to explore such issues as public opinion or the scientific merits of competing "definitions." Consequently, a judge's decision may be merely a rubberstamping of the opinions expressed by the medical experts who appear before him. . . .

Uncertainties in the law are, to be sure, inevitable at times and are often tolerated if they do not involve matters of general applicability or great moment. Yet the question of whether and when a person is dead plainly seems the sort of issue that cannot escape the need for legal clarity on these grounds. Therefore, it is not surprising that although they would be pleased simply to have the courts endorse their views, members of the medical profession are doubtful that the judicial mode of lawmaking offers them adequate protection in this area. There is currently no way to be certain that a doctor would not be liable, criminally or civilly, if he ceased treatment of a person found to be dead according to the Harvard Committee's criteria but not according to the "complete cessation of all vital functions" test presently employed by the courts. Although such "definitions" were adopted in cases involving inheritors' rights and survivorship rather than a doctor's liability for exercising his judgment about when a person has died, physicians have with good reason felt that this affords them little assurance that the courts would not rely upon those cases as precedent. On the contrary, it is reasonable to expect that the courts would seek precedent in these circumstances. Adherence to past decisions is valued because it increases the likelihood that an individual will be treated fairly and impartially; it also removes the need to relitigate every issue in every case. Most importantly, courts are not inclined to depart from existing rules because to do so may upset the societal assumption that one may take actions, and rely upon the actions of others, without fear that the ground rules will be changed retroactively.[6]

Considerations of precedent as well as other problems with relying on the judicial formulation of a new definition were made apparent in

Tucker v. *Lower,*[7] the first case to present the question of the "definition of death" in the context of organ transplantation. . . .

WHAT CAN AND SHOULD BE LEGISLATED?

Arguments both for and against the desirability of legislation "defining" death often fail to distinguish among the several different subjects that might be touched on by such legislation. As a result, a mistaken impression may exist that a single statutory model is, and must be, the object of debate. An appreciation of the multiple meanings of a "definition of death" may help to refine the deliberations.

Death, in the sense the term is of interest here, can be defined purely formally as the transition, however abrupt or gradual, between the state of being alive and the state of being dead. There are at least four levels of "definitions" that would give substance to this formal notion; in principle, each could be the subject of legislation: (1) basic concept or idea; (2) general physiological standards; (3) operational criteria; and (4) specific tests or procedures.

The *basic concept* of death is fundamentally a philosophical matter. Examples of possible "definitions" of death at this level include "permanent cessation of the integrated functioning of the organism as a whole," "departure of the animating or vital principle," or "irreversible loss of personhood." These abstract definitions offer little concrete help in the practical task of determining whether a person has died but they may very well influence how one goes about devising standards and criteria.

In setting forth the *general physiological standard(s)* for recognizing death, the definition moves to a level which is more medicotechnical, but not wholly so. Philosophical issues persist in the choice to define death in terms of organ systems, physiological functions, or recognizable human activities, capacities, and conditions. Examples of possible general standards include "irreversible cessation of spontaneous respiratory and/or circulatory functions," "irreversible loss of spontaneous brain functions," "irreversible loss of the ability to respond or communicate," or some combination of these.

Operational criteria further define what is meant by the general physiological standards. The absence of cardiac contraction and lack of movement of the blood are examples of traditional criteria for "cessation of spontaneous circulatory functions," whereas deep coma, the absence of reflexes, and the lack of spontaneous muscular movements and spontaneous respiration are among criteria proposed for "cessation of spontaneous brain functions" by the Harvard Committee.

Fourth, there are the *specific tests and procedures* to see if the criteria are fulfilled. Pulse, heartbeat, blood pressure, electrocardiogram, and examination of blood flow in the retinal vessels are among the specific tests of cardiac contraction and movement of the blood. Reaction to painful stimuli, appearance of the pupils and their responsiveness to light, and observation of movement and breathing over a specified time period are among specific tests of the "brainfunction" criteria enumerated above.

There appears to be general agreement that legislation should not seek to "define death" at either the most general or the most specific levels (the first and fourth). In the case of the former, differences of opinion would seem hard to resolve, and agreement, if it were possible, would provide little guidance for practice. In the case of the latter, the specific tests and procedures must be kept open to changes in medical knowledge and technology. Thus, arguments concerning the advisability and desirability of a statutory definition of death are usually confined to the two levels we have called "standards" and "criteria," yet often without any apparent awareness of the distinction between them. The need for flexibility in the face of medical advance would appear to be a persuasive argument for not legislating any specific operational criteria. Moreover, these are almost exclusively technical matters, best left to the judgment of physicians. Thus, the kind of "definition" suitable for legislation would be a definition of the general physiological standard or standards. Such a definition, while not immutable, could be expected to be useful for a long period of time and would therefore not require frequent amendment.

There are other matters that could be comprehended in legislation "defining" death. The statute could specify who (and how many) shall make the determination. In the absence of a compelling reason to change past practices, this may continue to be set at "a physician," [8] usually the doctor attending a dying patient or the one who happens to be at the scene of an accident. Moreover, the law ought probably to specify the "time of death." The statute may seek to fix the precise time when death may be said to have occurred, or it may merely seek to define a time that is clearly after "the precise moment," that is, a time when it is possible to say "the patient is dead," rather than "the patient has just now died." If the medical procedures used in determining that death has occurred call for verification of the findings after a fixed period of time (for example, the Harvard Committee's recommendation that the tests be repeated after twenty-four hours), the statute could in principle assign the "moment of death" to either the time when the criteria were first met or the time of verification. The former has been the practice with the traditional criteria for determining death.

Finally, legislation could speak to what follows upon the determination. The statute could be permissive or prescriptive in determining various possible subsequent events, including especially the pronouncement and recording of the death, and the use of the body for burial or other purposes.

It is our view that these matters are best handled outside of a statute which has as its purpose to "define death."

PRINCIPLES GOVERNING THE FORMULATION OF A STATUTE

In addition to carefully selecting the proper degree of specificity for legislation, there are a number of other principles we believe should guide the drafting of a statute "defining" death. First, the phenomenon of interest to physicians, legislators, and laymen alike is human death. Therefore, the statute should concern the death of a human being, not the death of his cells, tissues, or organs, and not the "death" or cessation of his role as a fully functioning member of his family or community. This point merits considerable emphasis. There may be a proper place for a statutory standard for deciding when to turn off a respirator which is ventilating a patient still clearly alive, or, for that matter, to cease giving any other form of therapy. But it is crucial to distinguish this question of "when to allow to die?" from the question with which we are here concerned, namely, "when to declare dead?" Since very different issues and purposes are involved in these questions, confusing the one with the other clouds the analysis of both. The problem of determining when a person is dead is difficult enough without its being tied to the problem of whether physicians, or anyone else, may hasten the death of a terminally ill patient, with or without his consent or that of his relatives, in order to minimize his suffering or to conserve scarce medical resources. Although the same set of social and medical conditions may give rise to both problems, they must be kept separate if they are to be clearly understood.

Distinguishing the question "is he dead?" from the question "should he be allowed to die?" also assists in preserving continuity with tradition, a second important principle. By restricting itself to the "is he dead?" issue, a revised "definition" permits practices to move incrementally, not by replacing traditional cardiopulmonary standards for the determination of death but rather by supplementing them. These standards are, after all, still adequate in the majority of cases, and are the ones that both physicians and the public are in the habit of employing and relying on. The supplementary standards are needed primarily for those cases in which artificial means of support of comatose patients render the traditional standards unreliable.

Third, this incremental approach is useful for the additional and perhaps most central reason that any new means for judging death should be seen as just that and nothing more—a change in method dictated by advances in medical practice, but not an alteration of the meaning of "life" and "death." By indicating that the various standards for measuring death relate to a single phenomenon, legislation can serve to reduce a primary source of public uneasiness on this subject. Once it has been established that certain consequences—for example, burial, autopsy, transfer of property to the heirs, and so forth—follow from a determination of death, definite problems would arise if there were a number of "definitions" according to which some people could be said to be "more dead" than others.

There are, of course, many instances in which the law has established differing definitions of a term, each framed to serve a particular purpose. One wonders, however, whether it does not appear somewhat foolish for the law to offer a number of arbitrary definitions of a natural phenomenon such as death. Nevertheless, legislators might seek to identify a series of points during the process of dying, each of which might be labeled "death" for certain purposes. Yet so far as we know, no arguments have been presented for special-purpose standards except in the area of organ transplantation. Such a separate "definition of death," aimed at increasing the supply of viable organs, would permit physicians to declare a patient dead before his condition met the generally applicable standards for determining death if his organs are of potential use in transplantation. The adoption of a special standard risks abuse and confusion, however. The status of prospective organ donor is an arbitrary one to which a person can be assigned by relatives[9] or physicians and is unrelated to anything about the extent to which his body's functioning has deteriorated. A special "definition" of death for transplantation purposes would thus need to be surrounded by a set of procedural safeguards that would govern not only the method by which a person is to be declared dead but also those by which he is to be classified as an organ donor. Even more troublesome is the confusion over the meaning of death that would probably be engendered by multiple "definitions." Consequently, it would be highly desirable if a statute on death could avoid the problems with a special "definition." Should the statute happen to facilitate organ transplantation, either by making more organs available or by making prospective donors and transplant surgeons more secure in knowing what the law would permit, so much the better.

If, however, more organs are needed for transplantation than can be legally obtained, the question whether the benefits conferred by transplantation justify the risks associated with a broader "definition" of death should be addressed directly rather than by attempting to subsume it under the question "what is death?" Such a direct confrontation with the issue could lead to a discussion about the standards and procedures under which organs might be taken from persons near death, or even those still quite alive, at their own option or that of relatives, physicians, or representatives of the state. The major advantage of keeping the issues separate is not, of course, that this will facilitate transplantation, but that it will remove a present source of concern: it is unsettling to contemplate that as you lie slowly dying physicians are free to use a more "lenient" standard to declare you dead if they want to remove your organs for transplantation into other patients.

Fourth, the standards for determining death ought not only to relate to a single phenomenon but should also be applied uniformly to all persons. A person's wealth or his "social utility" as an organ donor should not affect the way in which the moment of his death is determined.

Finally, while there is a need for uniformity of application at any one time, the fact that changes in medical technology brought about the present need for "redefinition" argues that the new formulation should be flexible. As suggested in the previous section, such flexibility is most easily accomplished if the new "definition" confines itself to the general standards by which death is to be determined and leaves to the continuing exercise of judgment by physicians the establishment and application of appropriate criteria and specific tests for determining that the standards have been met.

THE KANSAS STATUTE

The first attempt at a legislative resolution of the problems discussed here was made in 1970 when the State of Kansas adopted "An Act relating to and defining death." [10] The Kansas statute has received a good deal of attention; similar legislation was enacted in the spring of 1972 in Maryland and is presently under consideration in a number of other jurisdictions.[11] The Kansas legislation, which was drafted in response to developments in organ transplantation and medical support of dying patients, provides "alternative definitions of death," [12] set forth in two paragraphs. Under the first, a person is considered "medically and legally dead" if a physician determines "there is the absence of spontaneous respiratory and cardiac function and . . . attempts at resuscitation are considered hopeless." [13] In the second "definition," death turns on the absence of spontaneous brain function if during "reasonable attempts" either to "maintain or restore spontaneous circulatory or respiratory function," it appears that "further attempts at resuscitation or supportive maintenance will not succeed." [14] The purpose of the latter "definition" is made clear by the final sentence of the second paragraph:

> Death is to be pronounced before artificial means of supporting respiratory and circulatory function are terminated and *before any vital organ is removed for the purpose of transplantation.*[15]

The primary fault with this legislation is that it appears to be based on, or at least gives voice to, the misconception that there are two separate phenomena of death. This dichotomy is particularly unfortunate because it seems to have been inspired by a desire to establish a special definition for organ transplantation, a definition which physicians would not, however, have to apply, in the draftsman's words, "to prove the irrelevant deaths of most persons." [16] Although there is nothing in the Act itself to indicate that physicians will be less concerned with safeguarding the health of potential organ donors, the purposes for which the Act was passed are not hard to decipher, and they do little to inspire the average patient with confidence that his welfare (including his not being prematurely declared dead) is of as great concern to medicine and the State of Kansas as is the facilitation of organ transplantation. . . .[17]

A STATUTORY PROPOSAL

As an alternative to the Kansas statute we propose the following:

> A person will be considered dead if in the announced opinion of a physician, based on ordinary standards of medical practice, he has experienced an irreversible cessation of spontaneous respiratory and circulatory functions. In the event that artificial means of support preclude a determination that these functions have ceased, a person will be considered dead if in the announced opinion of a physician, based on ordinary standards of medical practice, he has experienced an irreversible cessation of spontaneous brain functions. Death will have occurred at the time when the relevant functions ceased.

This proposed statute provides a "definition" of death confined to the level of *general physiological standards,* and it has been drafted in accord with the five principles set forth above. First, the proposal speaks in terms of the *death* of a *person.* The determination that a person has died is to be based on an evaluation of certain vital bodily functions, the permanent absence of which indicates that he is no longer a living human being. By concentrating on the death of a human being as a whole, the statute rightly disregards the fact that some cells or organs may continue to "live" after this point, just as others may have ceased functioning long before the determination of death. This statute would leave for resolution by other means the question of when the absence or deterioration of certain capacities, such as the ability to communicate, or functions, such as the cerebral, indicates that a person may or should be allowed to die without further medical intervention.

Second, the proposed legislation is predicated upon the single phenomenon of death. Moreover, it applies uniformly to all persons, by specifying the circumstances under which each of the standards is to be used rather than leaving this to the unguided discretion of physicians. Unlike the Kansas law, the model statute does not leave to arbitrary decision a choice between two apparently equal yet different "alternative definitions of death." [18] Rather, its second standard is applicable only when "artificial means of support preclude" use of the first. It does not establish a separate kind of death, called "brain death." In other words, the proposed law would provide two standards gauged by different functions, for measuring different manifestations of the same phenomenon. If cardiac and pulmonary functions have ceased, brain functions cannot continue; if there is no brain activity and respiration has to be maintained artificially, the same state (i.e., death) exists. Some people might prefer a single standard, one based either on cardiopulmonary or brain functions. This would have the advantage of removing the last trace of the "two deaths" image, which any reference to alternative standards may still leave. Respiratory and circulatory indicators, once the only touchstone, are no longer adequate in some situations. It would be possible, however, to adopt the alternative, namely that death is *always* to be established by assessing spontaneous brain functions. Reliance only on brain activity, however, would represent a sharp and unnecessary break with tradition. Departing from continuity with tradition is not only theoretically unfortunate in that it violates another principle of good legislation suggested previously, but also practically very difficult, since most physicians customarily employ cardiopulmonary tests for death and would be slow to change, especially when the old tests are easier to perform, more accessible and acceptable to the lay public, and perfectly adequate for determining death in most instances.

Finally, by adopting standards for death in terms of the cessation of certain vital bodily functions but not in terms of the specific criteria or tests by which these functions are to be measured, the statute does not prevent physicians from adapting their procedures to changes in medical technology.

A basic substantive issue remains: what are the merits of the proposed standards? For ordinary situations, the appropriateness of the traditional standard, "an irreversible cessation of spontaneous respiratory and circulatory functions," does not require elaboration. Indeed, examination by a physician may be more a formal than a real requirement in determining that most people have died. In addition to any obvious injuries, elementary signs of death such as absence of heartbeat and breathing, cold skin, fixed pupils, and so forth, are usually sufficient to indicate even to a layman that the accident victim, the elderly person who passes away quietly in the night, or the patient stricken with a sudden infarct has died. The difficulties arise when modern medicine intervenes to sustain a patient's respiration and circulation. . . . [T]he indicators of brain damage appear reliable, in that studies have shown that patients who fit the Harvard criteria have suffered such extensive damage that they do not recover. Of course, the task of the neurosurgeon or physician is simplified in the common case where an accident victim has suffered such gross, apparent injuries to the head that it is not necessary to apply the Harvard criteria in order to establish cessation of brain functioning.

The statutory standard, "irreversible cessation of spontaneous brain functions," is intended to encompass both higher brain activities and those of the brainstem. There must, of course, also be no spontaneous respiration; the second standard is applied only when breathing is being artificially maintained. The major emphasis placed on brain functioning, although generally consistent with the common view of what makes man distinctive as a living creature, brings to the fore a basic issue: What aspects of brain function should be decisive? The question has been reframed by some clinicians in light of their experience with patients who have undergone what they term "neocortical death" (that is, complete destruction of higher brain capacity, demonsrated by a flat EEG). "Once neocortical death has been unequivocally established and the possibility of any recovery of consciousness and intellectual activity [is] thereby excluded, . . . although [the] patient breathes spontaneously, is he or she alive?" [19] While patients with irreversible brain damage from cardiac arrest seldom survive more than a few days, cases have recently been reported of survival for up to two and one-quarter years.[20] Nevertheless, though existence in this state falls far short of a full human life, the very fact of spontaneous respiration, as well as coordinated movements and reflex activities at the brainstem and spinal-cord levels, would exclude these patients from the scope of the statutory standards. The condition of "neocortical death" may well be a proper justification for interrupting all forms of treatment and allowing these patients to die, but this moral and legal problem cannot and should not be settled by "defining" these people "dead."

The legislation suggested here departs from the Kansas statute in its basic approach to the problem of "defining" death: the proposed statute does not set about to establish a special category of "brain death" to be used by transplanters. Further, there are a number of particular points of difference between them. For example, the proposed statute does not speak of persons being "medically and legally dead," thus avoiding redundancy and, more importantly, the mistaken implication that the "medical" and "legal" definitions could differ. Also, the proposed legislation does not include the provision that "death is to be pronounced before" the machine is turned off or any organs removed. Such a *modus operandi,* which was incorporated by Kansas from the Harvard Committee's report, may be advisable for physicians on public relations grounds, but it has no place in a statute "defining" death. The proposed statute already provides that "Death will have occurred at the time when the relevant functions ceased." If supportive aids, or organs, are withdrawn after this time, such acts cannot be implicated as having caused death. The manner in which, or exact time at which, the physician should articulate his finding is a matter best left to the exigencies of the situation, to local medical customs or hospital rules, or to statutes on the procedures for certifying death or on transplantation if the latter is the procedure which raises the greatest concern of medical impropriety. The real safeguard against doctors' killing patients is not to be found in a statute "defining" death. Rather, it inheres in physicians' ethical and religious beliefs, which are also embodied in the fundamental professional ethic of *primum non nocere* and are reinforced by homicide and "wrongful death" laws and the rules governing medical negligence applicable in license revocation proceedings or in private actions for damages. . . .

CONCLUSION

Changes in medical knowedge and procedures have created an apparent need for a clear and acceptable revision of the standards for determining that a person has died. Some commentators have argued that the formulation of such standards should be left to physicians. The reasons for rejecting this argument seem compelling: the "definition of death" is not merely a matter for technical expertise, the uncertainty of the present law is unhealthy for society and physicians alike, there is a great potential for mischief and harm through the possibility of conflict between the standards applied by some physicians and those assumed to be applicable by the community at large and its legal system, and patients and their relatives are made uneasy by physicians' apparently being free to shift around the meaning of death without any societal guidance. Accordingly, we conclude the public has a legitimate role to play in the formulation and adoption of such standards. This article has proposed a model statute which bases a determination of death primarily on the traditional standard of final respiratory and circulatory cessation; where the artificial maintenance of these functions precludes the use of such a standard, the statute authorizes that death be determined on the basis of irreversible cessation of spontaneous brain functions. We believe the legislation proposed would dispel public confusion and concern and protect physicians and patients, while avoiding the creation of "two types of death," for which the statute on this subject first adopted in Kansas has been justly criticized. The proposal is offered not as the ultimate solution to the problem, but as a catalyst for what we hope will be a robust and well-informed public debate over a new "definition." Finally, the proposed statute leaves for future resolution the even more difficult problems concerning the conditions and procedures under which a decision may be reached to cease treating a terminal patient who does not meet the standards set forth in the statutory "definition of death."

Notes

1. KAN. STAT. ANN. § 77–202 (Supp. 1971); see notes 10–18 *infra* and accompanying text for a discussion of this statute.
2. See *Thomas* v. *Anderson,* 96 Cal. App. 2d 371, 215 P.2d 478 (1950).
3. *Smith* v. *Smith,* 229 Ark. 579, 587, 317 S.W.2d 275, 279 (1958) (quoting 41 AM. JUR. *Husbands and Wives* § 244 (1938)).

4. *Irreversible Coma,* Harvard Committee Report, at 337.

5. S.J. Res. 75, 92d Cong., 1st Sess. (1971), in *Congressional Record,* 117, S20,090 (daily ed. Dec. 2, 1971).

6. [R]ules of law on which men rely in their business dealings should not be changed in the middle of the game. . . ." *Woods* v. *Lancet,* 303 N.Y. 349, 354, 102 N.E.2d 691, 695 (1951).

7. *Tucker* v. *Lower,* No. 2831 (Richmond, Va., L. & Eq. Ct., May 23, 1972).

8. Cf. Uniform Anatomical Gift Act § 7(b).

9. Uniform Anatomical Gift Act § 2(c). For example, if a special standard were adopted for determining death in potential organ donors, relatives of a dying patient with limited financial means might feel substantial pressure to give permission for his organs to be removed in order to bring to a speedier end the care given the patient.

10. Law of Mar. 17, 1970, ch. 378, [1970] Kan. Laws 994 (codified at KAN. STAT. ANN. § 77–202 [Supp. 1971]).

11. In the Maryland law, which is nearly identical to its Kansas progenitor, the phrase "in the opinion of a physician" was deleted from the first paragraph, and the phrase "and because of a known disease or condition" was added to the second paragraph following "ordinary standards of medical practice." Maryland Sessions Laws, ch. 693 (1972).

12. Note 10 *supra.*

13. *Ibid.* In using the term "hopeless," the Kansas legislature apparently intended to indicate that the "absence of spontaneous respiratory and cardiac function" must be irreversible before death is pronounced. In addition to being rather roundabout, this formulation is also confusing in that it might be taken to address the "When to allow to die?" question as well as the "Is he dead?" question.

14. Note 10 *supra.*

15. *Ibid.* (emphasis added).

16. Taylor, at 296, in *Journal of the American Medical Association,* 215 (1971), Letter to the Editor.

17. Cf. Kass, "A Caveat on Transplants," *The Washington Post,* Jan. 14, 1968, § B, at 1, col. 1.

18. KAN. STAT. ANN. § 77-202 (Supp. 1971).

19. Brierley, Adams, Graham, and Simpsom, "Neocortical Death after Cardiac Arrest," *The Lancet* 2 (1971), 560, 565.

20. Brierley and his colleagues report two cases of their own in which the patients each survived in a comatose condition for five months after suffering cardiac arrest before dying of pulmonary complications. They also mention two unreported cases of a Doctor Lewis, in one of which the patient survived for 2¼ years. Brierley, *supra* note 19, at 565.

Robert M. Veatch spells out the policy implications of the earlier selection from his work by assessing the merits of the arguments presented by Capron and Kass. Veatch's argument provides an interesting blend of sympathetic appreciation of as well as constructive criticisms of their article. Furthermore, Veatch shows the difficulties faced by Kansas and other states in attempting to update the definition of death in a document with standing in law. Somewhat like the authors of the original Kansas statute, Veatch argues that "When dealing with a philosophical conflict so basic that it is literally a matter of life and death, the best solution may be individual freedom to choose between different philosophical concepts within the range of what is tolerable to all the interests involved." Veatch proposes model legislation where a cerebral locus rather than a whole-brain locus is allowed. There are two main features in his model program: the elimination of possible conflicts of interest and freedom of choice among competing criteria of death.

Robert M. Veatch

DEFINING DEATH ANEW: POLICY OPTIONS *

While we philosophize about the meaning of death in the age of the biological revolution, people are being pronounced dead (or alive) by physicians who choose one definition or another. The philosophical discussion becomes literally a matter of life and death. You may be pronounced dead by a randomly available physician even if you and your family believe (or have believed) you are still alive and even if you would be considered alive at another hospital down the block. Or you may be considered living by a physician who has chosen to reject the newer notions of death centered on the brain or some part of it, even if you have thought about the issue and decided in favor of a brain-oriented concept.

Doctors in the forty states that have not adopted specific legislation are taking it upon themselves to use a brain-oriented concept of death, although the laws in these states do not authorize them to. Other doctors are reluctant to use newer concepts of death, fearing they may offend the patient's family or some district attorney. The fact is, "There is currently no way to be certain that a doctor would not be liable, criminally or civilly, if he ceased treatment of a person found to be dead according to the Harvard Committee's criteria, but not according to the 'complete cessation of all vital functions' test presently employed by the courts." [1]

Some order must be brought out of this confusion. A public policy must be developed that will enable us to know who should be treated as alive and who should be treated as dead. . . .

Laying the responsibility on the individual physician or the profession as a whole for deciding what the definition of death should be is the result

---

* From *Death, Dying, and the Biological Revolution.* Copyright © 1976. Reprinted by permission of Yale University Press.

of inadequate analysis, of failing to distinguish adequately between the levels of the debate. The medical professional undoubtedly has special skills for determining and applying the specific criteria that measure whether particular body functions have irreversibly ceased. Whether the Harvard criteria taken together accurately divide those who are in irreversible coma from those who are not is clearly an empirical question (although the important consideration of just how sure we want to be takes us once again into matters that cannot be answered scientifically). But the crucial policy question is at the conceptual level: should the individual in irreversible coma be treated as dead? No medical answers to this question are possible. If I am to be pronounced dead by the use of a philosophical or theological concept that I do not share, I at least have a right to careful due process. Physicians in the states that do not authorize brain-oriented criteria for pronouncing death who take it upon themselves to use those criteria not only run the risk of criminal or civil prosecution but, in my opinion, should be so prosecuted.

A STATUTORY DEFINITION OF (WHOLE) BRAIN DAMAGE

When the *Tucker* case (in which the Virginia physicians defended their use of criteria for death not sanctioned by state law) reached court, it was the first case to test a *public* policy for defining death. Judge A. Christian Compton was not willing to have such a major question resolved in his court, saying, "If such a radical change is to be made in the law of Virginia, the application should be made therefore not to the courts but to the legislature wherein the basic concept of our society relating to the preservation and extension of life could be examined, and, if necessary, reevaluated." [2]

The Kansas Proposal

In 1968 Kansas was the first state to pass a law permitting the procuring of organs for transplantation. . . . Maryland next passed an almost identical bill.[3] Subsequently Alaska, California, Georgia, Illinois, Michigan, New Mexico, Oregon, and Virginia passed such legislation. States now considering changes include Florida, Minnesota, and New York. Others have legislators interested in new death definitions.

These statutory proposals have not gone without opposition. Probably the best focused and most widely known criticism has come from British law professor Ian McColl Kennedy.[4] "Let us have guidelines by all means. They are essential," he argues. "But let them be set down by the medical profession, not by the legislature." That the medical profession, as a profession, may have no special competence to set such guidelines is a possibility he completely misses. Like many others, he confuses medical and policy expertise. He goes on to outline six specific criticisms of the Kansas bill. Some of them seem to me more valid than others.

The first is probably the most critical and the most valid. The act, he observes, "seems to be drafted only with transplantation surgery in mind." Indeed, the bill incorporates explicit directions on this matter: "death is to be pronounced before artificial means of supporting respiratory and circulatory function are terminated and before any vital organ is removed for the purpose of transplantation." As Dr. Taylor has revealed in his 1971 article, the University of Kansas Medical Center was concerned about transplants when staff members began promoting the change in the law.

The relation between a new definition of death and transplantation is complex,[5] and Ian Kennedy's first critical point identifies a major cause of worry: "To draft a statute on death inspired apparently by the desire to facilitate what must still be considered experimental surgical procedures must serve to disturb the man in the street. . . . The Act in its present form does not serve to reassure the person who may fear that during his last hours on earth his doctors will be less concerned with his condition than with the person earmarked to receive one of his vital organs." [6]

Don Harper Mills, physician and lawyer, does not agree that the statute is so closely associated with transplant policy. He claims that it intentionally extends to questions of when the physician can terminate resuscitative efforts or discontinue artificial maintenance.[7] Whatever the intentions of the bill's authors, both the authors and Mills may be wrong in their assumptions of what purposes such a statutory definition should serve. It is dangerous to propose a statutory definition solely for the purpose of obtaining organs, but it is equally dangerous to confuse the issue of when resuscitation should be stopped with the one of when a patient is dead. Neither considers that a statutory definition may be needed to prevent the basic indignity of treating a corpse as if it were alive—of confusing a living human with one who has lost essential humanness. Kennedy is right in recognizing that the link between transplantation and the definition of death should not be as close as in the Kansas bill.

Second, Kennedy objects that the Kansas bill seems to propose two alternative definitions of death, implying a person may be simultaneously dead according to one criterion and alive according to the other. In a law review article agreeing with Kennedy on this point, Alexander Capron, law professor at the University of Pennsylvania, and Leon Kass, professor of bioethics at Georgetown University, pose a bizarre problem.[8] A patient who meets the brain-oriented criteria for death and is a good tissue match with a potential organ recipient is pronounced dead under a special "transplant definition." What would the patient's status be if the potential organ recipient died before the donor organs were removed? The donor would be alive according to the heart- and lung-oriented definitions but pronounced dead according to a definition no longer applicable. If it is the person who dies and not some organ or cells or function, then we need a single definition that can apply to all of us, independent of what someone may want to do with our parts. These two problems raised by Kennedy—the dangerous link with transplantation and the implication of alternative definitions of death—should be taken into account in any future bills dealing with a new definition of death.

Third, Kennedy senses something wrong with the requirement that death be pronounced before artificial means of supporting respiration and circulation are stopped. Here his instincts may be sounder than the reasons he uses to support them. The proposal that death be pronounced first is taken from the Harvard Committee report. Kennedy seems to agree with the policy but feels it should not be written into the legislation. He writes that the dilemma faced by physicians is "more imagined than real" and declares that "doctors" do this every day without legislative fiat and will continue to do so with impunity. . . ." I don't follow his reasoning. Does he mean that physicians declare death every day before turning off resuscitation equipment? The cry for legislative protection seems to contradict that. Or does he mean that physicians decide to stop supportive maintenance on dying patients every day? That is probably true, but an entirely different issue. Kennedy goes on to argue that the requirement that death be pronounced before stopping life support is "entirely redundant." He says, "Once the doctors decide that the conditions specified in the Act exist, and 'further attempts at resuscitation or supportive maintenance will not succeed,' death has already occurred." Indeed it has, according to the new definition, but to say that "death must be pronounced" is something else. If nothing more, this makes clear that the concept of death being used is radically new.

There is a more serious problem, which Kennedy does not mention. To say that death should be pronounced before supportive maintenance ceases (on a corpse) might imply to the less careful reader that it is never appropriate or legal to decide to stop life support on a dying individual. If anyone were to read that from the Kansas legislation, it would be a serious problem. The question of stopping treatment of the dying is a separate issue to be taken up later.

Kennedy's fourth objection to the Kansas bill is that it does not require a confirmatory judgment of a second physician before pronouncing death according to brain-oriented criteria. He criticizes others who find this "commendable." [9] Whether the requirement of a second judgment is reasonable will depend upon the purpose and context of the legislation. In the context of organ-transplant practices, a second judgment may indeed control aggressive transplanters. But if Kennedy is also right that the redefinition should not be limited to the transplantation context, then a confirmatory judgment seems less crucial. Is his position that the brain criteria are so much more complicated than the older heart and lung criteria that two technically competent individual judgments are necessary? I doubt that this is true now, and surely it will become completely unlikely, as experience is gained during the life of the legislation. There seems no plausible reason to have two experts involved in the general task of pronouncing death unless the techniques used are so complex that one cannot handle them adequately.

Kennedy's fifth criticism is that the act should require the physician pronouncing death to be a different one from the transplant physician. He calls for "safeguards" to protect the patient from potential conflict of interest. This is important and valid, particularly in the context of legislation explicitly for transplantation. Even better would be a more general ban on conflict of interest as part of a more general redefinition of death. No physician who has any interest beyond the patient's own welfare should be permitted to pronounce death.

Kennedy's final criticism is the most confusing. He claims that the act implicitly incorporates "the detailed clinical procedures that serve to determine 'brain death'," and he is rightly concerned that the law is no place to spell out in great detail the technical procedures for measuring whether a death has occurred. But it is impossible to read any such specification into the Act, which simply says that the diagnosis of absence of spontaneous brain function is to be "based upon ordinary standards of medical practice." These standards will vary from place to place and from time to time. New technical innovations or empirical data will change the tests to be used or the way they are used. The length of time an electroencephalogram has to be flat may change. Virtually all others who have criticized the Kansas bill [10] have thought that it does avoid the trap of overspecificity. The problem seems to be one of confusing the levels of the definition debate. Whatever Kennedy is taking exception to, "the absence of spontaneous brain function" certainly seems a rather general term. It specifies a function or a "locus" in the body, not empirical criteria or tests.[11]

A Better (Whole) Brain Statute

Capron and Kass are not happy with the Kansas statute for some of the same reasons as Kennedy: they do not like the close link with the transplantation issue, and they are particularly distressed at the implication that there are alternative forms of death appropriate for different situations. But they are still in favor of legislation. The questions at stake, in their opinion, are crucial matters that call for public involvement. "Physicians *qua* physicians are not expert on these philosophical questions nor are they expert on the question of which physiological functions decisively identify the 'living, human organism'." [12] The legislative route, they argue, would permit the public to play a more active role in decision making. It would also dispel both lay and professional doubt and provide needed assurance for physicians and patients' families that the new definition could be used without fear of a legal suit. They propose five "principles governing the formulation of a statute."

1. The statute should concern the death of a human being, not the death of cells, tissues, or organs, and not the "death or cessation of his role as a fully functioning member of his family or community."
2. It should move incrementally, supplementing rather than replacing the older cardiopulmonary standards.
3. It should avoid serving as a special definition for a special function such as transplantation.
4. It should apply uniformly to all persons.
5. It should be flexible, leaving specific criteria to the judgment of physicians. [13]

On the basis of these guidelines they propose a new draft statute as an alternative to the laws in Kansas and Maryland:

A person will be considered dead if in the announced opinion of a physician, based on ordinary standards of medical practice, he has experienced an irreversible cessation of spontaneous respiratory and circulatory functions. In the event that artificial means of support preclude a determination that these functions have ceased, a person will be considered dead if in the announced opinion of a physician, based on ordinary standards of medical practice, he has experienced an irreversible cessation of spontaneous brain functions. Death will have occurred at the time when the relevant functions ceased. [14]

Capron and Kass have captured all of the virtues and none of the problems of the Kansas statute. Their bill fails to meet two of Kennedy's objections—it does not require two physicians to participate in determining death and it does not provide that the death-pronouncing physician be separate from the physician interested in the potential cadaver's organs— but these requirements seem superfluous for a general public policy for determining when we are dead. Nevertheless, in holding to the principle of making the definition independent of transplantation concerns, Capron and Kass may have missed an important protection for the patient potentially dead because his brain has completely and irreversibly ceased functioning. They argue, "if particular dangers lurk in the transplantation setting, they should be dealt with in legislation on that subject, such as the Uniform Anatomical Gift Act." [15] That is reasonable, but it is also reasonable that there be observed a general requirement that the physician pronouncing death should be free of significant conflict of interest (whether interest in a respiring "patient," research, continued treatment fees, or transplantation). That there must be no such conflict is obviously essential, whether or not it should be banned by the statute itself.

Critics of the proposals for statutes setting out new standards for determining death have either dealt with technical wording difficulties or made misguided appeals for vesting decision-making authority in physicians or medical professional groups. These, however, are not the only problems. In order to accept the Kansas statute or the preferable Capron-Kass revision, it is first necessary to accept the underlying policy judgment that irreversible destruction of the brain is indeed death—that individuals should be treated as dead when, and only when, their brains will never again be able to function. Some of us continue to have doubts about that basic judgment.

A STATUTORY DEFINITION OF CEREBRAL DEATH

There has been great concern that statutes designed to legalize and regularize the use of brain-oriented criteria may not be sufficiently flexible to keep up with changes in this rapidly developing area. Kennedy and others who place their faith in medical discretion fear that a statute would not permit adoption of new techniques and procedures. For the most part they are wrong, since none of the proposed statutes specifies any particular criteria, techniques, or procedures. Techniques and procedures are changing rapidly; with that the proposed laws can cope. But our concepts, our philosophical sophistication, are evolving rapidly, too. Even today most people writing in the field, including competent scientists and physicians, are careless in distinguishing between the whole brain and the cerebrum and the functions of each. Here may arise a significant problem, for under even the highly generalized statutory proposals it may not be possible to make wanted distinctions between lower brain functions, such as those that control spontaneous respiration, and those giving rise to consciousness and individual personality.

If it is decided that a person without the capacities which are thought to reside in the higher brain (cerebral) centers should really be considered dead, then an amendment to the brain-death statutes might be in order. The change could be a simple one: simply strike the word *brain* and replace it with *cerebral.* This change in specifying the locus or the general standards for determining death may or may not have practical significance to the clinician who pronounces death. The question of criteria is an empirical one and the answer will change periodically. It may be that the only way of knowing for sure that the cerebrum has irreversibly lost its ability to function is to use exactly the same tests as for determining that the whole brain has lost its power to function, that is, the Harvard Committee criteria or something similar. But it may also be that other tests—such as EEG alone—could predict with certainty when individuals have irreversibly lost cerebral function even if they retain some lower brain functions, even if, say, they are still breathing spontaneously. The question of criteria can and must be left to the neurological experts.

There may be reasons for sticking with the old-fashioned statutes based on whole-brain conceptions of death. Only a few people will be dead according to a cerebral concept but alive according to a whole-brain concept. There may be some risk of making an empirical error in applying cerebral criteria and pronouncing someone dead who could still regain some form of consciousness. Some moral doubt may remain about the legitimacy of pronouncing someone dead who retains lower brain function. But these same problems arise with the whole-brain-oriented statutes as well. Once the judgment has been made that false positive diagnoses of life are a serious problem, serious enough to overcome any empirical or moral doubts, there is a strong case for moving on from the whole brain to a cerebral focus.

A STATUTE FOR A CONFUSED SOCIETY

There is still another option. Part of the current confusion reflects sincere and reasonable disagreements within society over which philosophical concept of death is the proper one. As with many philosophical questions, the conflict will not easily be resolved. In a democratic society, however, we have a well-established method for dealing with a diversity of religious, moral, or philosophical perspectives. It is to allow free and individual choice as long as it does not directly infringe on the freedom of others and does not radically offend the common morality.

When dealing with a philosophical conflict so basic that it is literally a matter of life and death, the best solution may be individual freedom to choose between different philosophical concepts within the range of what is tolerable to all the interests involved. There have been rare and tentative hints at this solution in the literature. In 1968 proposed by the general definition of human death Halley and Harvey had an apparent option clause:

> Death is irreversible cessation of *all* of the following: (1) total cerebral function, (2) spontaneous function of the respiratory system, and (3) spontaneous function of the circulatory system.

> Special circumstances may, however, justify the pronouncement of death when consultation consistent with established professional standards have (sic) been obtained and when valid consent to withhold or stop resuscitation measures has been given by the appropriate relative or legal guardian.[16]

They abandoned this "consent" formula, however, in later versions of their proposal.[17]

Halley and Harvey have been criticized for their "mistake in making the state of being dead (rather than the acceptance of imminent death) depend on the 'consent' of a relative or guardian." [18] It seems likely that they did indeed confuse the state of being dead with the state of being so close to death that a decision could justifiably be made by a relative or guardian to stop resuscitation. But I do not see that their perhaps naive formulation makes "the state of being dead" dependent upon consent of a relative. It makes the state of being *pronounced* dead dependent upon consent. Being dead or alive may be quite independent of the wishes of relatives, but the treatment of persons as if they were dead or alive can logically still be a matter of choice of a relative or even a prior choice of the individual. For those who believe that metaphysical states are to some extent independent of personal choice (as I do), this will mean that in some cases we shall continue to treat corpses as if they were alive or living people as if they were corpses, but we run that risk under any public policy alternative, whether or not it permits freedom of philosophical choice.

More recently Michael Sullivan, county probate judge in Milwaukee, had to make two critical legal decisions concerning whether patients have the right to refuse treatment. He has explained the basis of his decisions in the *New England Law Review*.[19] He writes in his article that he does not believe legislation defining death to be advisable "in this context." Since he is discussing whether dying patients have the right to refuse treatment, this attitude is perfectly plausible. But, although it is also irrelevant to his context, he goes on to state his opinion on who should decide what definition of death should be used: "The individual should decide whether he will employ the Harvard criteria, or some other definition for his death." According to Sullivan, it is the individual, not the physician, the medical society, or the state, who should have the "right to prescribe his death style" including the person's own definition of death. This obviously raises some problems, as in the cases of individuals in irreversible coma who have not recorded an opinion while conscious and competent. Some provision will have to be made for these cases.

There are two possibilities: (1) shifting decision making to the individual (or the next of kin or other legal guardians) and (2) setting up a definition to be followed unless otherwise instructed. As a practical matter both can probably be used. The law could specify a given general standard —oriented to heart or the whole brain or the cerebrum—with the proviso that the individual has the right to leave explicit instructions to the contrary. Further, as with the Uniform Anatomical Gift Act, the law could provide that, in those cases where the individual has left no instructions while conscious and competent, the right would be exercised by the next of kin or guardian appointed for the purpose. Many of these issues also arise in setting up mechanisms for refusing further medical treatment for the still living patient.

There is another problem, however. Has individualism run amok? Do we really want to be so antinomian, so anarchical, that any individual no matter how malicious or foolish can specify any meaning of death which the rest of society would be obliged to honor? What if Aunt Bertha says she knows Uncle Charlie's brain is completely destroyed and his heart is not beating and his lungs are not functioning, but she still thinks there is hope—she still thinks of him as her loving husband and does not want death pronounced for a few more days? Worse yet, what if a grown son who has long since abandoned his senile, mentally ill, and institutionalized father decides that his father's life has lost whatever makes it essentially human and chooses to have him called dead even though his heart, lungs, and brain continue to function? Clearly society cannot permit every individual to choose literally any concept of death. For the same reason, the shortsighted acceptance of death as meaning whatever physicians choose for it to mean is wrong. A physician agreeing with either Aunt Bertha or the coldhearted son should certainly be challenged by society and its judicial system.

There must, then, be limits on individual freedom. At this moment in history the reasonable choices for a concept of death are those focusing on respiration and circulation, on the body's integrating capacities, and on consciousness and related social interactions. Allowing individual choice among these viable alternatives, but not beyond them, may be the only way out of this social policy impasse.

To develop model legislation, we can begin with the Capron-Kass statutory proposal and make several changes to avoid the problems we have discussed. First, a cerebral locus for determining if a person is dead can be incorporated by simply changing the word *brain* to the narrower *cerebral*. Second, it seems to me a reasonable safeguard to insist, in general terms appropriate for a statutory definition, that there be no significant conflict of interest. Finally, wording should be added to permit freedom of choice within reasonable limits. These changes would create the following statute specifying the standards for determining that a person has died:

> A person will be considered dead if in the announced opinion of a physician, based on ordinary standards of medical practice, he has experienced an irreversible cessation of spontaneous respiratory and circulatory functions. In the event that artificial means of support preclude a determination that these functions have ceased, a person will be considered dead if in the announced opinion of a physician, based on

ordinary standards of medical practice, he has experienced an irreversible cessation of spontaneous cerebral functions. Death will have occurred at the time when the relevant functions ceased.

It is provided, however, that no person shall be considered dead even with the announced opinion of a physician solely on the basis of an irreversible cessation of spontaneous cerebral functions if he, while competent to make such a decision, has explicitly rejected the use of this standard or, if he has not expressed himself on the matter while competent, his legal guardian or next of kin explicitly expresses such rejection.

It is further provided that no physician shall pronounce the death of any individual in any case where there is significant conflict of interest with his obligation to serve the patient (including commitment to any other patients, research, or teaching programs which might directly benefit from pronouncing the patient dead).

Notes

1. Alexander Morgan Capron and Leon R. Kass, "A Statutory Definition of the Standards for Determining Human Death: An Appraisal and a Proposal," 121 *University of Pennsylvania Law Review* 97 (1972).

2. *Tucker* v. *Lower,* No. 2831 (Richmond, Va., Law and Equity Court, May 23, 1972), p. 10.

3. Maryland Sessions Laws, ch. 693 (1972). The phrase "in the opinion of a physician" was deleted from the first paragraph and the phrase "and because of a known disease or condition" was added in the second paragraph following "ordinary standards of medical practice." It is not clear why the irreversible loss of brain function must be caused by a known disease or condition unless this is thought to be a protection against falsely diagnosing irreversibility in cases where a central nervous system depressant is present, unknown to the medical personnel.

4. Kennedy, "The Kansas Statute," pp. 946–50.

5. See the discussion in chapter 1 [*Death, Dying, and the Biological Revolution*].

6. Kennedy, "The Kansas Statute," p. 947.

7. Don Harper Mills, "The Kansas Death Statute: Bold and Innovative," *New England Journal of Medicine,* 285 (1971), 968–69.

8. Capron and Kass, "A Statutory Definition," p. 197 n. 70.

9. Willam J. Curran, "Legal and Medical Death—Kansas Takes the First Step," *New England Journal of Medicine,* 284 (1971), 260–61. See also Capron and Kass, "A Statutory Definition," pp. 116–17.

10. See Mills, "The Kansas Death Statute," p. 969; Capron and Kass, "A Statutory Definition."

11. In order to clarify the problem of what can and should be legislated, Capron and Kass ("A Statutory Definition," pp. 102–3) have outlined four possible levels for legislative action. These parallel to some extent those in chap-

ter 1 of this book. While they also specify a purely formal definition ("the transition, however abrupt or gradual, between the state of being alive and the state of being dead"), the *basic concept* is the most general level of the four on the list. Not unlike my use of the term *concept,* they mean a philosophical specification of what it is that is the essential change in a person who is no longer considered alive. This, they argue, should not be legislated. I would agree, provided it is recognized that certain assumptions at the basic conceptual level will have to be made in order to move to the next level, which they call "the general physiological standard." They mean here something like what I called the locus: an area of the body whose functioning is critical. Here, we all agree, is the prime area for legislation. The third and fourth levels outlined by Capron and Kass are the operational criteria (e.g., absence of cardiac contraction and movement of the blood) and "specific tests and procedures" (e.g., pulse, heartbeat, blood pressure, etc.). All agree that there is no place in legislation for something as ephemeral as specific empirical tests. I also concur with Capron and Kass that "operational criteria" should not be incorporated into the law.

12. Capron and Kass, "A Statutory Definition," p. 94.

13. *Ibid.,* pp. 104–8.

14. *Ibid.,* p. 111.

15. *Ibid.,* p. 116.

16. M. M. Halley and W. F. Harvey, "Medical v. Legal Definitions of Death," *Journal of the American Medical Association,* 204 (1968), 423–25.

17. Halley and Harvey, "Law-Medicine Comment: The Definitional Dilemma of Death," *Journal of the Bar Association of the State of Kansas,* 39 (1968), 179.

18. Capron and Kass, "A Statutory Definition," p. 105 n. 66.

19. Michael T. Sullivan, "The Dying Person—His Plight and His Right," 8 *New England Law Review* 197–216 (1973).

SUGGESTED READINGS FOR CHAPTER 1

Books and Articles

"An Appraisal of the Criteria of Cerebral Death: A Summary Statement." *Journal of the American Medical Association,* 237 (March 7, 1977), 982–86.

BEAUCHAMP, TOM L., and WALTERS, LEROY. *Contemporary Issues in Bioethics.* Encino, Calif.: Dickenson Publishing Co., 1978. Chap. 6.

BEECHER, HENRY K. "After the 'Definition of Irreversible Coma.'" *New England Journal of Medicine,* 281 (November 6, 1969), 1070–71.

BEECHER, HENRY K. "Ethical Problems Created by the Hopelessly Unconscious Patient." *New England Journal of Medicine,* 278 (June 27, 1968), 1425–30.

BLACK, PETER McL. "Three Definitions of Death." *Monist,* 60 (January 1977), 136–46.

BRIERLEY, J. B., et al. "Neocortical Death after Cardiac Arrest." *Lancet,* 2 (September 11, 1971), 560–65.

California Medical Association, Committee on Evolving Trends in Society Affecting Life. *Death and Dying: Determining and Defining Death—A Compilation of Definitions, Selected Readings, and Bibliography.* San Francisco: California Medical Association, 1975.

Conference of Royal Colleges and Faculties of the United Kingdom. "Diagnosis of Brain Death." *Lancet,* 2 (November 13, 1976), 1069–70.

DWORKIN, ROGER B. "Death in Context." *Indiana Law Journal,* 48 (Summer 1973), 623–39.

GAYLIN, WILLARD. "Harvesting the Dead." *Harper's,* 249 (September 1974), 23–28ff.

HARP, JAMES R. "Criteria for the Determination of Death." *Anesthesiology,* 40 (April 1974), 391–97.

JENNETT, BRYAN. "The Donor Doctor's Dilemma: Observations on the Recognition and Management of Brain Death." *Journal of Medical Ethics,* 1 (July 1975), 63–66.

MARGOLIS, JOSEPH. *Negativities.* Columbus, Ohio: Charles E. Merrill Co., 1975. Chap. 1.

MORISON, ROBERT, and KASS, LEON. "Death—Process or Event?" *Science,* 173 (August 20, 1971), 694–702.

RAMSEY, PAUL. *The Patient as Person.* New Haven: Yale University Press, 1970. Chap. 2.

SKEGG, P. D. G. "Irreversibly Comatose Individuals: 'Alive' or 'Dead'?" *Cambridge Law Journal,* 33 (April 1974), 130–44.

VAN TILL, H. A. H. "Diagnosis of Death in Comatose Patients under Resuscitation Treatment: A Critical Review of the Harvard Report." *American Journal of Law and Medicine,* 2 (Summer 1976), 1–40.

"Study Suggests New, Less Rigid Criteria for Declaring Death." *Medical World News,* 16 (January 27, 1975), 26–27.

VEATCH, ROBERT M. "Brain Death: Welcome Definition or Dangerous Judgment?" *Hastings Center Report,* 2 (November 1972), 10–13.

VEATCH, ROBERT M. "Consideration about the Determination of Death." In *Philosophy and Public Policy.* Donnie J. Self, ed. Norfolk, Va.: Teagle & Little, Inc., 1977.

WALKER, A. EARL, and MOLINARI, GAETANO F. "Criteria of Cerebral Death." *Transactions of the American Neurological Association,* 100 (1975), 29–35.

Bibliographies

SOLLITTO, SHARMON, and VEATCH, ROBERT M., comps. *Bibliography of Society, Ethics, and the Life Sciences.* Hastings-on-Hudson, N.Y.: Institute of Society, Ethics, and the Life Sciences. Issued annually since 1973. See under "Defining Death."

WALTERS, LEROY, ed. *Bibliography of Bioethics.* Detroit: Gale Research Co. Issued annually since 1975. See under "Brain Death" and "Determination of Death."

Encyclopedia of Bioethics Articles

DEATH: Death in Western Societies—TALCOTT PARSONS

DEATH: ATTITUDES—RICHARD KALISH

DEATH: THE DEFINITION: Criteria for Death—G. F. MOLINARI

DEATH: THE DEFINITION: Pronouncing Death: Legal Aspects—ALEXANDER M. CAPRON

DEATH: THE DEFINITION: Philosophical and Theological Foundations—DALLAS M. HIGH

DEATH AND DYING: ETHICS: Death and Dying Policy—ROBERT M. VEATCH

LIFE SUPPORT DEVICES: Medical Perspective—KEITH REEMTSMA

LIFE SUPPORT DEVICES: Philosophical Perspective—A. G. M. VAN MELSEN

ORGAN DONATION: Ethical Issues—ANDREW JAMETON

ORGAN DONATION: Legal Aspects—JESSE DUKEMINIER, JR.

PERSON—A. G. M. VAN MELSEN

SUICIDE

INTRODUCTION

The major objective of this chapter is to evaluate critically certain moral and social views about suicide. However, the adequacy of our understanding of the nature of suicide is a necessary step in this evaluation process. For this reason the definition of suicide and causal models of suicidal behavior will first be discussed.

The Definition of Suicide

Definitions of suicide vary. There are two primary reasons for conceptual uncertainty regarding the nature of suicide. First, social attitudes are commonly reflected in linguistic definitions adopted by a culture. If suicide is socially disapproved, then the definition of suicide in that culture may reflect this disapproval by eliminating the possibility that any praiseworthy action may be considered a suicide. For example, if covering an exploding grenade with one's body in order to save others is regarded as praiseworthy, while suicide is generally disapproved, then a linguistic maneuver is to say that this action is sacrificial and not suicidal. Similarly, if suicide is highly approved in a culture, then actions that are very risky and that may eventuate in death might be considered suicides. For example, a doctor who experimented on herself for the benefit of her patients while knowing that she could easily die from the experiment, and who did die, might be considered a suicide.

A second, and related, reason for definitional confusion about suicide has to do with different assessments of suicidal *motives*. Sacrificial actions are perhaps the ones that most trouble us. For example, when a spy takes his life in order not to reveal secrets, or when a truck driver rams his truck into a hill (knowing he will die) in order to avoid killing others, or when a person terminates life-saving equipment attached to his body, we may be perplexed as to whether it is suicide or not, even if it is in a reasonable sense an *intentional* taking of one's life. In still other cases we may be similarly perplexed whether to call an action suicide or not. For example, when someone is playing Russian Roulette sheerly out of a motive to win money, but the gun fires and he dies, is it a suicide or not? Further, since the degree and awareness of the person's intention may vary, Shneidman has suggested that we classify all deaths, including natural, accidental, suicidal, and homicidal deaths, in terms of the role of the individual in his own demise. Three possible roles are (1) intentioned, (2) subintentioned (cases in which an individual has played partial, latent, covert, or unconscious roles in hastening his own death), or (3) unintended.

In recent years three kinds of definitions have been fairly popular. The first is simple and might be called the standard definition: there is a suicide if and only if there is intentional termination of one's life. The second supposedly does not rely on an awareness of intentions, and derives from Durkheim: suicide occurs when a person knows that he will die from his own positive or negative, direct or indirect action. The third is far broader in scope and is sometimes called the omnibus definition: suicide occurs when an individual engages in a style of life that he knows may kill him and it does kill him. Such definitions and still others are thoughtfully probed in the first two readings in this chapter.

Social and Psychological Models

Medically speaking, there is no sound evidence that suicide is a disease. In 1897, Durkheim first argued that suicide is a product of society that can be explained sociologically. In his model, the suicide rate fluctuates with the integration of an individual into his society. To try to predict which persons are most susceptible to suicide, Durkheim used the following three categories:

1. *Egoistic Suicide.*   A lack of meaningful social interaction subjects members of a society to personal isolation. For example, a single person who has few close personal friends is a greater risk of suicide than a married individual.

2. *Anomic Suicide.*   A lack of participation in the societal structure deprives persons of normative restraints. This phenomenon may occur when a person is deprived of position, wealth, spouse, etc.

3. *Altruistic Suicide.*   In the third, but minor, category social integration is actually excessive, and so suicide, as, e.g., in hara-kiri, under certain circumstances becomes an honorable and socially encouraged action.

Freud, in contrast to Durkheim, placed the emphasis more on a person's individual mental condition. He viewed suicide as created by the breakdown of ego defenses and the release of destructive forces that reflect the ambivalent relationship to those love objects with whom one identifies and makes part of oneself. Thus the hated parent with whom an individual identifies may be murdered symbolically in the act of self-killing. Recent modifications of Freud's thesis emphasize adaptational breakdowns in a social field: the failure to alter a destructive environment, on the one hand, and the apparent inability to conform, on the other. This breakdown may result in (retroflexed) rage in which the object for punishment becomes oneself. This coercive rage is fed by failure, and may assume the proportion of murderous wishes directed against another and oneself. Negative feelings about oneself and one's "world," along with helplessness and hopelessness, are important considerations in determining that suicide is the only available option.

Other theories emphasize the wish to die (particularly among the aged), in which suicide may be seen as a "release." Menninger, whose psychodynamic formulation reflects this view, regards suicide as a kind of death that entails three internal elements: the element of dying, the element of killing, and the element of being killed. Many suicides, however, apparently do not wish to die, or even to kill themselves; rather, they wish to interrupt intense anxiety and do so by "interrupting" their lives. In all these psychological models, impulsivity and ambivalence are prominent features. Furthermore, the carrying out of the act of suicide will be influenced by such situational variables as the availability of guns and pills, as well as by the overall influence of the psychological field.

Despite all these attempted explanations through models, it is probably fair to say that no theory—psychological or social—now suffices for the understanding of suicide.

The Morality and Rationality of Suicide

Strikingly diverse attitudes toward suicide have emerged in different societies, where the approval or disapproval of suicide is often influenced by ethical and religious considerations. Although the person who commits suicide is no longer diagnosed by competent investigators as psychotic purely on the basis of the act itself, a lively debate is still being carried on as to the possibility of making a rational decision to commit suicide; and on any presently accountable theory of compulsion, the degree to which a given act of suicide is voluntary is usually quite difficult to evaluate. Brandt argues in this chapter that suicide may be rational in certain circumstances, but only when such a decision follows exhaustive examination of other options. In discussing the blameworthiness of suicide, it is assumed that we are talking only about the class of *rational* suicides, for if a suicide were irrational, we would not judge the person to be blameworthy.

Moral arguments about the permissibility and impermissibility of suicide have typically revolved around the question whether or not suicide violates one or more of three obligations: to oneself, to others, and to God. This is precisely the framework used by St. Thomas Aquinas and by David Hume for the discussion of the morality of suicide in this chapter. Attempts to answer the question about moral permissibility usually appeal to one or more of three moral principles. The first is a principle of community responsibility: the suicide should consider not only his interests, but the interests of all affected. This principle does not demand, however, that society's interests are always overriding. Rather it demands a weighing and balancing of considerations by the person contemplating suicide. The second is a principle of self-determinism: the suicide is said to have the right to do whatever he wishes with his own life so long as his action does not seriously limit the rights of others. The third is a sanctity-of-life principle: the suicide is always wrong if he *intends* to take his life for his own sake, because nonsacrificial life-taking is always wrong.

There are many different reasons for invoking one or the other of these principles. The reasons might be utilitarian—as in Hume's case, and they lead him to strong views about the right to self-determination and to a weak sense of community obligations. The reasons might also be theological —as in Aquinas' case, and they lead him to strong views about the sanctity of life and also to views that there are strong obligations to the community.

Intervention to Prevent Suicide

Since persons in the process of committing suicide are often under the strain of a temporary crisis, under the influence of drugs or alcohol, and beset with considerable ambivalence (or simply wish to reduce or interrupt anxiety without wanting to die at all), the intervention of a second party to stop a person from killing himself seems to many persons for the most part reasonable, and even morally required. The community, furthermore, by not intervening, may seem not to care, may tend to dissuade people from seeing suicide as a social-psychological problem, and may, thereby, facilitate the actions of would-be suicides. Thomas Szasz' arguments, which are presented in this chapter, present reasons against intervening to prevent suicides. These arguments rest on the position that one ought not to interfere with the free acts of others insofar as those actions do not harm persons other than the actors. This position is often said to be antipaternalistic. Those who defend a paternalistic position contend that on at least some occasions we are morally obliged to intervene to prevent the person from doing harm to himself. It seems to such persons that we do not exhibit moral concern about others unless we intervene. Paternalists and antipaternalists usually agree that it is permissible to intervene where a person seems driven to suicide by an intense compulsion. Disagreement arises over cases where the suicidal person is capable of deliberating and choosing his own course of action, even though influenced in these deliberations by such factors as terminal illness and serious depression. The place of paternalism in suicide intervention (if any) remains a matter of considerable controversy.

In the following selection Joseph Margolis stresses the culturally variable character of suicide. He contrasts religious traditions with those nonreligious traditions that provide competing points of view. He also comments on the importance of cultural and personal value systems in labeling an act as suicide. For Margolis there is no "neutral" concept of suicide; what is allowed or disallowed is always based on some specific perspective taken by an individual observer.

Joseph Margolis

SUICIDE *

Suicide is thought to provide a telling test for a moral theory because, unlike murder, it is problematic whether and how it can be plausibly condemned. As far as linguistic usage goes, there is no clear sense in which characterizing an act as an act of suicide entails its being blameworthy, evil, sinful, or reprehensible. Not that suicide is not reprehensible: it may or it may not be. But that cannot be decided merely by labeling it as such.[1] . . .

An initial difficulty in deciding the issue concerns the sorting of specimen instances. A man may knowingly and willingly go to his death, be rationally capable of avoiding death, deliberately not act to save his life, and yet not count as a suicide. In this sense, we usually exclude the man who sacrifices his life to save another's, the religious martyr who will not violate his faith, the patriot who intentionally lays down his life for a cause. Not that men in such circumstances may not be suiciding; only that they cannot be said to be suiciding solely for those reasons. Some seem to have thought otherwise. "Suicide," says Emile Durkheim, "is applied to all cases of death resulting directly or indirectly from a positive or negative act of the victim himself, which he knows will produce this result."[2] So there may be an element of arbitrariness in including or excluding specimens. We can expect a theory of suicide to be applicable only relative to the cases admitted, but we may quarrel about the inclusion or exclusion of given cases. . . .

* From *Negativities: The Limits of Life*. Copyright © 1975, pp. 23–29, 34–35 (edited). Reprinted by permission of Charles E. Merrill Publishing Company.

Sometimes, quite reasonably, it is supposed that there is a fundamental difference between suicide religiously and nonreligiously construed. R. F. Holland, for instance, believes there is such a difference.[3] On his view, the suicide is religiously condemned because he is an ingrate respecting a gift his Creator has given him. Holland seems not to have taken seriously enough the fact that the Stoics, unlike the Christians, took their lives with ritual equanimity. The Stoics were hardly behaving as ingrates—on the contrary, they may have been celebrating their own divinity as fulgurations of the divine fire of Reason. . . . Holland also speaks of a so-called humanist, that is, nonreligious, attitude toward suicide: for him, it is embodied in the case of a man with terminal cancer, all his faculties intact, whose sense of the worth of life gave him a reason for suiciding when he "saw . . . no sense in prolonging his life beyond a certain point." The case is a fair and important one, of course; but in what sense, on the hypothesis, has an *ethical* justification been provided? We understand why the man acted as he did, but how did his sense of the worth of his life or of life itself justify his suiciding? And why should Holland insist that the "humanist" suicide had to view the world as he did? Could he not have decided that life was utterly meaningless? Could he not have found life to be utterly meaningless for him? If one could justify suicide in the terminal cancer case, how much more convincingly could a man justify suicide if he sincerely believed life to have no point at all? . . .

The point of pressing these obvious considerations is to bring home the culturally variable character of suicide. There is no bare religious or nonreligious view of suicide—there are many competing views, some religious, some not, some not even significantly so characterized. Every relevant instance collects a highly institutionalized tradition. There are paradigms of admissible Buddhist, Shinto, Stoic, Epicurean suicides; and, in terms that, for doctrinal reasons, cannot be construed as suicide but that involve very many of the same elements, there are, in the Christian and Muslim traditions, admissible ways of ending or yielding one's life that could be avoided on the option and action of the person affected. There is perhaps not that much difference between the action of the kamikaze pilot and the Christian crusader or the Muslim warrior seeking death in battle against the infidel. But in the Christian and Muslim traditions, to construe the activity involved as suicide would be to condemn the agent. So, for example, the martyr who yields his life to his tormentors is said not to be a suicide; though if, under the same pressure, he ended his life by his sword, he would have been a suicide. Socrates took his life by drinking the cup of hemlock and did not simply yield his life to others, and is said, in accord with another tradition, not to have suicided; yet, the Athenians were obviously hoping that Socrates would have taken the option open to him to leave the city forever. In Eskimo society, the elderly will take a small supply of food and leave their community never to return, anticipating that they will die in a matter of days. They will not take their own lives by a direct physical act but they will put themselves in the position of imminent and inevitable death; yet, they are usually not said to have committed suicide. Here, it seems undeniable that we either respect the favorable judgment or approval of the home culture and therefore refuse to label the act suicide in order not to raise the prospect (or the certainty) of condemning it in accord with our own conceptual preferences; or, viewing it favorably in terms of our own values, we refuse to label it such in order to avoid the same prospect. Socrates, we say, upheld the judgment of the Athenian court; and, having done so, he found the option of leaving the city meaningless, morally unacceptable, or repugnant. The Eskimo, we say, respected the implications of the marginal existence of his community and acted to permit others a more realistic distribution of food when he was no longer able to contribute useful labor; in doing so, he rejects as morally unacceptable whatever it would take to force others to provide for his own life under the general condition of mortality.

There is no reason to dispute these assessments. In fact, what is important is the force of their admission. There is no simple formula for designating, except trivially, an act of taking, or yielding, or making likely the end of one's life that will count, universally, as suicide. No, some selection of acts of this minimal sort will, in accord with an interpreting tradition, construe what was done as or as not suicide; and, so judging, the tradition will provide as well for the approval or condemnation of what was done. In short, suicide, like murder itself, is an act that can be specified only in a systematic way within a given tradition; and that specification itself depends on classifying the intention of the agent. We can say, therefore, that there is no minimal act of commission or omission that counts as suicide, except relative to some tradition; and, within particular traditions, the justifiability of particular suicides may yet be debatable.

There is, however, one way of characterizing suicide that, though it goes counter to some familiar judgments, manages to isolate as neutrally as possible the issue most in dispute: whether the deliberate taking of one's life in order simply to end it, not instrumentally for any ulterior purpose, can ever be rational or rationally justified. Durkheim's alternative characterization resolves the issue trivially, since, as in the case of a spy's taking his life to avoid capture or as in the case of sacrificing one's life for another, there could not but be, on Durkheim's criterion, ready cases of rational suicide. The trouble is that Durkheim's criterion does not enable us to focus the point of the serious charge that suicide is never rational or rationally justified. We shall, therefore, construe suicide as narrowly as possible in order to allow the issue a fair inning: we can thereafter, of course, always temper our classification in the direction of Durkheim's view—with the consequence of being increasingly unable to generalize meaningfully about the phenomenon itself. Thus construed, we shall take it that to characterize an act as an act of suicide is to describe it in a way that takes precedence over every alternative characterization. If Socrates is said not to have suicided, it is because what he did is described overridingly as adhering to the rules of Athenian justice: that characterization precludes his having suicided. We cannot hold consistently that Socrates suicided but was justified in doing so because, in so doing, he upheld Athenian justice overridingly. Obviously, in taking his life, he upheld Athenian justice. But to judge that he suicided is to render a verdict, all things considered, that disallows ascribing a merely *instrumental* purpose or intention to the act in question; to judge that, acting as he did, he supported Athenian justice is to assign Socrates an overriding and ulterior objective inconsistent with intending suicide. The suicide's overriding concern is to end his own life, not for the sake of any independent objective that, in principle, he might pursue in another way: he is persuaded there is no other commitment that, under the circumstances, would command his rational assent, and he knows that a successful act precludes any further commitment on his own part. . . .

The Buddhist monk who sets fire to himself in order to protest the war that he might have resisted in another way will not be said to have committed suicide if the *overriding* characterization of what he did fixes on the ulterior objective of influencing his countrymen. But he *may* be said to have suicided if resisting the war and influencing his countrymen are judged not to bear on what, all things considered, proves to be the overriding characterization of what he did; *and,* if he is said to have is no coherent way to view his act but as an act of protest-suicide, a suicided even though he took his life in order to protest the war, then there ritualized act of suiciding whose essential import, given the relevant doctrine, is that of protest. . . . Suicide supercedes every instrumental use of one's own life; only its intrinsic import remains to be considered. . . .

The critical distinctions are these: if an agent is presumed rational, then if he takes his own life or allows it to be taken for some further purpose that he serves instrumentally, we normally refuse to say he has suicided; and if he is presumed irrational, then taking his own life in some putatively instrumental way is normally taken as suicide. This is the reason that, in the clinical professions, suicide tends to be linked to illness, weakness of character, insanity, or the like: any scanning of the psychiatric literature, for instance, confirms this.[4] But such a view utterly ignores the kind of cases . . . in which people simply wish to put an end to their lives because life has ceased to have a sufficiently favorable significance or because taking one's life, under the circumstances, does have a sufficiently favorable significance. . . .

Suicide is an interpretive category imposed on acts, characterizable in relatively neutral ways, in accord with a relevant doctrine or ideology.

A rational suicide, then, may fairly be said to be a person who aims overridingly at ending his own life and who, in a relevant sense, performs the act. The manner in which he suicides may be said to be by commission or omission, actively or passively, directly or indirectly, consciously or unconsciously, justifiably or reprehensibly—in accord with the classificatory distinctions of particular traditions. Spinoza holds the drive to survive essential to human nature; reason, serving this *conatus* in man, cannot prefer suicide. Hence, he judges suicide to be inherently irrational. By a small adjustment, Freud, a true Spinozist, was inclined to view intended suicide as a form of illness. . . . In any event, the concept of a rational suicide is thought by them to be self-contradictory. On that view, the possibility of an ethical appraisal of suicide is either obviated or very seriously restricted; for if a given case is a genuine case of suicide, the agent must have been irrational and only his responsibility for being irrational could remain a relevant issue. Hence, the attractiveness of viewing suicide as an illness: it justifies full public and professional concern (and control) where the usual notions of responsibility are inapt. . . .

We have provided a sense in which a man may be a rational suicide, the sense in which a man has as his overriding concern the ending of his life. This permits us to preclude all cases in which a man ends his own life merely instrumentally, unless irrationally. Rational suicide invites an appraisal of the import or quality of the act, not of its ulterior objectives. In this sense, the terminal cancer patient behaves in a way comparable to that of the Muslim warrior, though their beliefs are different. The patient's interests in surviving are drained; life has lost its meaning or savor; there are no further prudential interests he means to pursue. Marginally, perhaps, reducing pain, for instance, by prolonged anesthesia, is prudentially preferable to enduring pain; but in itself this cannot justify construing suicide to end pain as a decision of a prudential sort. The defense or censure of suicide is undertaken, of course, in doctrinal terms—religiously (by Stoics and Christians), ethically (as in humanist and Kantian accounts), aesthetically (as in Nietzsche and, perhaps, Schopenhauer). But the hard case is the case of the suicide not committed to some *justificatory* doctrine. He takes his life only to end it, not, necessarily, to avoid evil or to secure some good. In a sense, we can only explain why he has suicided: life doesn't attract him any longer or sufficiently to go on living. Counsels of caution or patience are impertinent, for he does no more than fix the limit of his own mortality. We may condemn or applaud him on doctrinal grounds. In his own terms, however, we note only that he has acted rationally: believing overridingly that there is no point to going on, he acts consistently. In this sense, rationality is deeper than prudence or morality, and none is equivalent to any other. Finally, the very category of suicide interprets, in terms of some selective doctrine, the intentions and conduct of agents said to have taken or to have attempted to take their own lives and to provide for the appraisal of those actions: there is no neutral concept of suicide, and what is allowed or disallowed as a fair specimen reflects at least conditions that alternatively favored creeds would have to meet in order to be minimally coherent, if it does not already exhibit their actual preferences.

Notes

1. See David Daube, "The Linguistics of Suicide," *Philosophy and Public Affairs,* 1 (1972), 387–437. Karl Menninger takes suicide to be "obviously a *murder* . . . committed *by* the self as murderer"; see his comments in Edwin S. Shneidman, Norman L. Farberow, and Robert E. Litman, eds., *The Psychology of Suicide* (New York: Science House, 1970), p. 38.
2. *Suicide,* trans. John A. Spaulding and George Simpson (New York: Free Press, 1951), p. 44.
3. See "Suicide," in *Talk of God,* Royal Institute of Philosophy Lectures, vol. 2, 1967–68 (London: Macmillan, 1969).
4. Psychoanalytic resistance to the conception may be gauged in Joost A. M. Meerloo, *Suicide and Mass Suicide* (New York: E. P. Dutton, 1968), where considerable emphasis is placed on "the suicidal man within us," our inherent self-destructive urge.

In the following selection, Tom L. Beauchamp pursues the definitional question, "What is suicide?" He argues that it is not amenable to simple definitional analysis because of several kinds of cases that we tend to exclude from the realm of the suicidal. Unlike Durkheim, Beauchamp places considerable emphasis on *intention* and on the nature of the *cause* of death. Thus, Socrates is not considered a suicide, because his death, though intended by him, was decreed by others, who coerced him and who were causally responsible for his death. After treating the special cases of death by refusal of treatment and sacrificial deaths, Beauchamp formally defines suicide in terms of an intended, noncoerced death in circumstances where an agent plays a role in arranging the conditions which bring about his or her death. Although Beauchamp's analysis is of the ordinary, English-language meaning of suicide, he also argues that this ordinary-language meaning is tainted in that we tend to regard suicides as unjustified because of the very meaning of the term. His point is that we would be better off in discussing the moral justification of suicide if we had a more neutral concept than we in fact have.

Tom L. Beauchamp

WHAT IS SUICIDE? *

Although debate about the legality, rationality, and morality of suicide has increased in recent years, only fragmentary attention has been devoted to the development of an adequate definition of suicide. Because signifi-

* Copyright © 1977 by Tom L. Beauchamp.

cantly different moral, social, and legal sanctions will be implied by the classification of an act as suicide, euthanasia, murder, or accidental death, the development of an adequate definition will have important practical consequences. The way we classify actions is indicative of the way we think about them, and in the present case such classifications have immediate relevance for medicine, ethics, and law.

A start in the direction of a definition of "suicide" is the following: The death of a person is a suicide only if: (1) the person's own death is intentionally self-caused, and (2) the person's action is noncoerced. However, two special problems prevent this simple definition from being fully adequate.

THE PROBLEM OF TREATMENT REFUSAL

The first class of difficult cases for the above definition involve persons who suffer from a terminal illness or mortal injury, and who refuse some medical therapy without which they will die, but with which they could live for some period beyond the point they would die without the therapy. For example, refusal to allow a blood transfusion, or an amputation, or refusal of further kidney dialysis are now familiar facts of hospital life. But are they suicides? Two facts about such cases are noteworthy. First, these acts certainly *can* be suicides, because *any* means productive of death potentially can be used to the end of suicide. Pulling the plug on one's respirator is not relevantly different from plunging a knife into one's heart, if the reason for putting an end to life is identical in the two cases. Second, suicidal acts can also be sacrificial. For example, if a person were suffering from a costly terminal disease, then it would be an altruistic (even if perhaps misguided) action to take his own life in order to spare his family the inordinate cost of providing the care; but it would nonetheless be suicide.

Still, the seriously suffering person with end-stage renal disease who refuses to continue dialysis and dies a "natural" death does not strike most as a suicide. Why not? Three features of such situations need to be distinguished in order to answer this question:

1. whether the death is *intended* by the agent,
2. whether an *active* means to death is selected,
3. whether a *nonfatal condition* is present (no terminal disease or mortal injury exists).

The more we have unmistakable cases of actions by an agent that involve an *intentionally caused death* using an *active* means where there is a *nonfatal* condition, the more inclined we are to classify such acts as suicides, whereas the more such conditions are absent the less inclined we are to call the acts suicides. For example, if a seriously but not mortally wounded soldier turns his rifle on himself and intentionally brings about his death, it is a suicide. But what about the seriously ill patient of ambiguous intentions, suffering from a terminal illness, and refusing yet another blood transfusion?

Although considerations of terminal illness and of intention are important, the main source of our present definitional problem is the active/ passive distinction. A passively allowed, "natural" death seems foreign to the notion of suicide, both because the death is at least in part not caused by the agent and because the "cide" part of "suicide" entails "killing," which is commonly contrasted with allowing to die. In the face of this complex mixture of elements the following generalization may be offered about such cases: An act is *not* a suicide if the person who dies suffers from a terminal disease or from a mortal injury which, by refusal of treatment, he passively allows to cause his death—even if the person intends his death. However, this analysis does not seem adequate for all cases; for example, think of a patient with a terminal condition who could easily avoid dying for a long time but who chooses to end his life immediately by not taking cheap and painless medication. This counterexample might incline us toward the view that a time restriction is also needed. But this restriction probably could not be reasonably formulated, and I am inclined to think that we have reached the conceptual boundaries of our notion of suicide. We have come as close to an understanding as the concept permits. If in the end the analysis offered has become slightly reforming (one that requires that we change the ordinary meaning of "suicide" somewhat), the vagaries of the concept itself are perhaps responsible.

THE PROBLEM OF SACRIFICIAL DEATHS

There remains the problem of so-called "altruistically motivated (or other-regarding) suicide." Here the key notion responsible for our not classifying some intentional self-killings as suicides seems to some to be that of *sacrifice*. Perhaps those who sacrifice their lives are not conceived as "suicides" for an interesting reason: because we see such actions as from the suicide's point of view having plausible claim to being justified for *other-regarding*—not *self-regarding*—reasons, and hence we logically exclude them from the realm of the suicidal.

Sadly, exclusions based on self-sacrificial acts will not help much in structuring a definition of suicide unless further qualifications are introduced. The monk in Vietnam who pours gasoline over his body and burns himself to death as a protest against his government does not do so for his own sake but for the sake of his beloved countrymen, just as the father who kills himself in the midst of a famine so that his wife and children may have enough to eat acts from self-sacrificial motives. Many cases of this general description provide paradigms of suicidal actions but would have to be declared nonsuicides if the approach were taken that other-regarding, sacrificial acts fail to qualify as suicides.

In the face of this new complexity, a course paralleling the one for refusal-of-treatment cases may be taken: An act is *not* a suicide if the person is caused to die by a life-threatening condition he does not intend to bring about through his own actions. Interestingly, this approach does not turn on the notion of sacrifice, the original problem compelling consideration of these cases. It makes no difference whether the action is sacrificial or nonsacrificial, so long as the condition causing death is not brought about *by the agent* for the purpose of ending his life. This conclusion is somewhat troublesome, because the agent does intend his death in those cases of sacrifice where a person has the option either to save his life or to act in protection of others' lives, and then specifically chooses a course of action that brings about his own death. Nonetheless, in such cases *it cannot be said that he brings about the life-threatening condition causing his death in order to cause his death,* and that fact is the crucial matter.

There are further parallels between this kind of case and the refusal of treatment cases previously discussed. Three relevant ingredients can again be distinguished:

1. whether the death is *intended* by the agent,
2. whether the death is *caused by* the agent (or is caused to the agent),
3. whether the action is *self-regarding* (or is other-regarding).

Here the main source of confusion is not the "active/passive" distinction, but rather is the parallel "caused by/caused to" distinction. To cause one's own death in order to die is to kill oneself, but to have death caused by some alien condition in the course of an action with multiple objectives may not be. Here we might say that the killing/being killed distinction is involved, and that it functions rather like the killing/letting die distinction previously discussed. At any rate, we have again reached the boundaries of our concept of suicide, which is here being contrasted with the concept of an externally caused death. A person might be using an externally caused means as a socially acceptable and convenient way of ending his life, and hence it might be a suicide. But we have seen that this is true of any means to death whatsoever.

A good test case for the above analysis is the now classic case of Captain Oates, who walked into the Antarctic snow to die, because he was suffering from an illness that hindered the progress of a party attempting to make its way out of a severe blizzard.[1] According to R. F. Holland, Oates was not a suicide because: "in Oates's case I can say, 'No [he didn't kill himself]; the blizzard killed him.' Had Oates taken out a revolver and shot himself I should have agreed he was a suicide."[2] I cannot agree with Holland's estimate. On the analysis offered above, Oates' heroic sacrifice is a suicide because of the active steps that he took to bring about his death.

Although the climatic conditions proximately caused his death, he *brought about* the relevant life-threatening condition causing his death (exposure to the weather) in order that he die. There is no relevant difference between death by revolver and death by exposure to freezing weather when both equally are life-threatening conditions used to cause one's own death. However, the Oates case is not an easy one to declare a suicide. It is a close call precisely because there is both multiple causation and multiple intent: the action is an heroic way of being *causally responsible* for placing oneself in *conditions which cause* death, and death was intended as a merciful release from an intolerable burden, not only because of Oates' suffering but also because of his knowledge that he was imperilling the lives of his colleagues. Moreover, his release from these burdens is apparently his major objective. No wonder the Oates case has become a classic in literature on the definition of suicide; it is hard to imagine a case sitting more astride the boundaries between suicide and nonsuicide.

Although the analysis proposed above does not differ in some respects from that of Joseph Margolis', the point at which we part company is now evident, for he argues as follows:

> The Buddhist monk who sets fire to himself in order to protest the war that he might have resisted in another way will not be said to have committed suicide if the *overriding* characterization of what he did fixes on the ulterior objective of influencing his countrymen. . . . [If there is] some further purpose that he serves instrumentally, then we normally refuse to say he has suicided; . . .[3]

Margolis thinks there is a decisive difference between whether one's overriding reason is some sacrificial objective or the objective of ending one's life. In my view the matter is more complicated and has little to do with the notions of sacrifice, martyrdom, and patriotism. It has rather to do with whether death is caused by one's own arrangement of the life-threatening conditions causing death for the purpose of bringing about death (whether this purpose be the overriding reason or not). Since the monk arranges the conditions, precisely for this purpose (though for others as well), he is a suicide.

CONCLUSION

We have arrived, then, at an understanding of suicide that is fairly simple, even if somewhat more complicated than the definitions with which we began: An act is a suicide if a person intentionally brings about his own death in circumstances where others do not coerce him to the action, except in those cases where death occurs through an agent's intentional decision but is caused by conditions not specifically arranged by the agent for the purpose of bringing about his own death. However, in concluding, we should ask whether anything useful has been accomplished by this analysis, and especially whether such a definition of the ordinary language meaning of "suicide" is a proper one for moral philosophy. Terms in their ordinary meaning often contain evaluative accretions due to social attitudes that render them difficult for purposes of moral analysis; and the meaning we have located for "suicide" appears to be a premiere instance of this problem: Because self-caused deaths are often revolting and inexplicable, an emotive meaning of disapproval has been incorporated into our use of "suicide." More importantly, because of this already attached disapproval we find it hard to accept as "suicides" acts of which we approve, or at least do not disapprove. We thus by the very logic of the term prejudice any pending moral analysis of the action of a suicide as being right or wrong, let alone praiseworthy or blameworthy.

Notes

1. See *Scott's Last Expedition* (London: 1935), Vol. I, p. 462.
2. "Suicide," in J. Rachels, ed., *Moral Problems* (New York: Harper and Row, 1971), pp. 352–53.
3. Margolis, *"Suicide,"* in *Negativities* (Columbus, Ohio: Charles E. Merrill Co., 1975), pp. 27–28. Cf. his final definition on p. 33. [Reprinted above.]

In the following selection, Thomas Aquinas discusses the morality of suicide. He claims that suicide is an offense against self, an offense against society, and a violation of God's sovereignty. People belong to God, who is their creator; and suicide is, for that reason, analogous to theft: "Because life is God's gift to man . . . whoever takes his own life sins against God, even as he who kills another's slave, sins against that slave's master. . . ." While St. Thomas does appeal to explicit statements in the Bible, the core of his argument seems to be that suicide runs counter to the creator's general interest in human life and its flourishing. For Aquinas, there seems to be an absolute prohibition of suicide, unless it is directly commanded by God.

St. Thomas Aquinas

WHETHER IT IS LAWFUL TO KILL ONESELF *

FIFTH ARTICLE

Objection 1.   It would seem lawful for a man to kill himself. For murder is a sin insofar as it is contrary to justice. But no man can do an injustice to himself, as is proved in *Ethic.* v. 11. Therefore no man sins by killing himself.

---

* From *Summa Theologica* (1925 trans.). Copyright 1947, Part II-II, Q. 64, Art. 5. Reprinted by permission of Benziger Brothers.

Obj. 2. Further, it is lawful, for one who exercises public authority, to kill evildoers. Now he who exercises public authority is sometimes an evildoer. Therefore he may lawfully kill himself.

Obj. 3. Further, it is lawful for a man to suffer spontaneously a lesser danger that he may avoid a greater: thus it is lawful for a man to cut off a decayed limb even from himself, that he may save his whole body. Now sometimes a man, by killing himself, avoids a greater evil, for example an unhappy life, or the shame of sin. Therefore a man may kill himself.

Obj. 4. Further, Samson killed himself, as related in Judges xvi., and yet he is numbered among the saints (Heb. xi). Therefore it is lawful for a man to kill himself.

Obj. 5. Further, it is related (2 Mach. xiv. 42) that a certain Razias killed himself, *choosing to die nobly rather than to fall into the hands of the wicked, and to suffer abuses unbecoming his noble birth.* Now nothing that is done nobly and bravely is unlawful. Therefore suicide is not unlawful.

On the contrary, Augustine says (*De Civ. Dei* i. 20): *Hence it follows that the words "Thou shalt not kill" refer to the killing of a man;—not another man; therefore, not even thyself. For he who kills himself, kills nothing else than a man.*

I answer that, It is altogether unlawful to kill oneself, for three reasons. First, because everything naturally loves itself, the result being that everything naturally keeps itself in being, and resists corruptions so far as it can. Wherefore suicide is contrary to the inclination of nature, and to charity whereby every man should love himself. Hence suicide is always a mortal sin, as being contrary to the natural law and to charity.

Secondly, because every part, as such, belongs to the whole. Now every man is part of the community, and so, as such, he belongs to the community. Hence by killing himself he injures the community, as the Philosopher declares (*Ethic.* v. 11).

Thirdly, because life is God's gift to man, and is subject to His power, Who kills and makes to live. Hence whoever takes his own life, sins against God, even as he who kills another's slave, sins against that slave's master, and as he who usurps to himself judgment of a matter not entrusted to him. For it belongs to God alone to pronounce sentence of death and life, according to Deut. xxxii. 39, *I will kill and I will make to live.*

Reply Obj. 1. Murder is a sin, not only because it is contrary to justice, but also because it is opposed to charity which a man should have towards himself: in this respect suicide is a sin in relation to oneself. In relation to the community and to God, it is sinful, by reason also of its opposition to justice.

Reply Obj. 2. One who exercises public authority may lawfully put to death an evildoer, since he can pass judgment on him. But no man is judge of himself. Wherefore it is not lawful for one who exercises public authority to put himself to death for any sin whatever: although he may lawfully commit himself to the judgment of others.

Reply Obj. 3. Man is made master of himself through his free-will: wherefore he can lawfully dispose of himself as to those matters which pertain to this life which is ruled by man's free-will. But the passage from this life to another and happier one is subject not to man's free-will but to the power of God. Hence it is not lawful for man to take his own life that he may pass to a happier life, nor that he may escape any unhappiness whatsoever of the present life, because the ultimate and most fearsome evil of this life is death, as the Philosopher states (*Ethic.* iii. 6). Therefore to bring death upon oneself in order to escape the other afflictions of this life, is to adopt a greater evil in order to avoid a lesser. In like manner it is unlawful to take one's own life on account of one's having committed a sin, both because by so doing one does oneself a very great injury, by depriving oneself of the time needful for repentance, and because it is not lawful to slay an evildoer except by the sentence of the public authority. Again it is unlawful for a woman to kill herself lest she be violated, because she ought not to commit on herself the very great sin of suicide, to avoid the lesser sin of another. For she commits no sin in being violated by force, provided she does not consent, since *without consent of the mind there is no stain on the body,* as the Blessed Lucy declared. Now it is evident that fornication and adultery are less grievous sins than taking a man's, especially one's own, life: since the latter is most grievous, because one injures oneself, to whom one owes the greatest love. Moreover it is most dangerous since no time is left wherein to expiate it by repentance. Again it is not lawful for anyone to take his own life for fear he should consent to sin, because *evil must not be done that good may come* (Rom. iii. 8) or that evil may be avoided, especially if the evil be of small account and an uncertain event, for it is uncertain whether one will at some future time consent to a sin, since God is able to deliver man from sin under any temptation whatever.

Reply Obj. 4. As Augustine says (*De Civ. Dei* i. 21), *not even Samson is to be excused that he crushed himself together with his enemies under the ruins of the house, except the Holy Ghost, Who had wrought many wonders through him, had secretly commanded him to do this.* He assigns the same reason in the case of certain holy women, who at the time of persecution took their own lives, and who are commemorated by the Church.

Reply Obj. 5. It belongs to fortitude that a man does not shrink from being slain by another, for the sake of the good of virtue, and that he may avoid sin. But that a man takes his own life in order to avoid penal evils has indeed an appearance of fortitude (for which reason some, among whom was Razias, have killed themselves thinking to act from fortitude), yet is is not true fortitude, but rather a weakness of soul unable to bear penal evils, as the Philosopher (*Ethic.* iii. 7) and Augustine (*De Civ. Dei* i. 22, 23) declare.

Aquinas has presented an essentially theological argument. The following essay by David Hume rebuts the thrust of this point of view. Hume's views are antitheological and in support of a right to commit suicide. He argues that if God is the creator of the world, his will must be expressed in all events. Thus, if all events equally reflect God's will, then suicide cannot be a departure from that will. Hume further contends that suicide is not always harmful to society and may even contribute to the public good. He also believes that suicide may be consistent with our own interests and "with our duty to ourselves." He even finds some suicides "laudable."

David Hume

ON SUICIDE *

. . . So great is our horror of death that when it presents itself, under any form, besides that to which a man has endeavoured to reconcile his imagination, it acquires new terrors and overcomes his feeble courage: But when the menaces of superstition are joined to this natural timidity, no wonder it quite deprives men of all power over their lives, since even many pleasures and enjoyments, to which we are carried by a strong propensity, are torn from us by this inhuman tyrant. Let us here endeavour to restore men to their native liberty by examining all the common arguments against Suicide, and shewing that that action may be free from every imputation of guilt or blame, according to the sentiments of all the ancient philosophers.

If Suicide be criminal, it must be a transgression of our duty either to God, our neighbour, or ourselves. To prove that suicide is no transgression of our duty to God, the following considerations may perhaps suffice. In order to govern the material world, the almighty Creator has established general and immutable laws by which all bodies, from the greatest planet to the smallest particle of matter, are maintained in their proper sphere and function. To govern the animal world, he has endowed all living creatures with bodily and mental powers; with senses, passions, appetites, memory and judgment, by which they are impelled or regulated in that course of life to which they are destined. These two distinct principles of the material and

---

* Originally published in Edinburgh, Scotland, 1777.

animal world continually encroach upon each other, and mutually retard or forward each other's operations. The powers of men and of all other animals are restrained and directed by the nature and qualities of the surrounding bodies; and the modifications and actions of these bodies are incessantly altered by the operation of all animals. Man is stopped by rivers in his passage over the surface of the earth; and rivers, when properly directed, lend their force to the motion of machines, which serve to the use of man. But though the provinces of material and animal powers are not kept entirely separate, there results from thence no discord or disorder in the creation; on the contrary, from the mixture, union and contrast of all the various powers of inanimate bodies and living creatures, arises that surprising harmony and proportion which affords the surest argument of supreme wisdom. The providence of the Deity appears not immediately in any operation, but governs everything by those general and immutable laws, which have been established from the beginning of time. All events, in one sense, may be pronounced the action of the Almighty; they all proceed from those powers with which he has endowed his creatures. A house which falls by its own weight is not brought to ruin by his providence more than one destroyed by the hands of men; nor are the human faculties less his workmanship than the laws of motion and gravitation. When the passions play, when the judgment dictates, when the limbs obey; this is all the operation of God, and upon these animate principles, as well as upon the inanimate, has he established the government of the universe. Every event is alike important in the eyes of that infinite being, who takes in at one glance the most distant regions of space and remotest periods of time. There is no event, however important to us, which he has exempted from the general laws that govern the universe, or which he has peculiarly reserved for his own immediate action and operation. The revolution of states and empires depends upon the smallest caprice or passion of single men; and the lives of men are shortened or extended by the smallest accident of air or diet, sunshine or tempest. Nature still continues her progress and operation; and if general laws be ever broke by particular volitions of the Deity, 'tis after a manner which entirely escapes human observation. As, on the one hand, the elements and other inanimate parts of the creation carry on their action without regard to the particular interest and situation of men; so men are entrusted to their judgment and discretion, in the various shocks of matter, and may employ every faculty with which they are endowed, in order to provide for their ease, happiness, or preservation. What is the meaning then of that principle that a man, who, tired of life, and haunted by pain and misery, bravely overcomes all the natural terrors of death and makes his escape from this cruel scene; that such a man, I say, has incurred the indignation of his Creator by encroaching on the office of divine providence, and disturbing the order of the universe? Shall we assert that the Almighty has reserved to himself in any peculiar manner the disposal of the lives of men, and has not submitted that event, in common with others, to the general laws by which the universe is governed? This is plainly false; the lives of men depend upon the same laws as the lives of all other elements; and these are subjected to the general laws of matter and motion. The fall of a tower, or the infusion of poison, will destroy a man equally with the meanest creature; an inundation sweeps away every thing without distinction that comes within the reach of its fury. Since therefore the lives of men are for ever dependent on the general laws of matter and motion, is a man's disposing of his life criminal, because in every case it is criminal to encroach upon these laws, or disturb their operation? But this seems absurd; all animals are entrusted to their own prudence and skill for their conduct in the world, and have full authority, as far as their power extends, to alter all the operations of nature. Without the exercise of this authority they could not subsist a moment; every action, every motion of a man, innovates on the order of some parts of matter, and diverts from their ordinary course the general laws of motion. Putting together, therefore, these conclusions, we find that human life depends upon the general laws of matter and motion, and that it is no encroachment on the office of providence to disturb or alter these general laws: Has not everyone, of consequence, the free disposal of his own life? And may he not lawfully employ that power with which nature has endowed him? In order to destroy the evidence of this conclusion, we must shew a reason why this particular case is excepted; is it because human life is of so great importance, that 'tis a presumption for human prudence to dispose of it? But the life of a man is of no greater importance to the universe than that of an oyster. And were it of ever so great importance, the order of nature has actually submitted it to human prudence, and reduced us to a necessity in every incident of determining concerning it. Were the disposal of human life so much reserved as the peculiar province of the Almighty that it were an encroachment of his right for men to dispose of their own lives; it would be equally criminal to act for the preservation of life as for its destruction. If I turn aside a stone which is falling upon my head, I disturb the course of nature, and I invade the peculiar province of the Almighty by lengthening out my life beyond the period which by the general laws of matter and motion he had assigned it.

A hair, a fly, an insect is able to destroy this mighty being whose life is of such importance. Is it an absurdity to suppose that human prudence may lawfully dispose of what depends on such insignificant causes? It would be no crime in me to divert the Nile or Danube from its course, were I able to effect such purposes. Where then is the crime of turning a few ounces of blood from their natural channel? Do you imagine that I repine at providence or curse my creation, because I go out of life, and put a period to a being, which, were it to continue, would render me miserable? Far be such sentiments from me; I am only convinced of a matter of fact, which you yourself acknowledge possible, that human life may be unhappy, and that my existence, if further prolonged, would become ineligible: but I thank providence, both for the good which I have already enjoyed, and for the power with which I am endowed of escaping the ill that threatens me. To you it belongs to repine providence, who foolishly imagine that you have no such power, and who must still prolong a hated life, though loaded with pain and sickness, with shame and poverty. Do you not teach that when any ill befalls me, though by the malice of my enemies, I ought to be resigned to providence, and that the actions of men are the operations of the Almighty as much as the actions of inanimate beings? When I fall upon my own sword, therefore, I receive my death equally from the hands of the Deity as if it had proceeded from a lion, a precipice, or a fever. The submission which you require to providence in every calamity that befalls me excludes not human skill and industry, if possibly by their means I can avoid or escape the calamity: And why may I not employ one remedy as well as another? If my life be not my own, it were criminal for me to put it in danger, as well as to dispose of it; nor could one man deserve the appellation of *hero* whom glory of friendship transports into the greatest dangers, and another merit the reproach of *wretch* or *miscreant* who puts a period to his life for like motives. There is no being which possesses any power or faculty that it receives not from its Creator, nor is there any one which by ever so irregular an action can encroach upon the plan of his providence, or disorder the universe. Its operations are his works equally with that chain of events which it invades, and whichever principle prevails, we may for that very reason conclude it to be most favoured by him. Be it animate, or inanimate, rational, or irrational; 'tis all a case: Its power is still derived from the supreme creator, and is alike comprehended in the order of his providence. When the horror of pain prevails over the love of life; when a voluntary action anticipates the effects of blind causes; 'tis only in consequence of those powers and principles which he has implanted in his creatures. Divine providence is still inviolate and placed far beyond the reach of human injuries. 'Tis impious, says the old Roman superstition, to divert rivers from their course, or invade the prerogatives of nature. 'Tis impious, says the French superstition, to inoculate for the small-pox, or usurp the business of providence, by voluntarily producing distempers and maladies. 'Tis impious, says the modern European superstition, to put a period to our own life, and thereby rebel against our creator; and why not impious, say I, to build houses, cultivate the ground, or sail upon the ocean? In all these actions we employ our powers of mind and body to produce some innovation in the course of nature; and in none of them do we any more. They are all of them therefore equally innocent, or equally criminal. *But you are placed by Providence, like a sentinel in a particular station, and when you desert it without being recalled, you are equally guilty of rebellion against your Almighty Sovereign, and have incurred his displeasure.* I ask, why do you conclude that Providence has placed me in this station? For my part I find that I owe my birth to a long chain of causes, of which many depend upon voluntary actions of men. *But Providence guided all these causes, and nothing happens in the universe without its consent and cooperation.* If so, then neither does my death, however voluntary, happen without its consent; and whenever pain or sorrow so far overcome my patience as to make me tired of life, I may conclude that I am recalled from my station in the clearest and most express terms. 'Tis Providence surely that has placed me at this present moment in this chamber: But may I not leave it when I think proper, without being liable to the imputation of having deserted my post or station? When I shall be dead, the principles of which I am composed will still perform their part in the universe, and will be equally useful in the grand fabric, as when they composed this individual creature. The difference to the whole will be no greater than betwixt my being in a chamber and in the open air. The one change is of more importance to me than the other; but not more so to the universe.

'Tis a kind of blasphemy to imagine that any created being can disturb the order of the world or invade the business of providence! It supposes that that being possesses powers and faculties which it received not from its creator, and which are not subordinate to his government and authority. A man may disturb society no doubt, and thereby incur the displeasure of the Almighty: But the government of the world is placed far beyond his reach and violence. And how does it appear that the Almighty is displeased with those actions that disturb society? By the principles which he has implanted in human nature, and which inspire us with a sentiment of remorse if we ourselves have been guilty of such actions, and with that of blame and disapprobation, if we ever observe them in others. Let us now examine, according to the method proposed, whether Suicide be of this kind of action, and be a breach of our duty to our *neighbour* and to *society*.

A man who retires from life does no harm to society; He only ceases to do good; which, if it is an injury, is of the lowest kind. All our obligations to do good to society seem to imply something reciprocal. I receive the benefits of society and therefore ought to promote its interests, but when I withdraw myself altogether from society, can I be bound any longer? But, allowing that our obligations to do good were perpetual, they have certainly some bounds; I am not obliged to do a small good to society at the expense of a great harm to myself; why then should I prolong a miserable existence, because of some frivolous advantage which the public may perhaps receive from me? If upon account of age and infirmities I may lawfully resign any office, and employ my time altogether in fencing against these calamities, and alleviating as much as possible the miseries of my future life: Why may

I not cut short these miseries at once by an action which is no more prejudicial to society? But suppose that it is no longer in my power to promote the interest of society; suppose that I am a burden to it; suppose that my life hinders some person from being much more useful to society. In such cases my resignation of life must not only be innocent but laudable. And most people who lie under any temptation to abandon existence are in some such situation; those who have health, or power, or authority, have commonly better reason to be in humour with the world.

A man is engaged in a conspiracy for the public interest; is seized upon suspicion; is threatened with the rack; and knows from his own weakness that the secret will be extorted from him: Could such a one consult the public interest better than by putting a quick period to a miserable life? This was the case of the famous and brave Strozi of Florence. Again, suppose a malefactor is justly condemned to a shameful death; can any reason be imagined why he may not anticipate his punishment, and save himself all the anguish of thinking on its dreadful approaches? He invades the business of providence no more than the magistrate did, who ordered his execution; and his voluntary death is equally advantageous to society by ridding it of a pernicous member.

That suicide may often be consistent with interest and with our duty to ourselves, no one can question who allows that age, sickness, or misfortune may render life a burden, and make it worse even than annihilation. I believe that no man ever threw away life while it was worth keeping. For such is our natural horror of death that small motives will never be able to reconcile us to it; and though perhaps the situation of a man's health or fortune did not seem to require this remedy, we may at least be assured that any one who, without apparent reason, has had recourse to it, was curst with such an incurable depravity or gloominess of temper as must poison all enjoyment, and render him equally miserable as if he had been loaded with the most grievous misfortunes. If suicide be supposed a crime 'tis only cowardice can impel us to it. If it be no crime, both prudence and courage should engage us to rid ourselves at once of existence, when it becomes a burden. 'Tis the only way that we can then be useful to society, by setting an example, which, if imitated, would preserve to everyone his chance for happiness in life and would effectually free him from all danger or misery.

Tom Beauchamp puts the essays by Aquinas and Hume in perspective by presenting an interpretive thesis and a set of philosophical theses. *Interpretively* Beauchamp argues that Hume's essay is organized as a point-by-point reply to Thomas' three arguments against the moral acceptability of suicide. *Philosophically* he contends that Hume's arguments against Thomas' theological and natural-law reasons for the prohibition of suicide are careless and incomplete, although Beauchamp also maintains that Thomas' arguments fare no better. Beauchamp further maintains that Hume's utilitarian arguments favoring the moral acceptability of suicide provide important counterexamples to the moral claims advanced by Thomas concerning one's duty to the community.

Tom L. Beauchamp

AN ANALYSIS OF HUME
AND AQUINAS ON SUICIDE *

"On Suicide" is perhaps Hume's most influential and most widely reprinted essay.[1] I am interested here in the strengths and weaknesses of Hume's arguments. However, I have the subsidiary objective of placing his essay in an historical and interpretive framework that makes sense of its internal structure and at the same time rectifies certain past misunderstandings. Briefly, my *interpretive* suggestion is that the organization of the essay is that of a point-by-point reply to Thomas Aquinas' three arguments against the morality of suicide. *Philosophically,* I maintain that although Hume's main arguments against Aquinas contain serious weaknesses, some of his supporting arguments do successfully rebut central Thomistic contentions. On the whole, however, I find many of Hume's arguments less satisfactory than do those writers on suicide—such as R. B. Brandt [2]—who have been heavily influenced by them.

I

Most of Hume's essay is an intricate polemic against three arguments to the conclusion that suicide is immoral. He outlines his targets as follows: "If suicide be criminal [immoral], it must be a transgression of our duty either to God, our neighbor, or ourselves." A ready explanation exists for this choice of opposition. The most influential arguments against suicide in Hume's day were the Augustinian and Thomistic theories which informed the Church's position, and Aquinas' arguments directly parallel the content of Hume's essay. Here are slightly abbreviated versions of Aquinas' arguments, as found in the *Summa Theologica.*[3]

It is altogether unlawful to kill oneself, for three reasons:

[1] because everything naturally loves itself, the result being that every-

* Excerpted from "An Analysis of Hume's Essay 'On Suicide'," from *Review of Metaphysics,* 30, no. 1 (September 1976), 73–95. Reprinted by permission.

thing naturally keeps itself in being. . . . Wherefore suicide is contrary to the inclination of nature, and to charity whereby every man should love himself. Hence suicide is . . . contrary to the natural law and to charity.

[2] because . . . every man is part of the community, and so, as such, he belongs to the community. Hence by killing himself he injures the community. . . .

[3] because life is God's gift to man, and is subject to His power. . . . For it belongs to God alone to pronounce sentence of death and life. . . .

Although Hume never mentions Aquinas, the arguments he attacks are recognizably these arguments or close approximations of them. Characteristically Thomistic language is abandoned, but not the Thomistic content.

My evidence that Hume's essay is a point-by-point response to Aquinas is entirely internal and uncomplicated: (1) Hume individually attacks the three arguments advanced by Aquinas and only those three arguments; and (2) no other historical source known to me uses those three and only those three arguments against suicide.

Hume considers Aquinas' arguments in reverse order. I follow Hume's ordering except that his handling of the first Thomistic argument is best treated while considering one part of his criticism of the third Thomistic argument. I begin with this third argument.

II

Hume first attacks the third Thomistic argument, which, unlike the first two, is overtly theological. Roughly eighty percent of his essay is invested in his introductory paragraphs and in these arguments, which I shall refer to as his antitheological arguments.

Hume's strategy is not that of challenging belief in the existence of God. Rather, he isolates the following general theological proposition as the object of critical investigation: The act of suicide violates an obligation to God and provokes divine indignation *because it encroaches on God's established order for the universe.*[4] This proposition is a general and remote paraphrase of Aquinas' third argument. Hume gradually draws his analysis closer to Aquinas' exact contentions by substituting alternative but more specific meanings for the above italicized portion of the proposition under attack. His method is that of serially rejecting the several possible theological accounts that could be substituted—an eminently sensible approach, since it is not clear, even in Aquinas' philosophy, precisely what this phrase might mean. Each of Hume's arguments begins by specifying a variant account of "God's established order." Hume then argues that on the particular interpretation in question, the theology either is deficient or is perfectly compatible with the moral acceptance of suicide. While I have somewhat reordered Hume's presentation, the following seem to me the three main theological interpretations that he considers and subsequently rejects: (1) The Divine Ownership Interpretation, (2) The Natural Law Interpretation, and (3) The Divine Appointment Interpretation.

1. The Divine Ownership Interpretation

Hume first considers the possibility that encroaching on God's established order is wrong because "the Almighty has reserved to himself . . . the disposal of the lives of men, and has not submitted that event . . . to the general laws by which the universe is governed." This interpretation seems directly parallel to Aquinas' claim that "it belongs to God alone to provide sentence of death and life," while death "is subject not to man's free will but to the power of God." Plausibly Aquinas' first argument presumes that human life is God's property, because He created it. Aquinas specifically likens the "sin against God" to the sin committed against the master of a slave when the slave is killed by a third party. On this construal, the sin mentioned would be the sin of theft.

Hume sweeps aside the right-of-disposal contention as "plainly false" on grounds that human lives, like all matter in the universe, are subject to general causal laws. His point seems to be that since persons die of *natural* causes—as in the cases of being poisoned or swept away by a flood—it is gratuitous to maintain that there is an additional, nonnatural divine cause.

In isolation Hume's arguments are deficient, for it may be quite appropriately replied that natural causes are simply God's chosen means for the taking of human lives, yet the taking itself is a right God reserves and is an integral aspect of divine providence. Moreover, it does not follow from God's ownership of human lives that we ought not to endanger them any more than it follows from the entrusting of a life's savings to a speculative broker that (contingent upon our instructions) he ought not to risk it.

2. The Natural Law Interpretation

Hume's second accounting of the possible meanings of "encroaching on God's established order"—and of the wrongfulness of encroachment—is that it is wrong to disturb the operation of any general causal law, since the set of causal laws jointly defines the divine order. Hume construes this natural law thesis to mean that human beings must be absolutely passive in the face of natural occurrences, for otherwise they would disturb the operations of nature by their actions. Hume ridicules this theology as absurd, since unless we resisted some natural occurrences by counteractions, we "could not subsist for a moment." This overwhelmingly trivial objection to natural law ethics is quickly followed by a slightly more promising argument against the natural law interpretation. If it is morally permissible to disturb some operations of nature, Hume reasons, then would it not also be morally permissible to avert life by diverting blood from its natural course in human vessels? Does not this action relevantly resemble turning one's head aside to avoid a falling stone, since both alike simply divert the course of nature?

Hume apparently also thinks that he can, on this same basis, reject the claim that suicide is contrary to self-love, and therefore contrary to natural law—the *first* Thomistic argument, which may be reconstructed in the following form:

> *a.* It is a natural law that everything loves and seeks to perpetuate itself.
> *b.* Suicide is an act contrary to self-love and self-perpetuation.
> *c.* (Therefore) Suicide is contrary to natural law.
> *d.* Anything contrary to natural law is morally wrong.
> *e.* (Therefore) Suicide is morally wrong.

On the basis of his moral philosophy in general, Hume could be expected to dismiss both the first Thomistic argument and the natural law interpretation of the third as fallacious deductions of moral imperatives from mere empirical generalizations. Specifically, Hume could be expected to argue that Aquinas has illegitimately inferred the moral wrongness of suicide from the allegedly empirical law of self-preservation. Unfortunately, however, Hume does not pursue this line of argument. Instead he argues that it is *arbitrary* to prohibit intervention against the possible effects of some causal laws while permitting and even encouraging intervention against possible effects of other laws. His argument is unfortunate because it is both shabby and misdirected as an argument against natural law. Aquinas and natural law philosophers have always drawn a distinction between laws of nature and natural laws. Presumably the former are descriptive statements derived from scientific knowledge of universal regularities in nature, while the latter are prescriptive statements derived from philosophical knowledge of the essential properties of human nature. In this theory, natural laws do not empirically describe behavior but rather delimit the behavior that is morally appropriate for a human being. What is proper to a human differs from what is to be expected from other creatures insofar as their "natures" differ; and their natures differ because they possess different essences with different potentialities. Natural laws are the orderings of potentialities to their actualizations, and human goods are determined by reference to these orderings. Suicide is wrong precisely because it violates a natural inclination to live (and, as we shall see, because the person committing suicide does not exclusively intend a truly good outcome). This theory also permits the Thomist to admit that it is an empirical psychological fact that powerful inclinations to suicide do occur, while denouncing them as unnatural deprivations.

Hume's argument fails as an argument against Thomists (as do Brandt's and Hook's similar arguments [5]), because their contention that laws of nature and natural laws are distinct is not confronted. While it is true that this distinction is controversial and remains obscure even in current Thomistic literature, it is nonetheless an indispensable component in natural law ethics. If the distinction is observed, then there arguably is a morally relevant difference between diverting the Nile from its normal course and taking one's life by diverting blood from its normal channel; and the self-love argument also finds a plausible basis through this distinction. Hume's central contention—that it is arbitrary to permit resistance to the effects of some laws, while prohibiting intervention against the effects of others—would be acceptable *if the accusation of arbitrariness were demonstrated.* That is, his argument would be conclusive if he successfully showed the arbitrariness of accepting some law-governed natural processes as authoritative while excluding others. But Hume's conviction to this effect is only asserted, not argued, and hence begs the question against Thomists. This is not to say that Hume's conclusion is mistaken or even that the direction of his argument lacks all promise. But no fair-minded reader will find the arguments in this essay adequate, and it would not be easy to recast other regions of his philosophy in order to close the specific gap in the argument.

3. The Divine Appointment Interpretation

Hume's third accounting of "encroaching on God's established order" rests on the theological view that nothing in the universe happens without providential "consent and cooperation." He outlines this interpretation as follows:

> *You are placed by Providence, like a sentinel, in a particular station; and when you desert it without being recalled, you are equally guilty of rebellion against your Almighty Sovereign, and have incurred his displeasure. . . .*

With this interpretation—the only passage italicized in full sentences in the entire essay—Hume strikes at the heart of the theological matter. Hume's "rebellion" is Aquinas' "sin," and in general Hume's statement seems a paraphrase of a theology prominent in his time. The argument had appeared in Locke, and would later appear in strikingly similar form in Kant. But its popularity fails to impress Hume. He pronounces the argument absurd as an objection to suicide, because if this measure of divine causal control be exerted, then nothing in life happens without divine consent and "neither does my death, however voluntary, happen without its consent." He concludes with an appeal to the Stoic argument that whenever I no longer have a wish to live because of pain and exhaustion, and I want to die, it seems fair to "conclude that I am recalled from my station in the clearest and most express terms."

If Hume's third argument is sound, it has important implications for his first argument as well. Presumably Hume's first argument, even if unsuccessful, forces one to abandon the theological conviction that God *selectively* takes human lives. It drives one to the alternative view that he nonselectively takes those lives because everything happens by his design. One cannot have it both theological ways: either some things happen by special divine intervention into the natural order, or there is no special divine intervention and everything has its appointed place.

Despite the connections between the first and third arguments (and the theological dilemmas they jointly produce), even in combination they are unsuccessful as a case against all possible theological objections to suicide. Suppose a compatibilist position on the problem of freedom and determinism is espoused, a position Hume himself accepts. Assuming compatibilism, it is possible both to act freely and in accordance with God's instituted order, which, let us suppose, is causally deterministic. It follows that every event conforms to a causal law, including a human death; but it does not follow either that a human death need happen with God's moral approval, or that the suicide is being recalled from his station. The reason is simple: he may be acting out of the wrong motive in killing himself. For Hume to make good on his third antitheological argument, he would have to argue that no motive is morally better or worse than any other motive, since all motives are caused and in turn are the causes of action. This position Hume cannot consistently espouse, for he is himself a compatibilist on freedom and determinism and insists that some motives are blameworthy and others praiseworthy, even though all motives are caused. If this objection is sound, then Hume's first three antitheological arguments all fail. They may provide a powerful case against some theologies, but certainly not against all possible theologies. And if Aquinas' theology can accommodate the above argument, Hume's contentions fail to refute his thesis that suicide performed from certain motives is immoral.

Still, this conclusion does not take us to the end of the matter. Following his first two antitheological arguments, Hume suggests that everyone is rightfully free to dispose of his life as he sees fit because his free act of suiciding is no encroachment on the divine arrangement of general laws. Hume's conclusion that one is rightfully free to dispose of one's life would, of course, follow *if* it had been decisively shown that the action was not only free and in conformity with causal laws but also performed from the right motive—i.e., one that was divinely approved. Attention to right motives is essential to Aquinas' analysis. He excuses suicide if (and perhaps only if) one takes one's life because divinely commanded to do so. The principle of double effect allows him this conclusion. This principle may be formulated as follows: Whenever from a moral action there occur two effects, one good and the other evil, it is morally permissible to perform the action and to permit the evil if and only if:

1. The intention is to bring about the good effect and not to bring about the evil effect (which is merely foreseen).
2. The action intended must be truly good or at least not evil.
3. The good effect must bring at least as much good into the world as the evil effect brings evil into the world.

Aquinas clearly thinks that the immorality of suicide consists in acting from the wrong intention. The suicide intends evil effects except when specifically commanded by God to perform the act.[6] It is doubtful, however, that Aquinas' account can be consistently stated in such simple fashion, for he commits himself to a more substantive ethical conclusion than a mere divine command theory of the rightness of moral actions. This commitment can be seen by imagining the following dilemmatic situation, which I have reconstructed from an example of Kant's.[7] Suppose that a morally upright but violence-prone man is bitten by a rabid dog and that the man's condition is incurable. Knowing that he is almost certain to harm others when he becomes delirious, he kills himself. In doing so, he intends his action to protect others from harms he knows he would inflict. Under these conditions a Thomist might say that the man's action is sacrificial and therefore not a suicide because he intends a good outcome and does not intend his own death. However, suppose the man acts not out of the motive to save the lives of others but only to preserve his own moral integrity, which he devoutly believes to be a necessary condition of salvation. It seems to me inconceivable that Aquinas can, on a principled basis, condemn his act of suicide under either motive, since in each case the intention was to bring about a truly good effect, and Aquinas seems committed to the view that actions are right actions if they satisfy the conditions established by the principle of double effect.

If this interpretation of Aquinas be accepted (and it would be controversial), it is no longer clear whether or to what extent he and Hume have a serious moral disagreement. At bottom their disagreement seems to spring from what would count as a sufficiently good effect and what would count as a sufficiently good motive. Presumably Hume would no more approve a suicide done purely from cowardice than would Aquinas. It is most unfortunate that Hume, on the one hand, is not clearer concerning what range of reasons count as good motives in justification of suicide, and that Aquinas, on the other hand, is equally unclear and fails to appreciate that the principle of double effect commits him to the approval of all suicidal actions that satisfy the conditions of the principle. This failure by both philosophers seriously erodes the power of their respective arguments.

It would be most implausible, however, to suppose that there is not a serious disagreement, and perhaps even an unresolvable difference, between these two philosophers. In all likelihood Aquinas would demand that all of the conditions constituting the principle of double effect be satisfied, whereas Hume would not. It is not clear in Hume's ethics that he would accept any of these conditions, especially the first, which relates to a special role for intentions in ethics, and Hume is virtually silent on the matter of whether there is such an *independent* role for motives in ethical evaluation. Moreover, Aquinas specifically considers the possibility that a person might kill himself in order to avoid an utterly miserable life (*miseram vitam*), and rejects the action as unacceptable. His reason is based on a theory that grades good and evil effects.[8]

> . . . it is not lawful for man to take his own life . . . that he may escape any unhappiness whatsoever of the present life, because the ultimate and most fearsome evil of this life is death. . . . Therefore [suicide] is to adopt a greater evil in order to avoid a lesser.

Whatever Aquinas' value hierarchy may be, he here indicates that death is a most substantial evil. Hume's ethical theory and his views on *moral* arguments in "On Suicide" [9] would require rejection of this entire line of Thomistic thinking about the hierarchy of goods and evils. As we shall see momentarily, the miserable-life case rejected by Aquinas is for Hume a paradigm of justified suicide, and it is probably a difference in ethical theory concerning basic goods that in the end separates these two philosophers. Theological differences play a role only to the extent that a theory of human goods is or is not affected by a supporting theological position.

I do not conclude that either Aquinas or Hume is right or that either is wrong. My conclusion is the weaker one that Hume's antitheological arguments fail to refute Aquinas, except perhaps insofar as the offhand gratitude-in-death argument is reconstructed in terms of the importance of motives. It would be hard to reach a more critical or decisive conclusion, since the arguments of neither philosopher contain the requisite specificity. Still, it is disappointing to reach this conclusion, since so many writers have been so heavily influenced by both philosophers. For example, in one of the best essays on the moral justification of suicide in recent years, Brandt completely defers to Hume's antitheological arguments, claiming that Hume's arguments are "perspicacious" and that they "discuss at length" the difficulties and contradictions in theological arguments.[10] I cannot agree. To the extent Hume's arguments are perspicacious, the detail of argument is lacking; and to the extent there is detailed argument, perspicacity is lacking.

III

Hume turns his attention to the second Thomistic argument in two of the last three paragraphs in his essay. This is the moral argument that since every person belongs to a community as an integral part, to remove oneself from that community is to injure the community and hence to perform a moral wrong. Hume first tries to show that this claim is ill-supported by a proper account of moral and social obligation. This is his weak conclusion. He then argues that in some cases resignation of one's life from the community "must not only be innocent, but laudable." This is his strong conclusion. The strategy of the argument is that of analyzing hypothetical cases of suicide that stand as counterexamples to the Thomistic claim.

Hume begins with an analogy: Suppose a man retires from his work and from all social intercourse. He does not thereby harm society; he only ceases to do the good he formerly did by his productivity and amiability. Hume advances a general claim about the reciprocity of obligations that launches his argument:

> All our obligations to do good to society seem to imply something reciprocal. I receive the benefits of society, and therefore ought to promote its interests; but when I withdraw myself altogether from society, can I be bound any longer? But [even] allowing that our obligations to do good were perpetual, they have certainly some bounds; I am not obliged to do a small good to society at the expense of a great harm to myself: when then should I prolong a miserable existence, because of some frivolous advantage which the public may perhaps receive from me?

By means of this preface, Hume has already prepared the reader for his conclusion that suicide, if an injury at all (rather than simply a ceasing to do good), is small relative to the avoided harm to self.

In his first hypothetical case, Hume envisages a person still marginally productive in society. If his social contribution is small in proportion to the largeness of his misery, then Hume thinks (presuming the reciprocity axiom) there is no social obligation to continue in existence. The claim is utilitarian: if the value of taking one's own life in order to escape misery is greater than the value to the community of one's continued existence, then suicide is justified on utilitarian grounds. Hume seems to realize that one might attack his use of the reciprocity thesis, and he quickly protects himself by second and third hypothetical cases. In the second, the potential suicide's existence is so bleak that he is not only miserable and relatively unproductive, but a complete burden to society. In the third, a political patriot is spying in the public interest, is seized by enemies and threatened with the rack, and is aware that he is too weak to avoid divulging all he knows. In both cases Hume stipulates that the individuals can only be miserable for the remainder of their days. He then proclaims suicide under such conditions praiseworthy, because in the larger public interest. He even maintains that "most people who live under any temptation to abandon existence" act from such lofty motives—thus clearly indicating his belief that most suicides are "not only innocent, but laudable."

There are two relevant weaknesses in Hume's argument, neither insurmountable. First, Hume's probability estimate that most suicides are motivated by considerations of social utility is a factual claim that would be challenged both by Thomists and by suicidologists. They would argue that most suicides are the result of prolonged mental depression or some related psychic abnormality. Hume should have made at least two sets of distinctions: (1) between altruistic, egoistic, and anomic suicides (Durkheim's categories); and (2) between rational and irrational suicides. His probability estimate would have had claim to truth had he said that rational and altruistic suicides, and some egoistic and rational suicides, are blameless and perhaps even laudable—while not passing judgment on other combinations of categories. Second, if one accepts the liberal double-effect interpretation of Aquinas mentioned in the previous section, then it is not clear that Thomists would disagree with Hume, in which case his second argument would successfully reach its conclusion, but would fail as a refutation of Aquinas. This reservation simply reiterates the importance of the issues about good effects and intentions previously discussed.

These two objections seem to me to leave Hume's moral argument unaffected, especially as an argument against Aquinas, whose views depend on the thesis that the state is *injured* by removal of the part from the whole. Hume's examples point to the empirical possibility that a person might be so situated that everyone actually benefits from his suicide. Should this result occur, then the Thomist would seem compelled by his principle to require suicide in order to avoid injury to the state, or at the very least to permit suicide. More specifically, Hume's counterexamples show the Thomistic premises to be too feeble to support the desired conclusion in prohibition of suicide. Whether the state is advantaged or disadvantaged by citizen involvement is relative to the citizen's situation, and it is utterly implausible to insist that the state is always advantaged by the participation of all its members under all circumstances. Aquinas' real grounding principle, it seems, is the absolutistic one that it is *always* illegitimate to take one's own life when the motive is self-regarding. Accordingly, the Thomist must either beg the question or shift ground in order to satisfy the demands of Hume's counterexamples. The shift is from an argument governed by general considerations of social usefulness to an absolutistic prohibition against invasion of the sanctuary of the self.

For Hume, purely self-regarding acts of suicide (e.g., where one deliberately aims at taking one's own life purely to relieve one's own suffering) are justifiable, whereas they never are for Aquinas. Even on an extreme liberal construal (as sketched in the previous section), Aquinas' moral theory does not permit agreement with Hume's conviction that every person has a right to freely dispose of a miserable life whenever the act is not "prejudicial [harmful] to society." Nonetheless, the Thomistic objection we have been entertaining is illuminating in a most interesting way, because it reveals the most significant underlying source of disagreement between Hume and Aquinas: Hume's moral theory is utilitarian, while Aquinas' is not. This underlying disagreement in ethical theory dictates their differences over the justification of suicide. It was almost certainly a mistake on Aquinas' part to use what amounts to utilitarian premises in his second argument; and because he does, Hume's reply is rendered effective.

Notes

1. Throughout I use page references to the reprinting in *Of the Standard of Taste and Other Essays,* ed. John Lenz (Indianapolis: Bobbs-Merrill, 1965).
2. "The Morality and Rationality of Suicide," in Seymour Perlin, ed., *A Handbook for the Study of Suicide* (New York: Oxford University Press, 1975). Reprinted in this volume.
3. Part II-II, Q. 64, Art. 5. All references to the *Summa Theologica* are to the translation by the English Dominican Fathers (New York: Benziger Brothers, 1948).
4. Hume's exact words are: "What is the meaning of that principle, that a [suicide] . . . has incurred the indignation of his Creator by encroaching on the office of divine providence, and disturbing the order of the universe?"
5. Brandt, *op. cit.,* p. 66. Cf. Sidney Hook's distinctly Humean approach in "The Ethics of Suicide," *Ethics,* Vol. 37 (1927) and reprinted in Marvin Kohl, ed., *Beneficent Euthanasia* (Buffalo: Prometheus Books, 1975), p. 62.
6. Aquinas discusses the case of Samson as follows: ". . . not even Samson is to be excused . . . except the Holy Ghost . . . had secretly commanded him to do this." Reply Obj. 4. Cf. Reply Obj. 1 in Art 6.
7. *The Metaphysics of Morals,* Part II, published as *The Metaphysical Principles of Virtue,* trans. J. Ellington (Indianapolis: Bobbs-Merrill, 1964), pp. 84f.
8. Reply to Obj. 3.
9. Moral arguments are considered in the next section (III).
10. Brandt, *op. cit.,* p. 66.

In the following selection, R. B. Brandt discusses the moral blameworthiness of suicide, the moral reasons for and against suicide, and situations in which a suicide is *morally* excusable even if it is objectively wrong (e.g., suicide committed from a genuine sense of duty or suicide committed in an unsound state of mind). Brandt provides further criticism of the theological and natural-law arguments of Aquinas and also of arguments based on harm done to others and to society. If "suicide" is not committed by a pilot who crashes his plane to avoid civilians, he points out, innocent lives will be lost. Here there are opposing obligations, with greater harm occurring if "suicide" is not committed. Again, on the basis of the Introduction and the selections by Margolis and Holland, readers may wish to challenge the claim that this act is one of suicide.

Brandt also discusses the ramifications of teachings that suicide is morally wrong, by addressing himself to the issue of "whether or when suicide is best or rational for the agent."

R. B. Brandt

THE MORALITY AND RATIONALITY OF SUICIDE *

From the point of view of contemporary philosophy, suicide raises the following distinct questions: whether a person who commits suicide (assuming that there is suicide if and only if there is intentional termination of one's own life) is morally blameworthy, reprehensible, sinful in all circumstances; whether suicide is objectively right or wrong, and in what circumstances it is right or wrong, from a moral point of view; and whether, or in which circumstances, suicide is the best or the rational thing to do from the point of view of the agent's personal welfare.

The Moral Blameworthiness of Suicide

In former times the question of whether suicide is sinful was of great interest because the answer to it was considered relevant to how the agent would spend eternity. At present the practical issue is not as great, although a normal funeral service may be denied a person judged to have committed suicide sinfully. The chief practical issue now seems to be that persons may disapprove of a decedent for having committed suicide, and his friends or relatives may wish to defend his memory against moral charges.

* From *A Handbook for the Study of Suicide,* ed. Seymour Perlin, pp. 61–75. Reprinted by permission of Oxford University Press.

The question of whether an act of suicide was sinful or morally blame-worthy is not apt to arise unless it is already believed that the agent morally ought not to have done it: for instance, if he really had very poor reason for doing so, and his act foreseeably had catastrophic consequences for his wife and children. But, even if a given suicide is morally wrong, it does not follow that it is morally reprehensible. For, while asserting that a given act of suicide was wrong, we may still think that the act was hardly morally blameworthy or sinful if, say, the agent was in a state of great emotional turmoil at the time. We might then say that, although what he did was wrong, his action is *excusable,* just as in the criminal law it may be decided that, although a person broke the law, he should not be punished because he was *not responsible,* that is, was temporarily insane, did what he did inadvertently, and so on.

The foregoing remarks assume that to be morally blameworthy (or sinful) on account of an act is one thing, and for the act to be wrong is another. But, if we say this, what after all does it *mean* to say that a person is morally blameworthy on account of an action? We cannot say there is agreement among philosophers on this matter, but I suggest the following account as being safe from serious objection: "X is morally blameworthy on account of an action A" may be taken to mean "X did A, and X would not have done A had not his character been in some respect below standard; and in view of this it is fitting or justified for X to have some disapproving attitudes including remorse toward himself, and for some other persons Y to have some disapproving attitudes toward X and to express them in behavior." Traditional thought would include God as one of the "other persons" who might have and express disapproving attitudes.

In case the foregoing definition does not seem obviously correct, it is worthwhile pointing out that it is usually thought that an agent is not blame-worthy or sinful for an action unless it is a *reflection on him;* the definition brings this fact out and makes clear why.

If someone charges that a suicide was sinful, we may now properly ask, "What defect of character did it show?" Some writers have claimed that suicide is blameworthy because it is *cowardly,* and since being cowardly is generally conceded to be a defect of character, if an act of suicide is admitted to be both objectively wrong and also cowardly, the claim to blameworthiness might be warranted in terms of the above definition. Of course, many people would hesitate to call taking one's own life a cowardly act, and there will certainly be controversy about which acts are cowardly and which are not. But at least we can see part of what has to be done to make a charge of blameworthiness valid.

The most interesting question is the general one: which types of sui-cide in general are ones that, even if objectively wrong (in a sense to be explained below), are not sinful or blameworthy? Or, in other words, when is a suicide *morally excused* even if it is objectively wrong? We can at least identify some types that are morally excusable.

1. Suppose I *think* I am morally bound to commit suicide because I have a terminal illness and continued medical care will ruin my family financially. Suppose, however, that I am mistaken in this belief, and that suicide in such circumstances is not right. But surely I am not morally blameworthy; for I may be doing, out of a sense of duty to my family, what I would personally prefer not to do and is hard for me to do. What defect of character might my action show? Suicide from a genuine sense of duty is not blameworthy, even when the moral conviction in question is mistaken.

2. Suppose that I commit suicide when I am temporarily of unsound mind, either in the sense of the M'Naghten rule that I do not know that what I am doing is wrong, or of the Durham rule that, owing to a mental defect, I am substantially unable to do what is right. Surely, any suicide in an unsound state of mind is morally excused.

3. Suppose I commit suicide when I could not be said to be temporarily of unsound mind, but simply because I am not myself. For instance, I may be in an extremely depressed mood. Now a person may be in a very depressed mood, and commit suicide on account of being in that mood, when there is nothing the matter with his character—or, in other words, his character is not in any relevant way below standard. What are other examples of being "not myself," of emotional states that might be responsible for a person's committing suicide, and that might render the suicide excusable even if wrong? Being frightened; being distraught; being in almost any highly emotional frame of mind (anger, frustration, disappointment in love); perhaps just being terribly fatigued.

So there are at least three types of suicide which can be morally excused even if they are objectively wrong. The main point is this: Mr. X may commit suicide and it may be conceded that he ought not to have done so, but it is another step to show that he is sinful, or morally blameworthy, for having done so. To make out that further point, it must be shown that his act is attributable to some substandard trait of character. So, Mrs. X after the suicide can concede that her husband ought not to have done what he did, but she can also point out that it is no reflection on his character. The distinction, unfortunately, is often overlooked. St. Thomas Aquinas, who recognizes the distinction in other places, seems blind to it in his discussion of suicide.

The Moral Reasons for and Against Suicide

Persons who say suicide is morally wrong must be asked which of two positions they are affirming: Are they saying that *every* act of suicide is wrong, *everything considered;* or are they merely saying that there is always *some* moral obligation—doubtless of serious weight—not to commit suicide, so that very often suicide is wrong, although it is possible that there are *countervailing considerations* which in particular situations make it right or even a moral duty? It is quite evident that the first position is absurd; only the second has a chance of being defensible.

In order to make clear what is wrong with the first view, we may begin with an example. Suppose an army pilot's single-seater plane goes out of control over a heavily populated area; he has the choice of staying in the plane and bringing it down where it will do little damage but at the cost of certain death for himself, and of bailing out and letting the plane fall where it will, very possibly killing a good many civilians. Suppose he chooses to do the former, and so, by our definition, commits suicide. Does anyone want to say that his action is morally wrong? Even Immanuel Kant, who opposed suicide in all circumstances, apparently would not wish to say that it is; he would, in fact, judge that this act is not one of suicide, for he says, "It is no suicide to risk one's life against one's enemies, and even to sacrifice it, in order to preserve one's duties toward oneself." [1] St. Thomas Aquinas, in his discussion of suicide, may seem to take the position that such an act would be wrong, for he says, "It is altogether unlawful to kill oneself," admitting as an exception only the case of being under special command of God. But I believe St. Thomas would, in fact, have concluded that the act is right because the basic intention of the pilot was to save the lives of civilians, and whether an act is right or wrong is a matter of basic intention. [2]

In general, we have to admit that there are things with some moral obligation to avoid which, on account of other morally relevant considerations, it is sometimes right or even morally obligatory to do. There may be some obligation to tell the truth on every occasion, but surely in many cases the consequences of telling the truth would be so dire that one is obligated to lie. The same goes for promises. There is some moral obligation to do what one has promised (with a few exceptions); but, if one can keep a trivial promise only at serious cost to another person (i.e., keep an appointment only by failing to give aid to someone injured in an accident), it is surely obligatory to break the promise.

The most that the moral critic of suicide could hold, then, is that there is *some* moral obligation not to do what one knows will cause one's death; but he surely cannot deny that circumstances exist in which there are obligations to do things which, in fact, will result in one's death. If so, then in principle it would be possible to argue, for instance, that in order to meet my obligation to my family, it might be right for me to take my own life as the only way to avoid catastrophic hospital expenses in a terminal illness. Possibly the main point that critics of suicide on moral grounds would wish to make is that it is never right to take one's own life *for reasons of one's own personal welfare,* of any kind whatsoever. Some of the arguments used to support the immorality of suicide, however, are so framed that if they were supportable at all, they would prove that suicide is *never* moral.

One well-known type of argument against suicide may be classified as *theological.* St. Augustine and others urged that the Sixth Commandment ("Thou shalt not kill") prohibits suicide, and that we are bound to obey a divine commandment. To this reasoning one might first reply that it is arbitrary exegesis of the Sixth Commandment to assert that it was intended to prohibit suicide. The second reply is that if there is not some consideration which shows on the merits of the case that suicide is morally wrong, God had no business prohibiting it. It is true that some will object to this point, and I must refer them elsewhere for my detailed comments on the divine-will theory of morality.[3]

Another theological argument with wide support was accepted by John Locke, who wrote: ". . . Men being all the workmanship of one omnipotent and infinitely wise Maker; all the servants of one sovereign Master, sent into the world by His order and about His business; they are His property, whose workmanship they are made to last during His, not one another's pleasure. . . . Every one . . . is bound to preserve himself, and not to quit his station wilfully. . . ."[4] And Kant: "We have been placed in this world under certain conditions and for specific purposes. But a suicide opposes the purpose of his Creator; he arrives in the other world as one who has deserted his post; he must be looked upon as a rebel against God. So long as we remember the truth that it is God's intention to preserve life, we are bound to regulate our activities in conformity with it. This duty is upon us until the time comes when God expressly commands us to leave this life. Human beings are sentinels on earth and may not leave their posts until relieved by another beneficent hand."[5] Unfortunately, however, even if we grant that it is the duty of human beings to do what God commands or intends them to do, more argument is required to show that God does *not* permit human beings to quit this life when their own personal welfare would be maximized by so doing. How does one draw the requisite inference about the intentions of God? The difficulties and contradictions in arguments to reach such a conclusion are discussed at length and perspicaciously by David Hume in his essay "On Suicide," and in view of the unlikelihood that readers will need to be persuaded about these, I shall merely refer those interested to that essay.[6]

A second group of arguments may be classed as arguments *from natural law.* St. Thomas says: "It is altogether unlawful to kill oneself, for three reasons. First, because everything naturally loves itself, the result being that everything naturally keeps itself in being, and resists corruptions so far as it can. Wherefore suicide is contrary to the inclination of nature, and to charity whereby every man should love himself. Hence suicide is always a mortal sin, as being contrary to the natural law and to charity." [7] Here St. Thomas ignores two obvious points. First, it is not obvious why a human being is morally bound to do what he or she has some inclination to do. (St. Thomas did not criticize chastity.) Second, while it is true that most human beings do feel a strong urge to live, the human being who commits suicide obviously feels a stronger inclination to do something else. It is as natural for a human being to dislike, and to take steps to avoid, say, great pain, as it is to cling to life.

A somewhat similar argument by Immanuel Kant may seem better. In a famous passage Kant writes that the maxim of a person who commits suicide is "From self-love I make it my principle to shorten my life if its continuance threatens more evil than it promises pleasure. The only further question to ask is whether this principle of self-love can become a universal law of nature. It is then seen at once that a system of nature by whose law the very same feeling whose function is to stimulate the furtherance of life should actually destroy life would contradict itself and consequently could not subsist as a system of nature. Hence this maxim cannot possibly hold as a universal law of nature and is therefore entirely opposed to the supreme principle of all duty." [8] What Kant finds contradictory is that the motive of self-love (interest in one's own long-range welfare) should some-times lead one to struggle to preserve one's life, but at other times to end it. But where is the contradiction? One's circumstances change, and, if the argument of the following section in this chapter is correct, one sometimes maximizes one's own long-range welfare by trying to stay alive, but at other times by bringing about one's demise.

A third group of arguments, a form of which goes back at least to Aristotle, has a more modern and convincing ring. These are arguments to show that, in one way or another, a suicide necessarily does harm to other persons, or to society at large. Aristotle says that the suicide treats the *state* unjustly. [9] Partly following Aristotle, St. Thomas says: "Every man is part of the community, and so, as such, he belongs to the community. Hence by killing himself he injures the community." [10] Blackstone held that a suicide is an offense against the king "who hath an interest in the preservation of all his subjects," perhaps following Judge Brown in 1563, who argued that suicide cost the king a subject—"he being the head has lost one of his mystical members." [11] The premise of such arguments is, as Hume pointed out, obviously mistaken in many instances. It is true that Freud would perhaps have injured society had he, instead of finishing his last book, committed suicide to escape the pain of throat cancer. But surely there have been many suicides whose demise was not a noticeable loss to society; an honest man could only say that in some instances society was better off without them.

It need not be denied that suicide is often injurious to other persons, especially the family of a suicide. Clearly it sometimes is. But, we should notice what this fact establishes. Suppose we admit, as generally would be done, that there is some obligation not to perform any action which will probably or certainly be injurious to other people, the strength of the obligation being dependent on various factors, notably the seriousness of the expected injury. Then there is *some* obligation not to commit suicide, when that act would probably or certainly be injurious to other people. But, as we have already seen, many cases of *some* obligation to do something nevertheless are *not* cases of a duty to do that thing, *everything considered*. So it could sometimes be morally justified to commit suicide, even if the act will harm someone. Must a man with a terminal illness undergo excruciating pain because his death will cause his wife sorrow—when she will be caused sorrow a month later anyway, when he is dead of natural causes? Moreover, to repeat, the fact that an individual has some obligation not to commit suicide when that act will probably injure other persons does not imply that, everything considered, it is wrong for him to do it, namely, that in all circumstances suicide *as such* is something there is some obligation to avoid.

Is there any sound argument, convincing to the modern mind, to establish that there is (or is not) *some moral obligation* to avoid suicide *as such,* an obligation, of course, which might be overridden by other obligations in some or many cases? (Captain Oates may have had a moral obligation not to commit suicide as such, but his obligation not to stand in the way of his comrades' getting to safety might have been so strong that, everything considered, he was justified in leaving the polar camp and allowing himself to freeze to death.)

To present all the arguments necessary to answer this question convincingly would take a great deal of space. I shall, therefore, simply state one answer to it which seems plausible to some contemporary philosophers. Suppose it could be shown that it would maximize the long-run welfare of everybody affected if people were taught that there is a moral obligation to avoid suicide—so that people would be motivated to avoid suicide just because they thought it wrong (would have anticipatory guilt feelings at the very idea), and so that other people would be inclined to disapprove of persons who commit suicide unless there were some excuse (such as those mentioned in the first section). One might ask: how could it maximize utility to mold the conceptual and motivational structure of persons in this way? To which the answer might be: feeling in this way might make persons who are impulsively inclined to commit suicide in a bad mood, or a fit of anger or jealousy, take more time to deliberate; hence, some suicides that have bad effects generally might be prevented. In other words, it might be a good thing in its effects for people to feel about suicide in the way they feel about breach of promise or injuring others, just as it might be a good thing for people to feel a moral obligation not to smoke, or to wear seat belts. However, it might be that negative moral feelings about suicide as such would stand in the way of action by those persons whose welfare really is best served by suicide and whose suicide is the best thing for everybody concerned.

WHEN A DECISION TO COMMIT SUICIDE IS RATIONAL FROM THE PERSON'S POINT OF VIEW

The person who is contemplating suicide is obviously making a choice between future world-courses; the world-course that includes his demise, say, an hour from now, and several possible ones that contain his demise at a later point. One cannot have precise knowledge about many features of the latter group of world-courses, but it is certain that they will all end with death some (possibly short) finite time from now.

Why do I say the choice is between *world*-courses and not just a choice between future life-courses of the prospective suicide, the one shorter than the other? The reason is that one's suicide has some impact on the world (and one's continued life has some impact on the world), and that conditions in the rest of the world will often make a difference in one's evaluation of the possibilities. One *is* interested in things in the world other than just oneself and one's own happiness.

The basic question a person must answer, in order to determine which world-course is best or rational for him to choose, is which he *would* choose under conditions of optimal use of information, when *all* of his desires are taken into account. It is not just a question of what we prefer *now,* with some clarification of all the possibilities being considered. Our preferences change, and the preferences of tomorrow (assuming we can know something about them) are just as legitimately taken into account in deciding what to do now as the preferences of today. Since any reason that can be given today for weighting heavily today's preference can be given tomorrow for weighting heavily tomorrow's preference, the preferences of any time-stretch have a rational claim to an equal vote. Now the importance of that fact is this: we often know quite well that our desires, aversions, and preferences may change after a short while. When a person is in a state of despair—perhaps brought about by a rejection in love or discharge from a long-held position—nothing but the thing he cannot have seems desirable; everything else is turned to ashes. Yet we know quite well that the passage of time is likely to reverse all this; replacements may be found or other types of things that are available to us may begin to look attractive. So, if we were to act on the preferences of today alone, when the emotion of despair seems more than we can stand, we might find death preferable to life; but if we allow for the preferences of the weeks and years ahead, when many goals will be enjoyable and attractive, we might find life much preferable to death. So, if a choice of what is best is to be determined by what we want not only now but later (and later desires on an equal basis with the present ones)—as it should be—then what is the best or preferable world-course will often be quite different from what it would be if the choice, or what is best for one, were fixed by one's desires and preferences now.

Of course, if one commits suicide there are no future desires or aversions that may be compared with present ones and that should be allowed an equal vote in deciding what is best. In that respect the course of action that results in death is different from any other course of action we may undertake. I do not wish to suggest the rosy possibility that it is often or always reasonable to believe that next week "I shall be more interested in living than I am today, if today I take a dim view of continued existence." On the contrary, when a person is seriously ill, for instance, he may have no reason to think that the preference-order will be reversed—it may be that tomorrow he will prefer death to life more strongly.

The argument is often used that one can never be *certain* what is going to happen, and hence one is never rationally justified in doing anything as drastic as committing suicide. But we always have to live by probabilities and make our estimates as best we can. As soon as it is clear beyond reasonable doubt not only that death is now preferable to life, but also that it will be every day from now until the end, the rational thing is to act promptly.

Let us not pursue the question of whether it is rational for a person with a painful terminal illness to commit suicide; it is. However, the issue seldom arises, and few terminally ill patients do commit suicide. With such patients matters usually get worse slowly so that no particular time seems to call for action. They are often so heavily sedated that it is impossible for the mental processes of decision leading to action to occur; or else they are incapacitated in a hospital and the very physical possibility of ending their lives is not available. Let us leave this grim topic and turn to a practically more important problem: whether it is rational for persons to commit suicide for some reason other than painful terminal physical illness. Most persons who commit suicide do so, apparently, because they face a nonphysical problem that depresses them beyond their ability to bear.

Among the problems that have been regarded as good and sufficient reasons for ending life, we find (in addition to serious illness) the following: some event that has made a person feel ashamed or lose his prestige and status; reduction from affluence to poverty; the loss of a limb or of physical beauty; the loss of sexual capacity; some event that makes it seem impossible to achieve things by which one sets store; loss of a loved one;

disappointment in love; the infirmities of increasing age. It is not to be denied that such things can be serious blows to a person's prospects of happiness.

Whatever the nature of an individual's problem, there are various plain errors to be avoided—errors to which a person is especially prone when he is depressed—in deciding whether, everything considered, he prefers a world-course containing his early demise to one in which his life continues to its natural terminus. Let us forget for a moment the relevance to the decision of preferences that he may have tomorrow, and concentrate on some errors that may infect his preference as of today, and for which correction or allowance must be made.

In the first place, depression, like any severe emotional experience, tends to primitivize one's intellectual processes. It restricts the range of one's survey of the possibilities. One thing that a rational person would do is compare the world-course containing his suicide with his *best* alternative. But his best alternative is precisely a possibility he may overlook if, in a depressed mood, he thinks only of how badly off he is and cannot imagine any way of improving his situation. If a person is disappointed in love, it is possible to adopt a vigorous plan of action that carries a good chance of acquainting him with someone he likes at least as well; and if old age prevents a person from continuing the tennis game with his favorite partner, it is possible to learn some other game that provides the joys of competition without the physical demands.

Depression has another insidious influence on one's planning; it seriously affects one's judgment about probabilities. A person disappointed in love is very likely to take a dim view of himself, his prospects, and his attractiveness; he thinks that because he has been rejected by one person he will probably be rejected by anyone who looks desirable to him. In a less gloomy frame of mind he would make different estimates. Part of the reason for such gloomy probability estimates is that depression tends to repress one's memory of evidence that supports a nongloomy prediction. Thus, a rejected lover tends to forget any cases in which he has elicited enthusiastic response from ladies in relation to whom he has been the one who has done the rejecting. Thus his pessimistic self-image is based upon a highly selected, and pessimistically selected, set of data. Even when he is reminded of the data, moreover, he is apt to resist an optimistic inference.

Another kind of distortion of the look of future prospects is not a result of depression, but is quite normal. Events distant in the future feel small, just as objects distant in space look small. Their prospect does not have the effect on motivational processes that it would have if it were of an event in the immediate future. Psychologists call this the "goal-gradient" phenomenon; a rat, for instance, will run faster toward a perceived food box than a distant unseen one. In the case of a person who has suffered some misfortune, and whose situation now is an unpleasant one, this reduction of the motivational influence of events distant in time has the effect that present unpleasant states weigh far more heavily than probable future pleasant ones in any choice of world-courses.

If we are trying to determine whether we now prefer, or shall later prefer, the outcome of one world-course to that of another (and this is leaving aside the questions of the weight of the votes of preferences at a later date), we must take into account these and other infirmities of our "sensing" machinery. Since knowing that the machinery is out of order will not tell us what results it would give if it were working, the best recourse might be to refrain from making any decision in a stressful frame of mind. If decisions have to be made, one must recall past reactions, in a normal frame of mind, to outcomes like those under assessment. But many suicides seem to occur in moments of despair. What should be clear from the above is that a moment of despair, if one is seriously contemplating suicide, ought to be a moment of reassessment of one's goals and values, a reassessment which the individual must realize is very difficult to make objectively, because of the very quality of his depressed frame of mind.

A decision to commit suicide may in certain circumstances be a rational one. But a person who wants to act rationally must take into account the various possible "errors" and make appropriate rectification of his initial evaluations.

Notes

1. Immanuel Kant, *Lectures on Ethics* (New York: Harper Torchbook, 1963), p. 150.
2. See St. Thomas Aquinas, *Summa Theologica*, Second Part of the Second Part, Q. 64, Art. 5. In Article 7, he says: "Nothing hinders one act from having two effects, only one of which is intended, while the other is beside the intention. Now moral acts take their species according to what is intended, and not according to what is beside the intention, since this is accidental as explained above" (Q. 43, Art. 3: I-II, Q. 1, Art. 3, as 3). Mr. Norman St. John-Stevas, the most articulate contemporary defender of the Catholic view, writes as follows: "Christian thought allows certain exceptions to its general condemnation of suicide. That covered by a particular divine inspiration has already been noted. Another exception arises where suicide is the method imposed by the State for the execution of a just death penalty. A third exception is *altruistic* suicide, of which the best known example is Captain Oates. Such suicides are justified by invoking the principles of double effect. The act from which death results must be good or at least morally indifferent; some other good effect must result: The death must not be directly intended or the real means to the good effect: and a grave reason must exist for adopting the course of action" [*Life, Death and the Law* (Bloomington, Ind.: Indiana University

Press, 1961), pp. 250–51]. Presumably the Catholic doctrine is intended to allow suicide when this is required for meeting strong moral obligations; whether it can do so consistently depends partly on the interpretation given to "real means to the good effect." Readers interested in pursuing further the Catholic doctrine of double effect and its implications for our problem should read Philippa Foot, "The Problem of Abortion and the Doctrine of Double Effect," *The Oxford Review,* 5 (Trinity 1967), 5–15.

3. R. B. Brandt, *Ethical Theory* (Englewood Cliffs, N.J.: Prentice-Hall, Inc., 1959), pp. 61–82.

4. John Locke, *The Second Treatise on Civil Government,* Chap. 2.

5. Kant, *Lectures on Ethics,* p. 154.

6. This essay appears in collections of Hume's works.

7. For an argument similar to Kant's, see also St. Thomas Aquinas, *Summa Theologica,* II, II, Q. 64, Art. 5.

8. Immanuel Kant, *The Fundamental Principles of the Metaphysic or Morals,* trans. H. J. Paton (London: The Hutchinson Group, 1948), Chap. 2.

9. Aristotle, *Nicomachaean Ethics,* Bk. 5, Chap. 10, p. 1138a.

10. St. Thomas Aquinas, *Summa Theologica,* II, II, Q. 64, Art. 5.

11. Sir William Blackstone, *Commentaries,* 4:189; Brown in *Hales* v. *Petit,* I Plow. 253, 75 E.R. 387 (C.B. 1563). Both cited by Norman St. John-Stevas, *Life, Death and the Law,* p. 235.

Thomas Szasz rejects the argument that suicide is a manifestation of emotional illness. He believes this perspective is erroneous not only because he believes that mental illness is a myth, but also because psychiatric coercion (including involuntary hospitalization) is commonly justified by the notion that the psychiatrist is providing medical care. According to Szasz, successful suicide is generally an expression not of sickness but of an individual's desire for greater autonomy. The patient is seen as being deprived of freedom if society can apply coercive restraints to someone merely because he expresses the intention to commit suicide.

Szasz notes that refusal of treatment for physical illness is socially acceptable, whereas the threat of suicide is socially unacceptable. The consequence of this "imposed" value system is a struggle for power. Further, the "punishment" of psychiatric labeling and coercive care by the state may in fact "increase the desire for self-destruction."

Whereas Aquinas regards people as belonging to God, Szasz sees this ownership as resting more with the state and the individual. Whether or not suicide is morally wrong, he argues, moral wrongs should be punished neither by formal sanctions such as criminal or mental hygiene laws nor by the suicidologist. For all these reasons, he sees intervention and prevention of suicide as abridgements of individual liberty.

Thomas S. Szasz

THE ETHICS OF SUICIDE *

In 1967, an editorial in *The Journal of the American Medical Association* declared that "The contemporary physician sees suicide as a manifestation of emotional illness. Rarely does he view it in a context other than that of psychiatry" [March 6]. It was thus implied, the emphasis being the stronger for not being articulated, that to view suicide in this way is at once scientifically accurate and morally uplifting. I submit that it is neither; that, instead, this perspective on suicide is both erroneous and evil: erroneous because it treats an act as if it were a happening; and evil, because it serves to legitimize psychiatric force and fraud by justifying it as medical care and treatment. . . .

It is difficult to find "responsible" medical or psychiatric authority today that does not regard suicide as a medical, and specifically as a mental health, problem.

For example, Ilza Veith, the noted medical historian, writing in *Modern Medicine* [August 11, 1969], asserts that ". . . the act [of suicide] clearly represents an illness. . . ."

Bernard R. Shochet, a psychiatrist at the University of Maryland, offers a precise description of the kind of illness it is. "Depression," he writes, "is a serious systemic disease, with both physiological and psychological concomitants, and suicide is a part of this syndrome." And he articulates the intervention he feels is implicit in this view: "If the patient's safety is in doubt, psychiatric hospitalization should be insisted on." [1]

Harvey M. Schein and Alan A. Stone, both psychiatrists at the Harvard Medical School, are even more explicit about the psychiatric coercion justified, in their judgment, by the threat of suicide. "Once the patient's suicidal thoughts are shared," they write, "the therapist must take pains to make clear to the patient that he, the therapist, considers suicide to be a maladaptive action, irreversibly counter to the patient's sane interests and goals; that he, the therapist, will do *everything* [emphasis mine, T.S.] he can to prevent it; and that the potential for such an action arises from the patient's illness. It is equally essential that the therapist believe in the professional stance; if he does not he should not be treating the patient within the delicate human framework of psychotherapy." [2]

* From *The Antioch Review*, 31, no. 1 (Spring 1971), 7–17. Copyright ©
1971, Thomas S. Szasz. Reprinted by permission of the author.

Schein and Stone do not explain why the patient's confiding in his therapist to the extent of communicating his suicidal thoughts to him should *ipso facto* deprive the patient from being the arbiter of his own best interests. The thrust of their argument is prescriptive rather than logical. They seek to justify depriving the patient of a basic human freedom—the freedom to grant or withhold consent for treatment: "The therapist must insist that patient and physician—*together* [italics in the original]—communicate the suicidal potential to important figures in the environment, both professional and family. . . . Suicidal intent must not be part of therapeutic confidentiality." And further on they write: "Obviously this kind of patient must be hospitalized. . . . The therapist must be prepared to step in with hospitalization, with security measures, and with medication. . . ."

Schein and Stone thus suggest that the "suicidal" patient should have the right to choose his therapist; and that he should have the right to agree with his therapist and follow the latter's therapeutic recommendation (say, for hospitalization). At the same time, they insist that if "suicidal" patient and therapist disagree on therapy, then the patient should *not* have the right to disengage himself from the first therapist and choose a second—say, one who would consider suicidal intent a part of therapeutic confidentiality.

Many other psychiatric authorities could be cited to illustrate the current unanimity on this view of suicide.

Lawyers and jurists have eagerly accepted the psychiatric perspective on suicide, as they have on nearly everything else. . . .

When a person decides to take his life, and when a physician decides to frustrate him in this action, the question arises: Why should the physician do so?

Conventional psychiatric wisdom answers: Because the suicidal person (now called "patient" for proper emphasis) suffers from a mental illness whose symptom is his desire to kill himself; it is the physician's duty to diagnose and treat illness; *ergo,* he must prevent the "patient" from killing himself and, at the same time, must "treat" the underlying "disease" that "causes" the "patient" to wish doing away with himself. This looks like an ordinary medical diagnosis and intervention. But it is not. What is missing? Everything. This hypothetical, suicidal "patient" is not ill: he has no demonstrable bodily disorder (or if he does, it does not "cause" his suicide); he does not assume the sick role: he does not seek medical help. In short, the physician uses the rhetoric of illness and treatment to justify his forcible intervention in the life of a fellow human being—often in the face of explicit opposition from his so-called "patient."

I do not doubt that attempted or successful suicide may be exceedingly *disturbing* for persons related to, acquainted with, or caring for the ostensible "patient." But I reject the conclusion that the suicidal person is, *ipso facto,* disturbed, that being disturbed equals being *mentally ill,* and that being mentally ill *justifies* psychiatric hospitalization or treatment. I have developed my reasons for this elsewhere, and need not repeat them here.[3] For the sake of emphasis, however, let me state that I consider counseling, persuasion, psychotherapy, or any other *voluntary measure,* especially for persons troubled by their own suicidal inclinations and seeking such help, unobjectionable, and indeed generally desirable, interventions. However, physicians and psychiatrists are usually not satisfied with limiting their help to such measures—and with good reason: from such assistance the individual may gain not only the desire to live, but also the strength to die.

But we still have not answered the question: Why should a physician frustrate an individual from killing himself? As we saw, some psychiatrists answer: Because the physician values the patient's life, at least when the patient is suicidal, more highly than does the patient himself. Let us examine this claim. Why should the physician, often a complete stranger to the suicidal patient, value the patient's life more highly than does the patient himself? He does not do so in medical practice. Why then should he do so in psychiatric practice, which he himself insists is a form of medical practice? Let us assume that a physician is confronted with an individual suffering from diabetes or heart failure who fails to take the drugs prescribed for his illness. We know that this often happens, and that when it does the patient may become disabled and die prematurely. Yet it would be absurd for a physician to consider, much less to attempt, taking over the conduct of such a patient's life, confining him in a hospital against his will in order to treat his disease. Indeed, any attempt to do so would bring the physician into conflict with both the civil and the criminal law. For, significantly, the law recognizes the medical patient's autonomy despite the fact that, unlike the suicidal individual, he suffers from a real disease; and despite the fact that, unlike the nonexistent disease of the suicidal individual, his illness is often easily controlled by simple and safe therapeutic procedures.

Nevertheless, the threat of alleged or real suicide, or so-called dangerousness to oneself, is everywhere considered a proper ground and justification for involuntary mental hospitalization and treatment. Why should this be so?

Let me suggest what I believe is likely to be the most important reason for the profound antisuicidal bias of the medical profession. Physicians are committed to saving lives. How, then, should they react to people who are committed to throwing away their lives? It is natural for people to dislike, indeed to hate, those who challenge their basic values. The physician thus reacts, perhaps "unconsciously" (in the sense that he does not articulate the problem in these terms), to the suicidal patient as if the patient had affronted, insulted, or attacked him: The physician strives valiantly, often at the cost of his own well-being, to save lives; and here comes a person who not only does not let the physician save him, but, *horribile dictu,* makes the physician an unwilling witness to that person's deliberate self-destruction. This is more than most physicians can take. Feeling assaulted in the very center of their spiritual identity, some take to flight, while others fight back.

Some nonpsychiatric physicians will thus have nothing to do with suicidal patients. This explains why many people who end up killing themselves have a record of having consulted a physician, often on the very day of their suicide. I surmise that these persons go in search of help, only to discover that the physician wants nothing to do with them. And, in a sense, it is right that it should be so. I do not blame the doctors. Nor do I advocate teaching them suicide prevention—whatever that might be. I contend that because physicians have a relatively blind faith in their life-saving ideology —which, moreover, they often need to carry them through their daily work —they are the wrong people for listening and talking to individuals, intelligently and calmly, about suicide. So much for those physicians who, in the face of the existential attack which they feel the suicidal patient launches on them, run for *their* lives. Let us now look at those who stand and fight back.

Some physicians (and other mental health professionals) declare themselves not only ready and willing to help suicidal patients who seek assistance, but all persons who are, or are alleged to be, suicidal. Since they, too, seem to perceive suicide as a threat, not just to the suicidal person's physical survival but to their own value system, they strike back and strike back hard. This explains why psychiatrists and suicidologists resort, apparently with a perfectly clear conscience, to the vilest methods: they must believe that their lofty ends justify the basest means. Hence the prevalent use of force and fraud in suicide prevention. The consequence of this kind of interaction between physician and "patient" is a struggle for power. The patient is at least honest about what he wants: to gain control over his life *and* death—by being the agent of his own demise. But the (suicide-preventing) psychiatrist is completely dishonest about what he wants: he claims that he only wants to help his patient, while actually he wants to gain control over the patient's life in order to save himself from having to confront his doubts about the value of his own life. Suicide is medical heresy. Commitment and electro-shock are the appropriate psychiatric-inquisitorial remedies for it. . . .

But there is another aspect of the moral and philosophical dimensions of suicide that must be mentioned here. I refer to the growing influence of the resurgent idea of self-determination, especially the conviction that men have certain inalienable rights. Some men have thus come to believe (or perhaps only to believe that they believe) that they have a right to life, liberty, and property. This makes for some interesting complications for the modern legal and psychiatric stand on suicide. . . .

A man's life belongs to himself. Hence, he has a right to take his own life, that is, to commit suicide. To be sure, this view recognizes that a man may also have a moral responsibility to his family and others, and that, by killing himself, he reneges on these responsibilities. But these are moral wrongs that society, in its corporate capacity as the State, cannot properly punish. Hence the State must eschew attempts to regulate such behavior by means of formal sanctions, such as criminal or mental hygiene laws. . . .

The suicidologist has a literally schizophrenic view of the suicidal person: He sees him as two persons in one, each at war with the other. One-half of the patient wants to die; the other half wants to live. The former, says the suicidologists, is wrong; the latter is right. And he proceeds to protect the latter by restraining the former. However, since these two people are, like Siamese twins, one, he can restrain the suicidal half only by restraining the whole person.

The absurdity of this medical-psychiatric position on suicide does not end here. It ends in extolling mental health and physical survival over every other value, particularly individual liberty. . . .

I submit, then, that the crucial contradiction about suicide viewed as an illness whose treatment is a medical responsibility is that suicide is an action but is treated as if it were a happening. As I showed elsewhere, this contradiction lies at the heart of all so-called mental illnesses or psychiatric problems. However, it poses a particularly acute dilemma for suicide, because suicide is the only fatal "mental illness.". . .

Whether those who so curtail other people's liberties act with complete sincerity, or with utter cynicism, hardly matters. What matters is what happens: the abridgement of individual liberty, justified, in the case of suicide prevention, by psychiatric rhetoric; and, in the case of emigration prevention, by political rhetoric.

In language and logic we are the prisoners of our premises, just as in politics and law we are the prisoners of our rulers. Hence we had better pick them well. For if suicide is an illness because it terminates in death, and if the prevention of death by any means necessary is the physician's therapeutic mandate, then the proper remedy for suicide is indeed liberticide.

Notes

1. "Recognizing the Suicidal Patient," *Modern Medicine* (May 18, 1970).
2. "Psychotherapy Designed to Detect and Treat Suicidal Potential," *American Journal of Psychiatry* (March 1969).
3. T. S. Szasz, *Law, Liberty, and Psychiatry* (1963); *Ideology and Insanity* (1970), especially chaps. 9 and 12.

SUGGESTED READINGS FOR CHAPTER 2

Books and Articles

AUGUSTINE *The City of God,* trans. Marcus Dods. New York: Modern Library, Random House, 1950. Bk. I, secs. 17–27, esp. secs. 21–22, 26.

BEAUCHAMP, TOM L. "Suicide and the Sanctity of Life," in *The Value of Life,* ed. Tom Regan. New York: Random House, 1978.

BROOKE, EILEEN M., ed. *Suicide and Attempted Suicide.* Public Health Papers, no. 58. Geneva: World Health Organization, 1974.

CAIN, ALBERT C., ed. *Survivors of Suicide.* Springfield, Ill.: Charles C Thomas, 1972.

CHODOFF, PAUL. "The Case for Involuntary Hospitalization of the Mentally Ill." *American Journal of Psychiatry,* 133 (1976), 496–501.

DOUGLAS, JACK D. *Social Meanings of Suicide.* Princeton, N.J.: Princeton University Press, 1967.

DURKHEIM, EMILE. *Suicide: A Study in Sociology,* trans. John A. Spaulding and George Simpson. New York: Free Press, 1966.

FARBEROW, NORMAN L., ed. *Suicide in Different Cultures.* Baltimore: University Park Press, 1975.

GREENBERG, DAVID F. "Involuntary Psychiatric Commitments to Prevent Suicide." *New York University Law Review,* 49 (1974), 227–69.

HOOK, SIDNEY. "Ethics of Suicide." *International Journal of Ethics,* 37 (1927), 173–89.

KANT, IMMANUEL. *Lectures on Ethics,* trans. Louis Infield. New York: Harper & Row, 1963. Pp. 148–54.

————, *The Metaphysics of Morals,* Part II, published as *The Metaphysical Principles of Virtue,* trans. James Ellington. Indianapolis: Bobbs-Merrill, 1964.

LANDSBERG, P. L. *The Experience of Death and the Moral Problem of Suicide.* London: Rockcliff, 1963.

MENNINGER, KARL A. *Man Against Himself.* New York: Harcourt Brace Jovanovich, 1938.

MONTAIGNE, MICHEL DE. "A Custom of the Isle of Cea," *Essays,* trans. John F. Florio. 3 vols. London: J. M. Dent & Sons, 1928. Bk. 2, chap. 3.

MOSSNER, ERNEST CAMPBELL. "Hume's *Four Dissertations:* An Essay in Biography and Bibliography." *Modern Philology,* 48 (1950), 37–57.

NOVAK, DAVID. *Suicide and Morality: The Theories of Plato, Aquinas, and Kant and Their Relevance for Suicidology.* New York: Scholars Studies Press, 1975.

PERLIN, SEYMOUR, ed. *A Handbook for the Study of Suicide.* New York: Oxford University Press, 1975.

ST. JOHN-STEVAS, NORMAN. *Life, Death and the Law: Law and Christian*

Morals in England and the United States. Bloomington: Indiana University Press, 1961.

SCHOPENHAUER, ARTHUR. "On Suicide," *Studies in Pessimism,* trans. T. B. Saunders. London: George Allen & Unwin, 1890, 1962.

SENECA. "On Suicide," *Epistles,* trans. E. Barker. Oxford: Clarendon Press, 1932.

SHNEIDMAN, EDWIN S., ed. *Suicidology: Contemporary Developments.* Seminars in Psychiatry, ed. Milton Greenblatt. New York: Grune & Stratton, 1976.

SPROTT, S. E. *The English Debate on Suicide.* LaSalle, Ill.: Open Court, 1961.

STENGEL, ERWIN. *Suicide and Attempted Suicide.* Studies in Social Pathology. Harmondsworth, England: Penguin Books, 1973. Reprint, New York: J. Aronson, 1974.

VARAH, CHAD, ed. *The Samaritans: To Help Those Tempted to Suicide or Despair.* London: Constable & Co., 1965.

————, ed. *Samaritans in the '70's.* London: Constable & Co., 1973.

Bibliographies

FARBEROW, NORMAN L. *Bibliography on Suicide and Suicide Prevention, 1897–1957, 1958–1970.* DHEW Publication no. (HSM) 72–9080. Rockville, Md.: National Institute of Mental Health; Washington: Government Printing Office, 1972.

SOLLITTO, SHARMON, and ROBERT M. VEATCH, comps. *Bibliography of Society, Ethics, and the Life Sciences.* Hastings-on-Hudson, N.Y.: Institute of Society, Ethics, and the Life Sciences. Issued annually since 1973. See "Death and Dying: Suicide."

WALTERS, LEROY, ed. *Bibliography of Bioethics.* Detroit: Gale Research Co. Issued annually since 1975. See "Suicide."

Encyclopedia of Bioethics Articles

AGING AND THE AGED: Hearth Care and Research in the Aged— ERNLÉ YOUNG

LIFE: Value of Life—PETER SINGER

LIFE: Quality of Life—WARREN T. REICH

PAIN AND SUFFERING: Philosophical Perspective—JEROME SHAFFER

PAIN AND SUFFERING: Religious Perspective—JOHN BOWKER

SUICIDE—DAVID H. SMITH and SEYMOUR PERLIN

RIGHTS OF THE DYING PATIENT

An interesting array of professional obligations and patients' rights emerges from the practice of medicine. Professional obligations to patients, whether dying or not, have long been recognized in medical codes of ethics. The central affirmation of such codes is that, in treating the (frequently vulnerable and dying) patient, health professionals must not exploit their position of controlling influence. Recently, for perhaps the first time, systematic thought has been given to the moral and legal rights of patients. In this chapter some problems in the relationship between the professional and the dying patient are explored. These problems center on problems of providing or withholding both information and therapies.

Patients' Rights

The right of a patient to autonomous choice has often been neglected in medical practice. This neglect, together with newly emerging treatments for prolonging life, has led in recent years to explicit declarations of patients' rights. Perhaps the best known of these declarations is the American Hospital Association's "Statement on a Patient's Bill of Rights." This Bill was intended as a means of informing hospital patients that they have a right to critical information concerning their condition and do not have to endure certain treatments. It asserts, for example, a right to refuse life-saving therapy. Such documents, along with court cases, have brought to our attention a need to specify the conditions under which full disclosure should be given to patients, and also when they should be free to use such information in order to control the time of their own death. The rights most frequently asserted as fundamental rights are the right to be told the truth, the right to receive adequate information so that a responsible decision may be made, and the right to refuse therapy. We shall consider in turn each of these alleged rights.

The Dying Patient

A major reaction to dying by both professionals and lay persons in our society has been denial—the refusal to face honestly the process of dying. In a profession that teaches life-saving (such as medicine), a patient's death is frequently regarded as a professional failure. It is reacted to with hostility, and even with recrimination. Ethical issues surrounding such a response have been increased by the advent of new medical technology. Into the increasing isolation that emerges from decreased kinship systems has come a new site for dying—the hospital or other care facility. Approximately 70 percent of the people in the United States now die in such a facility. At the bedside may be a physician unknown to the patient, or a busy specialist. Thus the physician-patient relationship may vary with the duration of prior contact, the state of the patient, and the style the physician chooses for relating to the family. Given the large and influential context of the hospital setting, the often unknown physician, the state of the patient, and problems of patient-family interaction, it is important to scrutinize the patient's *right* to know the truth and the physician's *obligation* to tell it.

Truth-Telling

In general, both physicians and dying patients seem to have a tendency to deny the truth in their formal communications, whenever the truth concerns a fatal disease. However, in different stages of dying, patients (according to Kübler-Ross and others) are in fact aware of the seriousness of their illness, whether they are told or not. They may or may not share this information with their doctor or family.

Few moral philosophers regard truth-telling as an absolute obligation, especially where telling the truth may itself cause someone's condition to worsen. By contrast, except for patients who do not want the truth, some ethicists have argued that the intentional suppression of truth takes away a patient's rights. Yet most physicians believe that some circumstances of dying patients justify departures from the general principle of truth-telling. They have been especially sensitive to the Hippocratic principle that they should do no harm to patients by revealing too starkly what their condition is. Also, when they are told the truth and by whom (as it need not be the physician) will be important variables.

Children have posed special problems in the area of truth-telling. They often understand the gravity of their situation, even though the truth is unspoken. Increasingly, it has seemed desirable to develop environments for children in which questions can be asked and answers provided as a means of helping a child cope with problems of consent to procedures, serious illness, and death. In many situations the child is old enough to question the purpose and nature of a procedure or treatment, but too young to give legal consent. This leads to the general topic of informed consent and the dying patient.

Informed Consent

It is universally believed that the physician has a moral obligation to make it possible for dying patients to decide what shall and what shall not be done to them in their final days. The ability, however, to "make a decision" is largely dependent upon the information made available to the patient. A patient's consent to a medical procedure would be insignificant if relevant information were withheld. For example, suppose doctors believe, but have not confirmed, that a patient has cancer. If this patient is asked to submit to dangerous exploratory surgery, it may be of fundamental importance to him that he understands *that he has cancer* before consenting to the surgery. If he is merely informed that exploratory surgery is needed, a piece of *true but incomplete* information has been provided to him. Unless additional information is supplied, the consent should probably be regarded as invalid. But, even if the consent were genuinely informed, we would insist that it also be noncoercively obtained. Hence, it is often said that before a physician performs a medical procedure on a competent patient, the patient's voluntary informed consent must be obtained. This principle has become virtually an axiom of medical ethics, though it has by no means always been put into practice in difficult cases.

There are three main problems of informed consent. The first problem is conceptual. What is the proper meaning of "informed consent"? The *consent* element refers to an uncoerced decision. It is relatively unproblematic, if comprehending subjects are assumed. But what is it to give *informed* consent, as distinct from either partially informed or uninformed consent? Physicians cannot give patients a primer in medicine as a way of explaining their condition. But how can patients make an informed decision if they incompletely comprehend their medical diagnosis? Most medical decisions moreover are made by doctors on what *they* know to be incomplete information, because not all the desired information can be obtained. Since neither patient nor doctor can have full information in most situations, the notion of informed consent might seem an ideal that is not fully realizable and can only be approximated. Still, even if "informed consent" functions as an ideal, the question remains how much information must be provided for an approximation to informed consent, in any realistic sense, to be present.

The second problem has to do with the proper function of informed consent, or, as it is sometimes put, with the purpose and justification of informed consent. Two positions have dominated the literature. One maintains that the purpose and justification for obtaining informed consent is to protect persons from various harms that might be done to them. Those who subscribe to a justification that turns on *protection from harm* are inclined to protect patients whether or not it is the patient's choice that leads to an "unwise" taking of a risk. The other maintains that the purpose and justification for obtaining informed consent is to respect the autonomy of patients by granting them the right to choose what shall happen to them. Those who subscribe to a justification that turns on *protection of autonomy* are not inclined to protect patients against their own choices, on grounds that such constraint would be an overprotection that violates their autonomy. Justice Cardozo once maintained, in a famous legal pronouncement, that "every human being of adult years and sound mind has a right to determine what shall be done with his own body." This pronouncement favors the second purpose of informed consent over the first, but many who treat dying patients do not believe that Cardozo's model should apply to dying patients.

The third problem concerns how to ascertain that informed consent has been given. The requirement of informed consent is often regarded simply as a matter of obtaining the signature of a patient on a line of a so-called "consent form." But is the signature alone sufficient evidence of informed consent? It might be argued that the proper standard of informed consent is the prevailing standard used in any given community. Yet this standard may be unacceptably low or vague, and hence itself ethically unacceptable. In confronting this and other problems, some courts and institutional review boards have adopted the standard of the "reasonable person": the physician must have informed the patient to the extent that *any reasonable person* would have to be informed in order to make a decision about their case. Yet it is undetermined precisely what this standard requires, and even whether it is morally satisfactory.

Refusal of Treatment

Problems of informed *consent* to therapies are closely related to problems of informed *refusal* of therapies, where the patient makes an informed decision to refuse treatment with the knowledge that his or her own death will ensue. Patients have refused treatments such as blood transfusions because their religious convictions require rejection of such treatment; but ethical problems of patient refusal involve broader issues than those of freedom of religious exercise. A patient might refuse these same treatments for nonreligious reasons, and the case might, or might not, involve emergency measures. Refusal of treatment also encompasses problems of proxy refusal in the case of children and certain classes of incompetent patients, though in this chapter the primary focus is on refusal by competent adult patients.

A major moral and legal question is whether in life-and-death situations a patient should be judicially compelled to accept such treatment. If, as suggested above, the moral requirement of informed consent is a basic moral principle governing medical procedure, it might seem that a patient's informed refusal would be decisive, whether the decision was reached on religious or nonreligious grounds. Many regard such a right to refuse as fundamental in a free society, and there is a long tradition in the law that invasion of a person's body without valid consent is an assault.

On the other hand, others do not think that patients' rights include a right intentionally to "allow themselves to die." According to those who share this view, there are at least some circumstances where competent, nonconsenting patients should be *required* to accept life-saving medical therapies. Different reasons have been cited in defense of this view: Some regard a refusal of life-saving treatment as patently unreasonable, even if "competently" decided. Their arguments are similar to those of opponents of suicide. (Cf. Chapter 2.) Others think the state often has a "compelling interest" in preventing such deaths. Another reason for forcing therapy, closely connected to that of unreasonableness, is paternalistic: the competent adult person's liberty of choice is limited for his or her own good in order to prevent harm from befalling the person. This kind of paternalistic intervention occurred in the interesting case of Dr. Symmers, who—with complete information on his own case—asked his colleagues to take no steps to prolong his life if he suffered another cardiovascular collapse, yet was resuscitated against his wishes. Still another reason for coercive treatment challenges the *validity* of the patient's refusal on the grounds that patients in life-and-death situations may not possess the requisite mental or emotional stability to make an informed choice.

Of special interest are persons of *questionable competence,* where such persons definitely indicate *refusal* of therapy. For example, do those who are mentally ill have a right to refuse chemotherapy if it is determined by a physician that this treatment is the most efficacious treatment? And do children who understand what is contemplated for them have a right to refuse therapies when their parents and physicians determine that these therapies are in their own best interest? Such questions often seem to be more difficult even than those involving refusal of life-saving therapy, perhaps because we do not quite know how to assess a refusal by persons of questionable competence.

Many physicians believe that in all of these cases they are morally required (perhaps by the Hippocratic Oath) to prevent harm to patients. On the other hand, they also believe that it is a moral obligation to grant a patient's request whenever it is a true exercise of liberty. In the "Patient's Bill of Rights" mentioned earlier it is said that "The patient has the right to refuse treatment to the extent permitted by law and to be informed of the medical consequences of his action." It is the clash between these two convictions that creates the dilemma of whether to treat patients who may do the "ultimate harm" to themselves by refusing therapy, or to give priority instead to patient choice. In some interesting law cases involving refusal of therapy, courts have decided sometimes in favor of the patient and sometimes in favor of those who override patient wishes by administering the therapy. Several of these decisions are surveyed in the readings in this chapter.

The selections in this chapter provide only a few samples of the rich literature on the relationship between patients and those who attend them in the process of dying. In the past this literature was written largely by health professionals for health professionals. It proclaimed their own sense of their *obligations* to the patient. It seems likely that in the future most of the literature on this topic will originate outside the health professions and will emphasize the *rights* of patients.

In the context of the doctor-patient relationship, Joseph Fletcher discusses two issues about truth-telling: "First, has the patient a *right* to know the truth about himself? Next, has the doctor an *obligation* to tell it?" Fletcher regards human limitations in telling the truth as irrelevant to the continued obligation. The truth told is "truth" according to our best knowledge. Withholding the truth is seen as demeaning the personhood of the patient; and furthermore, he argues, evasion of the truth may be a protective device for the physician. Moreover, Fletcher argues that medical experience by no means lends support to the idea that telling the truth will aggravate a serious condition. As we will see, there is disagreement between Fletcher and Bernard Meyer as to the wishes of patients to know the truth and, for that matter, as to whether physicians would want to know the truth, were the roles of physician and patient to be reversed.

Joseph Fletcher

MEDICAL DIAGNOSIS:
OUR RIGHT TO KNOW THE TRUTH *

The Truth Can Hurt

. . . Dr. [John M.] Birnie concluded that "in hopeless cases, it is cruel and harmful to tell the patient the truth," and even if the doctor tells some member of the family it will be necessary for both "to lie like gentle-

* In Joseph Fletcher's *Morals and Medicine*. Copyright 1954 by Princeton University Press, pp. 36–63 (edited). Reprinted by permission of Princeton University Press.

men." [1] It is a hoary old problem of conscience in medical care. For our purposes we may attempt to explore it by posing two questions between which to shuttle back and forth. They are really obverse sides of the same coin, but they represent two distinguishable issues involved. First, has the patient a *right* to know the truth about himself? Next, has the doctor an *obligation* to tell it? Most of us upon occasion are patients, but only a few are physicians. The discussion, therefore, will naturally and properly tend to emphasize the first viewpoint and its question, namely, the *patient's right.*

If the doctor is thus obliged to tell the truth, what difference would it make if the patient is not sure he wants to know it, or if he actually does not want to know it? This question raises a matter of almost crucial importance for psychotherapy, and even for the less pathological areas of clinical counselling. And (most difficult of all) what if the doctor cannot know whether the patient wants to know? Is there a valid principle of therapeutic reservation when it comes to truth-telling in medical diagnosis? Very good reason would have to be found—better, at least than has ever been brought forward—to justify us in avoiding the answer that follows from the premise that our moral stature is proportionate to our responsibility and that we cannot act responsibly without the fullest possible knowledge. The patient *has* a right to know the truth. We are morally obligated to pay others the rights due them. Therefore a doctor is obligated to tell the truth to his patient. He *owes* the patient the truth as fully and as honestly as he owes him his skill and care and technical powers. . . .

"WHAT IS TRUTH?"

To say, however, that the doctor owes the truth to his patient does not altogether cover the ground of conscience involved. First of all, we ought to recognize that this right to know the truth does not apply to all truths. There are secrets of others, for example, to which few if any of us have any right at all. Furthermore, the classic question put by Pilate to Jesus, "What is truth?" can be applied to the problem of medical diagnosis and truth-telling. As Pilate's question seems to have been intended to suggest, none of us has perfect knowledge; also, the human intelligence with which we try to make sense of what knowledge we have is not infallible. Given a doctor's willingness and desire to respect the patient's right to know the truth, how shall he convey it? How can he be *sure?* . . .

When it comes to telling the truth, we can never be sure that we know it, nor can we always be sure that we convey it as we *do* know it or believe it to be. Our modern sociology of knowledge, and psychology with its new understanding of the subtleties of communication and the role of the unconscious, have humbled us a great deal about our capacity either to grasp or to convey the truth. But these considerations are only cautionary; they have to do only with the negative defects of truth, due to human limitations, not with positive injuries to the truth, due to willful distortion and suppression. Problems of morality or of conscience in connection with truth-telling arise only in the case of moral truth (veracity), not with logical truth (accuracy).

It is presumed that inaccuracy or error, in the case of medical advice or in any other area, is unintentional and therefore by definition entirely outside the forum of conscience. In short, as far as morality is concerned (although not so far as science is concerned) what is at stake in telling the truth is, precisely, honesty. Dr. John Homans once protested, "There can be no universal rule to tell the brutal truth. And the first and best reason for not telling the truth is the impossibility of being certain what the truth is." [2] But this admitted fact is too often a red herring, drawn across the trail to confuse conscience, since it bears only upon the problem of accuracy, not upon the problem of honesty. Indeed, a part of the truth which the doctor owes the patient is just that: that the doctor cannot be absolutely correct. After all, doctors, like their patients, have to be prepared to meet frustration through knowledge. Their very science often gives them an insight into bitter realities which would leave the primitive medicine-man, who could not know, reasonably hopeful. To take refuge in finitude to avoid reality is only a sophisticated form of escapism, when it is used as an excuse for departing from honesty. No: the question before us really is: *are we obliged to tell the truth as we see it according to our best knowledge?* For this very reason it is a matter of simple justice that the law does not require a physician to be responsible for errors in judgment, or to possess any unusual skill beyond the average. This is the principle of law under which every issue of professional responsibility is adjudicated. Indefectibility of the person—whether in knowledge, skill, or strength—is assumed to be out of the question. Therefore, to deny the obligation of truth-telling by pointing to human limitations is neither here nor there. . . .

The indecision and evasion over the nature of a lie, which we all have felt and fought with, is seen in the public words of one practitioner, whom we shall leave unidentified even though his statement was part of a lecture to medical students: "Personally, I can, I think, truthfully say that in a practice of forty years I never, as far as I can remember, found it necessary to tell an outright lie to a patient about his condition. Tactful and skillful explanations with their if's and and's, side issues and suggestions of possibilities, always sufficiently befogged the issue, satisfied the patient, and left my conscience unseared. A sick man is not a well man and what would be injudicious to say to the one is often swallowed with almost a real relish by the other." Here, in these tortuous terms, are all the involutions of our problem!

From the earliest times it has been argued that a lie is not a lie if there is a just cause for it. Among such just causes men have included self-defense, military necessity, and even zeal for God's honor! . . .

IS IGNORANCE BLISS?

There are many ways by which a physician can deceive his patient, either by misrepresenting the facts as he sees them or by withholding them. Our opinion is that in either case such deceptions are morally speaking unlawful, being acts of theft because they keep from the patient what is rightfully his (the truth about himself), or acts of injustice because they deny to another what is his due as a free and responsible person. The most dramatic case of conscience in medical diagnosis and truth-telling has to do, of course, with the patient who is found to be the victim of a possibly or probably fatal disease, or one for whom no hope at all can be held out. In medical practice, as a matter of fact, there are many other diagnoses that entail sadness equal to or greater than the sadness that is caused by the malignant neoplasms; there are such conditions as brain damage in babies, leading to spastic paralysis, cardiovascular diseases with poor prognosis, and the like. Yet even in terminal diseases the reaction of patients to the truth is varied and unpredictable. Dr. Fred C. Shattuck relates that one cancer patient, a cheerful businessman, never smiled again after he was told the truth, apparently crushed in spirit. But another patient, fretful and troublesome, who complained constantly at the discomfort, pulled himself together and showed great courage and moral vigor to the last.[3] Experienced pastors can tell of episodes wherein their own faith has been deepened by the faith and assurance and joy with which terminal patients faced death, sometimes over a long period, and in some cases *not until* they were made fully aware of the truth. But fear of the truth is very strong in many people, including physicians, and this fear accounts for the fact that from ancient to modern times no universal or local code of medical ethics has ever attempted to regulate the doctor's conscience in matters of truth-telling. The first code on the tablets of Hammurabi, 2080 B.C., said nothing about it; the confessors' manuals of the Middle Ages dealing with the rules of shriving surgeons and leechers said nothing; the latest code of the American Medical Association, by its silence or equivocation, leaves the whole thing up to the individual practitioner.

Suppose we turn for a moment to the opinion set forth by Dr. Richard C. Cabot, who was for so many years a physician and teacher at the Massachusetts General Hospital. . . . In . . . *The Meaning of Right and Wrong,* Dr. Cabot put the matter along these lines: "How can we ever be sure where a conscientious liar will draw the line? It appears to me, therefore, that the doctrine that it is sometimes right to lie can never be effectively asserted. For our hearers take notice, and so make ineffective our subsequent attempts to lie. I recall a sick man who ordered his physician never to tell him the truth in case he should be seriously ill. Picture the state of that sick man's mind when later he hears his physician's reassurances. 'Perhaps he really doesn't consider this sickness a serious one. Then he will be telling me the truth!' How can the sick man know? If he asks the doctor whether he considers the disease serious and gets a negative answer, how is he to interpret that answer? If the doctor did consider the disease serious he would also have to say 'No.' His words have become mere wind. No one can interpret them. His reassuring manner, his smiles, his cheering tones may be true or they may be lies. Who can say?

"Suppose the disease comes to a point which demands operation. But to mention operation is to let the patient know that his trouble is serious, and that is forbidden. Shall the doctor therefore let the operation go and let the patient get worse? Whatever he does or says his patient has grounds for fearing the worst. No reassurance can be taken at its face value. The most trifling ailment must be suspect; good news may always mean bad.

"Here then is a self-enforcing moral law. 'Thou shalt not confess to a belief in occasional lies.' " [4]

Dr. Cabot then goes on to point out that if you *do not* admit that you tell conscientious lies, you make yourself an unconscientious liar. "For the very conscientiousness of conscientious lies depends on their being known to be exceptions to the rule. No one can be a universal conscientious liar." He was, in his own way, reaching the view put long ago in an old German proverb, *Wer einmal lügt dem glaubt man nicht, und wenn er auch die Warheit spricht* (he who once lies is never believed, even when he is telling the truth). [5] . . .

There is inescapably a subversive result of occasional lying. It makes no real difference whether it is perpetrated by a direct commission of an untruth, or indirectly through the omission of a truth. Lying troubles the waters of human relations and takes away the one element of mutual trust without which medical practice becomes a manipulation of bodies rather than the care of and for persons. The assumption made by the physician, when he has the *presumption* to withhold the truth, is that the patient is really no longer an adult, but rather either a child or an idiot, more an *it* than a *thou*. In this connection we should note that medical experience by no means lends support to the idea that telling the patient ominous truths will aggravate a serious condition. Some years ago the Division of Cancer in the Massachusetts Department of Public Health issued a bulletin in which it was said, "The fallacious argument [that lies are necessary] may be answered as follows. . . . [We find that] those physicians and hospitals making a practice of telling the patients frankly when they have the disease, report only the fullest cooperation of the patient in his treatment. But the physician who lies to his patient denies him a chance to show his common sense and helps him one step nearer to the undertaker." [6]

Dr. Cabot, as we have seen, put forward a number of good reasons for truth-telling in medical care. In much of what he had to say he was answering a statement by Dr. Joseph Collins, who had defended medical falsehoods in *Harper's Magazine* for August 1927 in an article entitled "Should Doctors Tell the Truth?" Dr. Cabot pointed out, among other things, that without the truth patients will often object to decisive and costly forms of treatment, surgical or otherwise, since their urgency will not be apparent while the cost will be. If the patient is not told of approaching death, or at least of its grave possibility, he may fail to make proper preparation for his death in wills and testaments, or in reparations and restorations of one kind or another, or in reconciliations with God and/or men. . . .

Furthermore, only a little experience with doctors, patients' families, and ministers of religion as they deal with terminal diseases or some other condition threatening death or helplessness is enough to show that a great deal of the time their evasion of the plain truth is a protective mechanism for themselves, a rationalization of their own embarrassment and dis-ease. Much of our human behavior, even among doctors, is aimed at satisfying our own needs, emotional and otherwise, not the needs of others. It is a fact to be faced that reservation or corruption of the truth is not always based on a genuine and maturely weighed decision that the patient "is just as well off if he (or she) doesn't know." Fear, we repeat, leads to lies. Fear and lies tend to require and presuppose each other, as do love and truth. Perhaps we need not feel so threatened emotionally by the truth. Dr. Walter Alvarez of the Mayo Clinic says, "Often it is the relatives who have fear and mental pain. . . . In forty-odd years of practice I cannot remember anyone's committing suicide because I told him the hopeless truth. Instead hundreds of persons thanked me from their hearts and told me I had relieved their minds." Who are we to choose ignorance for others? We *have* to make the choice for animals, because they are animals, incapable of receiving or making creative use of such knowledge. But *ought* we to make it for men?

These considerations apply with just as much force to illnesses of the kind that are far from fatal. Even in imaginary illnesses of a neurasthenic nature, the common practice of the medical lie called "placebo" or the bread pill, the "pink water" or the "water subcut" (a pretended hypodermic), can be shown to undermine a truly moral relationship between physician and patient. A false pill of sugar, or something of the sort to deceive the patient into thinking he receives treatment or medication, is a self-defeating practice. In the first place, it *is* a deception, however well meant. In the second place, it is amazing how few good liars (to use a curious and contradictory phrase) there are, especially in such intimate relationships as illness and medical care. A good many doctors would be well advised, in the light of what we know nowadays about the dynamics of personal relationships, to rely instead, for supportive therapy and encouragement, upon a confident and genuine empathy. In the third place, these practices encourage the idea among neurotic patients that drugs will cure most ailments, and thus serve to extend the patent-medicine evil.

It may be pointed out, of course, that psychiatrists *on principle* do not in all cases share their diagnoses with the patient. Sometimes ignorance is bliss in correcting mental and emotional disorders. It might be claimed that something of the same therapeutic principle may apply to the general practitioner in his work. But for one thing we can answer that the cases are not parallel, inasmuch as the psychiatrist withholds his knowledge precisely because he may prevent the patient's recovery by revealing it, at least if he does so too soon. It is by no means evident that the same is true if the truth has to do with a pink pill for an imaginary illness, or with a diagnosis of cancer disguised to the patient as a tumor, or a heart disease camouflaged as overweight or indigestion. And in any case, the psychiatrist's ministrations are not even relevant in cases where imminent death or its probability is a chief reality factor, or in cases of primarily physical pathology, surgery, and the like.

There is no good reason, merely out of rigid adherence to abstract principle, to be hard or brutally logical about the morality of truth-telling in illness and dying. On the other hand it seems fair to say that the right of the patient to know the truth is clear on moral grounds, and this is true whether or not our ultimate sanction for loyalty to truth and to personal rights is religious. . . .

THE MEDICAL CODE ON LYING

The A.M.A. *Code of Ethics,* 1940, says (in Chapter Two): "A physician should give timely notice of dangerous manifestations of the disease to the friends of the patient." Not, we should notice, to the patient himself! The Code goes on to say, still with patent uncertainty, that the doctor should "assure himself that the patient *or* his friends have such knowledge of the patient's condition as will serve the best interests of the patient and his family." It should be obvious that this is assuming much more knowledge of a family's affairs than medical care, as such, would normally provide. And again, how often the family's and the patient's idea of the best interests at stake are not the same! How often, by keeping the patient in ignorance, precisely the opposite of what the patient would want has in fact come about, perhaps through a consequent failure to change a will, or to add a codicil, or to make some explanation to a loved one—all of these being things which only the patient could have done had he known the true state of affairs. It is also ironical to observe how often doctors and families are mistaken in supposing that the patient can be fooled by evasion and suppression of the truth. . . .

A strange inconsistency is also to be found in the *Code of Ethics.* Following the equivocation we have already noted, it declares (Chapter Three, article three, section two) that in cases of medical consultation "all the physicians interested in the case should be frank and candid with the patient and his family." It is not at all clear why a medical consultant should thus be directly charged to be candid with the patient when the physician in charge is not. Yet even here the Code qualifies itself by remarking at another point that the consultant should "state the result of his study to the patient *or* his next friend in the presence of the physician in charge." And after all this temporizing about the doctor's obligation to tell the patient and his family." It is not at all clear why a medical consultant should physician should "constantly behave towards others as he desires them to deal with him." But can it really be that doctors who practice professional deception would, if the roles were reversed, want to be coddled or deceived? If this is actually the moral standard of those practitioners who deny their patients the truth, then one can only marvel to find so many who are themselves willing, as the Quaker lady expressed it, to have their feeling "poulticed," and willing to be denied knowledge of the most decisive events of their lives, whether it is a fact of health or the final fact of death itself.

The tradition in Western civilization allows for what the law calls "privileged communications" between patient and physician, as between people and pastor. This, indeed, is one of the few priestly aspects of the doctor's role left over from the ancient times. What we tell our doctors and our clergymen is private, personal, our own; and in that sense, secret. Now, as it bears upon truth-telling, the significant thing is that this ethical principle of the professional secret rests upon the conviction that knowledge of a person's private life gained in the course of professional services is a *trust,* the stewardly possession by a professional servant of what belongs to another. The secrets of the confessional box and pastor's study, and of the consulting room and clinic, *belong* to the person served, not to the priest or to the physician. They therefore have no *right* to pass them on to others *without the owner's consent.* By the nature of his office the priest has only that knowledge of a penitent's life which is already known to the penitent and shared by him with the priest. In the case of medicine, however, the physician, the diagnostician, gains knowledge of the patient which (in the nature of the case) the patient does not yet have. But it is still the patient's knowledge and information; it is his life and health which are at stake. The patient has "opened his books" to the doctor on the reasonable assumption that what is found there will be turned over to him, just as a business firm has a right to expect no deception or suppression from an auditor. In spite of all this, some doctors assume the god-like power to ignore the propriety or proper ownership of the secret. On their own behalf they will insist upon the rule of privileged communication, expressing righteous indignation when others attempt to pry or extort information from them; at the same time, however, what they have refused others as not rightfully theirs to give, they will also deny to the patient himself, the rightful owner! Or, with a strange further confusion of ethical reasoning, they will deny the patient the truth which belongs to him, and then proceed to give it to his family or friends, regardless of the principle of professional secrecy. . . .

DO PEOPLE WANT THE TRUTH?

By way of summary, we may say that in general we can validly assert our right as patients to know the medical facts about ourselves. Several reasons have been given for it, but perhaps the four fundamental ones are: first, that as persons our human, moral quality is taken away from us if we are denied whatever knowledge is available; second, that the doctor is *entrusted* by us with what he learns, but the facts are ours, not his, and to deny them to us is to steal from us what is our own, not his; third, that the highest conception of the physician-patient relationship is a personalistic one, in the light of which we see that the fullest possibilities of medical treatment and cure in themselves depend upon mutual respect and confidence, as well as upon technical skill; and, fourth, that to deny a patient knowledge of the facts as to life and death is to assume responsibilities which cannot be carried out by anyone but the patient, with his own knowledge of his own affairs. On the negative side, we have reasoned that the common excuse given for deceiving the patient—"after all, the doctors are fallible and make mistakes"—is not a valid excuse. In the first place, physicians are in conscience bound to indicate that they find pathological conditions and advise treatment only to the best of their knowledge and judgment, not with absolute certainty. In the second place, while the admission of human fallibility always qualifies any claims a doctor might make as to accuracy, *it does not qualify and cannot disqualify the obligation to be honest.* And, finally, we have rejected any distinction between lies (positive injuries to the truth) and concealment (merely negative failure to convey what is foreseen as prognosis and discovered by diagnosis). When moralists such as K. E. Kirk offer this distinction, condemning the former and justifying the latter, they have failed completely to grasp the foundation principles of the ethics of communication. We have argued, instead, that commission of untruth and suppression of truth are alike deprivations of a patient's right; and therefore theft, therefore unjust, therefore immoral.

The only remaining question is: what if the patient does not ask for the truth? This problem may arise either because he does not *want* the truth (perhaps out of fear, being threatened by what he suspects, or for some other reason), or because he does not realize that there is a truth not known to him but now discovered by the doctor. This problem, surely, cannot be regarded as a very difficult one in conscience. In the first case, when the patient has no desire to know the truth and the doctor has good reason to believe that the patient does not want to know it, the doctor should respect his wishes, even though it might well be a proper part of his role to help his patient to want the truth and to become able to accept it. It is no part of a doctor's duty to impose his diagnosis upon a patient or flout his wishes, unless, of course, he has reason to believe that he could not continue to treat the patient properly, according to the demands of the best medical care, without telling him. In such a case, surely, he should explain why he needs to tell (or at least that he feels obliged to tell), and if the patient still refuses to hear, then ask leave to withdraw from the case, urging that another physician be called in his place. In the second case, when the patient is too ignorant to ask for the information acquired by the doctor, it is clearly the doctor's moral obligation to supply it, together with an explanation of its meaning and importance. A person cannot refuse to return his neighbor's watch if he finds it, or at least to tell him where it is lying in the garden, merely because his neighbor does not know that he has lost it and has not asked the doctor if he found it or knows where it is.

Throughout this discussion of medical truth-telling our frame of reference has been physical rather than psychological diagnosis. A great many people naturally raise the question whether the reasoning here would be or could be applied equally to psychotherapy. In all probability it would not, and could not be without upsetting well-tested principles of therapy. In the first place, genuinely psychotic patients fall into Jeremy Taylor's category of "children and idiots," as far as competence to seek or to receive the truth is concerned. If it is judged to be in their best interests, surely the truth about them ("their" truth) can be withheld in the same way that a minor's or dependent's property can be withheld and rationed by a parent or guardian. Yet, even in the case of people who are far from psychotic, suffering some much less pathological disorder such as emotional or personality problems, there is a further consideration that makes a great difference between the right to know the truth in their case, and a patient's who has come, for example, for advice in internal medicine. In the latter case the doctor discovers a truth which is factually perceived. But in the case of psychiatric medicine and clinical psychology, apart from a physical analysis which may be related to it, the diagnosis is one of *evaluative judgment* about the patient's behavior and sentiments. However sound and wise the professional expert's diagnosis of behavior and motives and drives may be, it is, as far as honesty is at stake, in the area of *opinion*. Here, surely, the expert's obligation to tell the patient or client what is in or on his mind (i.e., the doctor's) is not as certain or compelling.

Notes

1. J. M. Birnie, "Ethics for Doctors," *New England Journal of Medicine,* 205, 1126.
2. *The Care of the Patient from the Surgeon's Standpoint* (Boston, 1934).
3. "Medical Ethics," address at Western Reserve College, April 25, 1908.
4. *The Meaning of Right and Wrong* (New York, 1933), pp. 167–68.
5. Cf. a supporting opinion by Edith M. Stern, *McCall's Magazine,* August 1951.
6. *Cancer Clinic Bulletin,* no. 41 (December 1936).

Meyer is concerned that others often advocate rigid adherence either to the formula of "always telling" or "never" doing so. In contrast to Fletcher, he notes that physicians *as* patients are not always eager to be told the truth. He decries the attention to an abstract principle rather than reliance upon the "humanity principle." For Meyer, the matter of the definition of truth and the problem of determining the patient's desires are seen as affecting the relationship between health-care provider and patient in a substantive manner. In keeping with the observations of Kübler-Ross and others, he points out the commonly made, but erroneous assumption that until someone has been formally told the truth he or she doesn't know it. Such an assumption may, he contends, block a therapeutic response to the needs of the dying, and he provides examples in which discussion of the known but unspoken truth may not be useful. For Meyer, "the precept that transcends the virtue of uttering truth for truth's sake" is "so far as possible do no harm."

Bernard C. Meyer

TRUTH AND THE PHYSICIAN *

ADHERENCE TO A FORMULA

In the dilemma created both by a natural disinclination to be a bearer of bad news [and by other considerations], many a physician is tempted to abandon personal judgment and authorship in his discourse with his patients, and to rely instead upon a set formula which he employs with dogged and indiscriminate consistency. Thus, in determining what to say to patients with cancer, there are exponents of standard policies that

---

* In *Ethical Issues in Medicine: The Role of the Physician in Today's Society,* E. Fuller Torrey, ed. Copyright © 1968, pp. 166–177 (slightly edited). Reprinted by permission of the author and Little, Brown and Company.

are applied routinely in seeming disregard of the overall clinical picture and of the personality or psychological makeup of the patient. In general, two such schools of thought prevail; i.e., those that always tell and those that never do. Each of these is amply supplied with statistical anecdotal evidence proving the correctness of the policy. Yet even if the figures were accurate—and not infrequently they are obtained via a questionnaire, itself a rather opaque window to the human mind—all they demonstrate is that more rather than less of a given proportion of the cancer population profited by the policy employed. This would provide small comfort, one might suppose, to the patients and their families that constitute the minority of the sample.

TRUTH AS ABSTRACT PRINCIPLE

At times adherence to such a rigid formula is dressed up in the vestments of slick and facile morality. Thus a theologian has insisted that the physician has a moral obligation to tell the truth and that his withholding it constitutes a deprivation of the patient's right; therefore it is "theft, therefore unjust, therefore immoral."[1] "Can it be," he asks, "that doctors who practice professional deception would, if the roles were reversed, want to be coddled or deceived?" To which, as many physicians can assert, the answer is distinctly *yes*. Indeed so adamant is this writer [Joseph Fletcher] upon the right of the patient to know the facts of his illness that in the event he refuses to hear what the doctor is trying to say, the latter should "ask leave to withdraw from the case, urging that another physician be called in his place."[2] . .

In this casuistry wherein so much attention is focused upon abstract principle and so little upon humanity, one is reminded of the no less specious arguments of those who assert that the thwarting of suicide and the involuntary hospitalization of the mentally deranged constitute violations of personal freedom and human right.[3] It is surely irregular for a fire engine to travel in the wrong direction on a one-way street, but if one is not averse to putting out fires and saving lives, the traffic violation looms as a conspicuous irrelevancy. No less irrelevant is the obsessional concern with meticulous definitions of truth in an enterprise where kindness, charity, and the relief of human suffering are the essential verities. "The letter killeth," say the Scriptures, "but the spirit giveth life."

Problem of Definition

Nor should it be forgotten that in the healing arts, the matter of truth is not always susceptible to easy definition. Consider for a moment the question of the hopeless diagnosis. It was not so long ago that such a designation was appropriate for subacute bacterial endocarditis, pneumococcal meningitis, pernicious anemia, and a number of other conditions which today are no longer incurable, while those diseases which today are deemed hopeless may cease to be so by tomorrow. Experience has proved, too, the unreliability of obdurate opinions concerning prognosis even in those conditions where all the clinical evidence and the known behavior of a given disease should leave no room for doubt. To paraphrase Clemenceau, to insist that a patient is hopelessly ill may at times be worse than a crime; it may be a mistake.

Problem of Determining Patient's Desires

There are other pitfalls, moreover, that complicate the problem of telling patients the truth about their illness. There is the naïve notion, for example, that when the patient asserts that what he is seeking is the plain truth he means just that. But as more than one observer has noted, this is sometimes the last thing the patient really wants. Such assertions may be voiced with particular emphasis by patients who happen to be physicians and who strive to display a professional or scientifically objective attitude toward their own condition. Yet to accept such assertions at their face value may sometimes lead to tragic consequences, as in the following incident.

> A distinguished urological surgeon was hospitalized for a hypernephroma, which diagnosis had been withheld from him. One day he summoned the intern into his room, and after appealing to the latter on the basis of we're-both-doctors-and-grown-up-men, succeeded in getting the unwary younger man to divulge the facts. Not long afterward, while the nurse was momentarily absent from the room, the patient opened a window and leaped to his death.

Role of Secrecy in Creating Anxiety

Another common error is the assumption that until someone has been formally told the truth he doesn't know it. Such self-deception is often present when parents feel moved to supply their pubertal children with the sexual facts of life. With much embarrassment and a good deal of backing and filling on the subjects of eggs, bees, and babies, sexual information is imparted to a child who often not only already knows it but is uncomfortable in hearing it from that particular source. There is indeed a general tendency to underestimate the perceptiveness of children not only about such matters but where graver issues, notably illness and death, are concerned. As a consequence, attitudes of secrecy and overprotection designed to shield children from painful realities may result paradoxically in creating an atmosphere that is saturated with suspicion, distrust, perplexity, and intolerable anxiety. Caught between trust in their own intuitive perceptions and the deceptions practiced by the adults about them, such children may suffer greatly from a lack of opportunity of coming to terms emotionally with some of the vicissitudes of existence that in the end are inescapable. A refreshing contrast to this approach has been presented in a paper entitled "Who's Afraid of Death on a Leukemia Ward?"[4] Recognizing that most of the children afflicted with this disease had some knowledge of its seriousness, and that all were worried about it, the hospital staff abandoned the traditional custom of protection and secrecy, providing instead an atmosphere in which the children could feel free to express their fears and their concerns and could openly acknowledge the fact of death when one of the group passed away. The result of this measure was immensely salutary.

Similar miscalculations of the accuracy of inner perceptions may be noted in dealing with adults. Thus, in a study entitled "Mongolism: When Should Parents Be Told?"[5] it was found that in nearly half the cases the mothers declared they had realized before being told that something was seriously wrong with the child's development, a figure which obviously excludes the mothers who refused consciously to acknowledge their suspicions. On the basis of their findings the authors concluded that a full explanation given in the early months, coupled with regular support thereafter, appeared to facilitate the mother's acceptance of and adjustment to her child's handicap.

A pointless and sometimes deleterious withholding of truth is a common practice in dealing with elderly people. "Don't tell Mother" often seems to be an almost reflex maxim among some adults in the face of any misfortune, large or small. Here, too, elaborate efforts at camouflage may backfire, for, sensing that he is being shielded from some ostensibly intolerable secret, not only is the elderly one deprived of the opportunity of reacting appropriately to it, but he is being tacitly encouraged to conjure up something in his imagination that may be infinitely worse.

Discussion of Known Truth

Still another misconception is the belief that if it is certain that the truth is known it is all right to discuss it. How mistaken such an assumption may be was illustrated by the violent rage which a recent widow continued to harbor toward a friend for having alluded to cancer in the presence of her late husband. Hearing her outburst one would have concluded that until the ominous word had been uttered, her husband had been ignorant of the nature of his condition. The facts, however, were different, as the unhappy woman knew, for it had been her husband who originally had told the friend what the diagnosis was.

DENIAL AND REPRESSION

The psychological devices that make such seeming inconsistencies of thought and knowledge possible are the mechanisms of repression and denial. It is indeed the remarkable capacity to bury or conceal more or less transparent truth that makes the problem of telling it so sticky and difficult a matter, and one that is so unsusceptible to simple rule-of-thumb formulas. For while in some instances the maintenance of denial may lead to severe emotional distress, in others it may serve as a merciful shield. For example,

> A physician with a reputation for considerable diagnostic acumen developed a painless jaundice. When, not surprisingly, a laparotomy revealed a carcinoma of the head of the pancreas, the surgeon relocated the biliary outflow so that postoperatively the jaundice subsided. This seeming improvement was consistent with the surgeon's explanation to the patient that the operation had revealed a hepatitis. Immensely relieved, the patient chided himself for not having anticipated the "correct" diagnosis. "What a fool I was!" he declared, obviously alluding to an earlier, albeit unspoken, fear of cancer.

Among less sophisticated persons the play of denial may assume a more primitive expression. Thus a woman who had ignored the growth of a breast cancer to a point where it had produced spinal metastases and paraplegia, attributed the latter to "arthritis" and asked whether the breast would grow back again. The same mental mechanism allowed another woman to ignore dangerous rectal bleeding by ascribing it to menstruation, although she was well beyond menopause.

In contrast to these examples is a case reported by Winkelstein and Blacher of a man who, awaiting the report of a cervical node biopsy, asserted that if it showed cancer he wouldn't want to live, and that if it didn't he wouldn't believe it.[6] Yet despite this seemingly unambiguous willingness to deal with raw reality, when the chips were down, as will be described later, this man too was able to protect himself through the use of denial.

From the foregoing it should be self-evident that what is imparted to a patient about his illness should be planned with the same care and executed with the same skill that are demanded by any potentially therapeutic measure. Like the transfusion of blood, the dispensing of certain information must be distinctly indicated, the amount given consonant with the needs of the recipient, and the type chosen with the view of avoiding untoward reactions. This means that only in selected instances is there any justification for telling a patient the precise figures of his blood pressure, and that the question of revealing interesting but asymptomatic congenital anomalies should be considered in light of the possibility of evoking either hypochondriacal ruminations or narcissistic gratification.

Under graver circumstances the choices confronting the physician rest upon more crucial psychological issues. In principle, we should strive to make the patient sufficiently aware of the facts of his condition to facilitate his participation in the treatment without at the same time giving him cause to believe that such participation is futile. "The indispensable ingredient of this therapeutic approach," write Stehlin and Beach, "is free communication between [physician] and patient, in which the latter is sustained by hope within a framework of reality."[7] What this may mean in many instances is neither outright truth nor outright falsehood but a carefully modulated formulation that neither overtaxes human credulity nor invites despair. Thus a sophisticated woman might be expected to reject with complete disbelief the notion that she has had to undergo mastectomy for a benign cyst, but she may at the same time accept postoperative radiation as a prophylactic measure rather than as evidence of metastasis. . . .

THE DYING PATIENT

The general point of view expressed in the foregoing pages has been espoused by others in considering the problem of communicating with the dying patient. Aldrich stresses the importance of providing such persons with an appropriately timed opportunity of selecting acceptance or denial of the truth in their efforts to cope with their plight.[8] Weisman and Hackett believe that for the majority of patients it is likely that there is neither complete acceptance nor total repudiation of the imminence of death.[9] "To deny this 'middle knowledge' of approaching death," they assert,

> . . . is to deny the responsiveness of the mind to both internal perceptions and external information. There is always a psychological sampling of the physiological stream; fever, weakness, anorexia, weight loss and pain are subjective counterparts of homeostatic alteration. . . . If to this are added changes in those close to the patient, the knowledge of approaching death is confirmed.

Other observers agree that a patient who is sick enough to die often knows it without being told, and that what he seeks from his physician are no longer statements concerning diagnosis and prognosis, but earnest manifestations of his unwavering concern and devotion. As noted earlier, it is at such times that for reason of their own psychological makeup some physicians become deeply troubled and are most prone to drift away, thereby adding, to the dying patient's physical suffering, the suffering that is caused by a sense of abandonment, isolation, and emotional deprivation.

In contrast, it should be stressed that no less potent than morphine nor less effective than an array of tranquilizers is the steadfast and serious concern of the physician for those often numerous and relatively minor complaints of the dying patient. . . .

If what has been set down here should prove uncongenial to some strict moralists, one can only observe that there is a hierarchy of morality, and that ours is a profession which traditionally has been guided by a precept that transcends the virtue of uttering truth for truth's sake; that is, "So far as possible, do no harm." Where it concerns the communication between the physician and his patient, the attainment of this goal demands an ear that is sensitive to both what is said and what is not said, a mind that is capable of understanding what has been heard, and a heart that can respond to what has been understood.

Notes

1. J. Fletcher, *Morals and Medicine* (Princeton, N.J.: Princeton University Press, 1954).
2. The same writer relaxes his position when it concerns psychiatric patients. Here he would sanction the withholding of knowledge "precisely because he may prevent the patient's recovery by revealing it." But in this, too, the writer is in error, in double error, it would seem, for, first, it is artificial and inexact to make a sharp distinction between psychiatric and nonpsychiatric patients —the seriously sick and the dying are not infrequently conspicuously emotionally disturbed; and second, because it may at times be therapeutically advisable to acquaint the psychiatric patient with the facts of his illness.
3. Proponents of these views have seemingly overlooked the unconscious elements in human behavior and thought. Paradoxical though it may seem, the would-be suicide may wish to live: what he seeks to destroy may be restricted to that part of the self that has become burdensome or hateful. By the same token, despite his manifest combativeness, a psychotic individual is often inwardly grateful for the restraints imposed upon his dangerous aggression. There can be no logical objection to designating such persons as "prisoners," as Szasz would have it, provided we apply the same term to breathless individuals who are "incarcerated" in oxygen tents.
4. J. Vernick and M. Karon, "Who's afraid of death on a leukemia ward?" *American Journal of Diseases of Children,* 109 (1965), 393.
5. C. M. Drillien and E. M. Wilkinson, "Mongolism: When should parents be told?" *British Medical Journal,* 2 (1964), 1306.
6. C. Winkelstein and R. Blacher, Personal communication, 1967.
7. J. S. Stehlin and K. A. Beach, "Psychological aspects of cancer therapy," *Journal of the American Medical Association,* 197 (1966), 100.
8. C. K. Aldrich, "The dying patient's grief," *Journal of the American Medical Association,* 184 (1963), 329.
9. A. D. Weisman and T. Hackett, "Predilection to death: Death and dying as a psychiatric problem," *Psychosomatic Medicine,* 23 (1961), 232.

In the following article Paul Ramsey seeks to discover the moral limits that ought properly to surround efforts to save life and to recover the meaning of "only" caring for the dying. Ramsey draws two pivotal conclusions: (1) that there is no duty to employ useless means, however natural or ordinary in practice, (2) that human acts of caring should focus exclusively on the patient, not on the diseases. Ramsey argues from the general perspective that the "correct" medical practice is one which provides those who are dying with the care they need in their final passage, and not simply with the first available technology. The best "care," he points out, is often given outside the hospital.

Ramsey also discusses other conditions that can make it morally right to stop the use of medical means, although the decision may not be strictly medical judgment.

Paul Ramsey

ON (ONLY) CARING FOR THE DYING *

In 1964 Dr. Belding H. Scribner, pioneer in the use of the kidney machine at the University of Washington School of Medicine and the Swedish Hospital, Seattle, Washington, delivered the presidential address at the annual meeting of the American Society for Artificial Internal Organs.[1] In his remarks on that occasion there is a striking passage in which Dr. Scribner addressed himself to the problem of a patient on chronic hemodialysis himself overtly terminating treatment (which Dr. Scribner, mistakenly I believe, describes as "a form of suicide"). We should expect, Dr. Scribner said, that as chronic kidney dialysis becomes a normal exigency of life for an increasing number of people there will be a proportionate increase in the number of those persons who will stop or simply omit this means of their survival. This led to speculation concerning the "death with dignity" which medical practice might extend to such patients. Death from chronic uremia is one of the most horrible known, involving intense suffering, vomiting, prolongation of the dying process, and great costs. "How much more humane and less expensive it would be to offer such a dying patient a weekly hemodialysis for a limited period"—instead of the bi-weekly or tri-weekly blood washings needed to keep a chronic uremia patient alive. "Then he could live a normal life right up to the end and die quickly and without prolonged suffering." Such a "maneuver to provide hemodialysis for a limited period" would avoid all the suffering, but Dr. Scribner described this as "utterly impossible under existing moral, ethical and religious guidelines." That judgment was, I believe, a completely mistaken and uninstructed verdict. Nothing in our moral tradition or religious teachings sustains the conclusion that such care cannot be extended to the dying. The proposed maneuver may or may not be illegal; it is certainly not immoral. Attending and companying with the patient in his dying is, in fact, the oldest medical ethics there is.

* From *The Patient as Person: Explorations in Medical Ethics,* pp. 113–44. Copyright © 1970 by Yale University. Reprinted by permission of Yale University Press.

THE PROBLEM

Shall a patient suffering from terminal illness be given life-sustaining procedures? Should he be placed on a respirator, and is there reason for ever turning off the respirator if such treatment was hopefully begun? Is there any moral difference between not starting the respirator, compared to turning it off once started? Are we bound to begin and continue the use of the intravenous drip because it is so standard a procedure? The "essentially isolated heart" can be kept beating for weeks; should this be begun or continued? Alternatively, the heart can be stopped for surgery or transplantation, while circulation of the blood is shunted around the heart and maintained, along with artificial respiration, by a heart-lung machine: are we obliged to use these means, and, if sometimes not, when not? Should a hopelessly paralyzed person be placed in an iron lung for the rest of his life? Must a terminal cancer patient be urged to undergo major surgery for the sake of a few months' palliation? What of fragmented creatures in deep and prolonged coma from severe brain damage, whose spontaneous cerebral activities have been reduced to those arising from the brainstem (diencephalon, mesencephalon, pons, and medulla) but who can be maintained "alive" for years by a combination of artificial activators and by nourishment? How much blood are we going to give a terminal patient, or how many successive organ transplants? Should transfusions for the treatment of hemorrhage from a gastrointestinal cancer be discontinued, when an operation to relieve this condition is not contemplated or feasible? Is there no end to the doctor's vocation to maintain life until the matter is taken out of his hands?

Alternatively expressed, ought there to be any relief for the dying from a physician's search for exquisite triumphs over death in a sort of salvation by works? Is a quadruple amputee absolutely obliged to choose existence on such terms? If not, what right has a doctor to save his life forcibly (apart from the general benefit of pushing back the frontiers of medical science); and then by what right should medical practice advance through achieving this success by means of him? Should cardiac surgery be performed to remove the lesions that are part of the picture in cases of mongolism, from which many mercifully died before the brilliant developments of recent years?

The same sort of question can be raised about many quite standard or routine procedures. Suppose that a diabetic patient long accustomed to self-administration of insulin falls victim to terminal cancer, or suppose that a terminal cancer patient suddenly develops diabetes. Is he in the first case obliged to continue, and in the second case obliged to begin, insulin treatment and die painfully of cancer, or in either or both cases may the patient choose rather to pass into diabetic coma and a earlier death? The same question can be raised in case of the onset of diabetes in a patient who has lived to old age in an institution for the severely retarded. What of the conscious patient suffering from painful incurable disease who suddenly gets pneumonia? Or an old man slowly deteriorating who from simply being inactive and recumbent gets pneumonia: are we to use antibiotics in a likely successful attack upon this disease which from time immemorial has been called "the old man's friend"? If this is the judgment to be made in regard to the aged, what shall we say of an infant who has hydrocephalus and develops pneumonia which could cause death in a short time? Should a baby born with serious congenital defect be respirated and saved from normal dying by advanced incubator procedures, or protected from the compensating abnormality which nature has somehow provided in the form of lower resistance to ordinary infections? Shall the child who is gravely impaired by mongolism be saved by a simple treatment from an infection that could cause his death?

The question whether it is right to withhold routine procedures in these cases may remain to haunt us even if we agree with Dr. Edward Rynearson that a combination of the heroic measures that are now possible may deprive many a patient of a fulfillment of the wish to have a death of one's own. The scene Dr. Rynearson describes is one of patients with an "untreatable" disease being "kept alive indefinitely by means of tubes inserted into their stomachs, or into their veins, or into their bladders, or into their rectums—and the whole sad scene thus created is encompassed within a cocoon of oxygen which is the next thing to a shroud"[2]—separated from family, from friends, and from themselves—the victims, this physician believes, of massive and unwarranted medical interventions upon their own particular death that has seized them.

One cannot hope to resolve the legitimate disagreement of conscientious men over every one of these questions. These cases suffice to show the importance of the problem raised by asking whether, beyond many present-day efforts to rescue the perishing, there does not arise a medical duty to (only) care for the dying. . . .

THE MORALITY OF (ONLY) CARING FOR THE DYING

In discussions of ordinary and extraordinary means it is commonly assumed by physicians and moralists alike that the use of all "ordinary" remedies is morally required of everyone, and that the failure to provide or use ordinary means of preserving life is the equivalent of euthanasia. The crucial question to be asked of traditional medical ethics is whether ordinary, imperative procedures can, in a proper moral judgment, become "extraordinary" and elective only. Can a patient morally refuse ordinary remedies? Can a physician morally fail to supply them or fail to continue ordinary remedies in use?

This is an unavoidable question, and one that goes to the heart of the morality of *caring,* but *only* caring, for the dying. Whoever raises this question lightly, or with a concern to disprove or dismiss past moral reflection, can only deny himself one possible source of helpful insights. Our inquiry shall concern whether and in what sense traditional medical ethical concepts and distinctions should be ethically regulative of present-day medical practice in regard to the fatally ill and the dying. During this brief journey into the meanings of the moralists, our "method" of doing medical ethics will not be to propose *replacing* definitions. Instead, our search will be for an understanding of past moral wisdom, and in this to locate places at which a *reforming* definition of one or another relevant moral concept suggests itself. In this section two such important qualifications or creative lines of development will be brought into focus which are needed to complete an ethics of caring for the dying. Then in the following section we shall ask whether, understood in terms of these reforming definitions, the ancient distinctions between ordinary and extraordinary (as a way of telling the difference between mandatory and elective efforts to save life) do not in sum reduce to the obligation to determine when a person has begun to undergo irreversibly the process of his own particular dying; and whether with *the process of dying* (all other terms aside) there does not arise the duty only to care for the dying, simply to comfort and company with them, to be present to them. This is the positive object of our search.

Then, in subsequent sections, we shall have to ask whether, over and above only caring for the dying, there is significant meaning still remaining in the distinction between ordinary and extraordinary means as specifications of our human obligation to continue or to discontinue life-sustaining procedures in the case of persons seriously or perhaps fatally ill, but not yet irreversibly dying. In addition to positing or enforcing the duty to respect with simple acceptance the dying process of a fellow man, the question then will be: Do these terms have any relevance for the medical care of persons not yet seized by their own dying? . . .

To give a cup of cold water to a man who has entered upon the course of his own particular dying is to slack the thirst of a man who will soon thirst again, and thirst unto death. When a man is irreversibly in the process of dying, to feed him and to give him drink, to ease him and keep him comfortable—these are no longer given as means of preserving life. The use of glucose drip should often be understood in this way. This keeps a patient who cannot swallow from feeling dehydrated, and is often the only remaining "means" by which we can express our present faithfulness to him during his dying (since to give him water intravenously would destroy his red blood cells and directly weaken and kill him). If a glucose drip prolongs this patient's dying because of the calories that are also introduced into his system, it is not done for that purpose or as a means in a continuing useless effort to save his life.

The administration of increased dosages of pain-killing drugs in the care of the dying is, as it were, the "mirror image" of the glucose drip: these drugs are judged to be life-shortening (to an immeasurable degree, because to suffer extreme pain would also be debilitating), but they are properly to be given in order to keep the patient as comfortable as possible, to show that we understand his need for succor, and not as a "useful" means to push him beyond our love and care. All these procedures, some "natural," others "artificial," are appropriate means—if "means" they should be called —of only caring for the dying, of physically companying with the dying. They are the embodied and effective gestures of soul to soul. As such, these acknowledgments of solidarity in mortality are due to the dying man from any of us who also bear flesh. Thus do men give answer by their presence and comfort to the faithfulness-claims of persons who are passing through the acceptable death of all flesh. If death should be accepted and treatment can no longer affect it, one might even raise the question whether *glucose* water should be used to keep the dying patient comfortable. I understand that there are certain sugars which it might be possible to use to give water for hydration without metabolizing calories and prolonging the dying process.

A second place at which a liberalizing definition of our obligation to care for the dying begins to suggest itself is in Kelly's answer to the question, "Is a person who suffers from two lethal diseases obliged to take ordinary means of checking one of them when there is no hope of checking the other?" The question at issue is whether a person suffering from incurable cancer who develops diabetes is obliged to begin insulin treatment, or a diabetic who develops an incurable cancer obliged to continue on insulin, and die slowly of the cancer instead of sooner in coma. Other moralists had answered that the patient must use the insulin since that is an "ordinary" means of checking the *disease* diabetcs. Kelly doubts whether a patient is bound to "prescind from the cancer in determining her obligation of using the insulin." The latter depends on two factors: that it is an ordinary means and that it offers a reasonable hope of success. The simultaneous presence of cancer throws doubt on the second stipulation. But then Kelly observes: "I think the doubt would be even stronger were there some connection between the two diseases."[3] An illustration of this would be the need for intravenous feeding *connected with* the fatal disease from which a patient is dying. Presumably Kelly would be more certain about the judgment that it is permissible to withdraw intravenous feeding in this case, although nowadays a drip is surely per se an ordinary procedure for sustaining life. Thus, in assessing mandatory and only elective remedies, Kelly moves away from judging this in terms of *single* diseases only, to connected diseases, and only hesitantly beyond that. His reasoning should be faulted only for this hesitation.

The patient is not exhaustively characterized by one disease, two separate diseases, or the interconnected diseases from which he may be suffering, both incurable, one involving prolonged dying. Ideally, Kelly wanted the description of the human act of caring for this patient to terminate in a texture of related diseases. But a proper description of the human acts of caring for mortal man terminates in that man. He is the unity of the diseases he suffers when one his quietus makes. Doctors do not treat diseases, though often they conquer them. They treat patients, and here finally all fail. If a diabetic patient need not prescind from the cancer in determining her obligation to start or to continue to use insulin, the reason is that she is the one flesh in which both diseases inhere. If to use insulin is for her quite useless, it is surely contraindicated. To move beyond the interrelation of the ills to which all flesh is heir requires that we move to *the flesh* that is heir to all its ills, indifferent to whether these ills are themselves connected or physiologically unrelated. It is this flesh, and not diseases one by one, that is the subject of medical treatment. This truth is enough to undercut the bondage of conscience to the imperativeness of "customary" or "usual" procedures for treating single diseases. . . .

THE PROCESS OF DYING

In the foregoing analysis we have drawn two pivotal conclusions: (1) that there is no duty to use useless means, however natural or ordinary or customary in practice; and (2) that the description of human acts of caring for the dying (or caring for the not yet dying) terminates in the man who is the patient of these ministrations and not in the disease or diseases he has. These are related points: in judging whether to try a given treatment one has to estimate whether there is a reasonable hope of success in saving the man's life.

A recent essay reviewing the distinction of extraordinary from ordinary means, and the different ways in which particular cases have been judged by traditional moralists, concludes that in the final analysis "the one general positive guideline from the past that will remain" may prove to be the directive that "the use of any means should be based on what is commonly termed a 'reasonable hope of success.' "[4] The residue of the distinctions we have reviewed, this author seems to suggest, is the test of usefulness. If so, the moral meaning of dispensable means would seem to reduce without remainder to a determination of an irreversible "process of dying."

This is certainly a principal component of the medical-moral imperative. It can certainly be said that our duties to the dying differ radically from our duties to the living or to the potentially still living. Just as it would be negligence to the sick to treat them as if they were about to die, so it is another sort of "negligence" to treat the dying as if they were going to get well or might get well.[5] The right medical practice will provide those who may get well with the assistance they need, and it will provide those who are dying with the care and assistance they need in their final passage. To fail to distinguish between these two sorts of medical practice would be to fail to act in accord with the facts. It would be to act in accord with some rule-book medicine. It would be to act without responsivity to those who have no longer any responsivity or recuperative powers.

Thus would we fail to care for them as the dying men they are, just as surely as if we failed to take account of the responsivity that the living sick or the not yet dying still have. Only a physician can determine the onset of the process of dying. For all the uncertainty, he must surely make this determination. He is bound to distinguish so far as he can between that time span in which his treatment of a patient is still a part of diagnosis and treatment—diagnosis and treatment not of the disease but of a patient's particular responsivity—and a subsequent time in which the patient is irreversibly doing his own dying. The "treatment" for that is care, not struggle. The claims of the "suffering-*dying*"[6] upon the human community are quite different from the claims of those who, through suffering, still may live, or who are incurably ill but not yet dying.

In connection with all that has just been said we should not have in mind only those patients who are in deep and prolonged coma. A conscious patient as well may have begun irreversibly the process of his particular dying; and, precisely because conscious, his claims are strong upon the human community that only care and comfort and company be given him and that pretended remedies or investigative trials or palliative operations be not visited upon him as if these were hopeful therapy. Therefore, to all of the foregoing the words of David Daube, Professor of Law at Oxford University, are pertinent. "The question of at what moment it is in order to discontinue extraordinary—or even ordinary—measures to keep a person alive," Professor Daube writes, "should not be confused with the question at what moment a man is dead" or with the question whether he is conscious or unconscious. "Discontinuation of such measures is often justifiable even while the patient is conscious."[7]

This risk-filled decision concerning the onset of a man's own process of dying can be and is made by physicians. The problem is to find the courage (and perhaps legal protection) to act upon it. Dr. John R. Cavanagh defines the "dying process" as "the time in the course of an irreversible illness when treatment will no longer influence it."[8] The patient has entered a covenant with the physician for his complete *care,* not for continuing useless efforts to *cure*. Therefore, Dr. H. P. Wasserman calls for "a program of 'pre-mortem care,' " and for the training of doctors in this, and in the diverse ways in which they may fulfill their vocation to cure sometimes, to relieve often, and to comfort always.[9]

If the sting of death is sin, the sting of dying is solitude. What doctors should do in the presence of the process of dying is only a special case of what should be done to make a human presence felt to the dying. Desertion is more choking than death, and more feared. The chief problem of the dying is how not to die alone. To care, if only to care, for the dying is, therefore, a medical-moral imperative; it is a requirement of us all in exhibiting faithfulness to all who bear a human countenance. In an extraordinary article, Dr. Charles D. Aring says flatly that "it is not to be surmised that under the most adverse circumstances the patient is not aware."[10] That may be to say too much, but it strongly suggests that the sound of human voices and the clasp of the hand may be as important in keeping company with the dying as the glucose-drip "drink of cool water" or relieving their pain.

Dr. Aring tells of the case of a man who, under continuing exotic treatments, kept asking to be returned to his ward and be within the presence of his three ward companions. Instead, "he died alone, denied what he most wanted, the unspoken comfort of people—any people—around him." This physician's judgment is that this man's "want of his friends and familiar surroundings, new though they were, should have been an imperative and taken precedence over any and all technical matters." That would have been proper "pre-mortem care" of the dying. To do this, the physician needs to become aware of his own feelings about death, and to lean against his possible proneness to visit cursorily or to pass hurriedly by the room in which lies one of his "failures." And all of us in the "age of the enlightenment" need to recognize "death's growing remoteness and unfamiliarity," the masks by which it is suppressed, the fantastic rituals by which we keep the presence of death at bay and our own presence from the dying, the inferiority assigned to the dying because it would be a human accomplishment not to do so, the ubiquity of the fear of dying that is one sure product of a secular age.[11]

There is a final entailment of caring for the dying that is required of priests, ministers, rabbis, and every one of us, and not only or not even mainly of the medical profession. "The process of dying" needs to be got out of the hospitals and back into the home and in the midst of family, neighborhood, and friends. This would be a "systemic change" in our present institutions for caring for the dying as difficult to bring about as some fundamental change in foreign policy or the nation-state system. Still, any doctor will tell you that by no means does everyone need to die in a hospital who today does so. They are there because families want them there, or because neighbors might think not everything was done in efforts to save them. They are there because hospitals are well equipped to "manage death," and families are ill equipped to do so.

If the "systemic change" here proposed in caring for the dying were actually brought about, ministers, priests, and rabbis would have on their hands a great many shattered families and relatives. But for once they would be shattered by confrontation with reality, by the claims of the dying not to be deserted, not to be pushed from the circle that specially owes them love and care, not to be denied human presence with them. Then God might not be as dead as lately He is supposed to be. The "sealing up of metaphysical concerns," Peter Berger recently pointed out, is one of the baneful results of a "happy" childhood—a childhood unhappily sheltered from the dying in all our advanced societies.[12]

CARING FOR THE SERIOUSLY ILL AND THE IRREVERSIBLY ILL

Nevertheless, it would not be correct to suggest that the distinction of extraordinary from ordinary treatments—of elective from imperative remedies—and the subtle ethical judgments falling under these heads can be reduced without significant remainder to the twin concepts of "reasonable hope of success" (usefulness) and "the process of dying." That, as we have seen, is an important component. It is, in fact, the component encompassing the duty of only caring for the dying. In this respect, the moral imperative and the medical imperative are the same. For medicine to do more or otherwise would be blameworthy. But this is not all the meaning of ordinary-extraordinary—of imperative and only elective efforts to save life.

In the remaining meaning of these concepts, the moral imperative may be more extensive than the medical imperative. The "process of dying" is not the only condition for stopping the use of medical means, although when present it is a sufficient and a morally obliging condition. Other conditions can make it morally right to stop the use of medical means, although the decision to do so may not be a strictly medical judgment. "No reasonable hope of success" (uselessness) is not the only warrant for stopping the use of medical means, although where present it is a sufficient and a morally obliging condition. Other grounds than hopelessness can make it morally right to stop the use of medical means, although the decision to cease using them is not a strictly medical judgment. Fr. Kelly speaks of "the recognized principle that an extraordinary means is not per se obligatory even when success would be certain."[13] The true humanity of moralists of the past led them unanimously to say that there are conditions that could make efforts to save life only elective even if they are certain to be successful. When a physician yields or—better still—himself makes room for these more extensive moral and human judgments, he likely does so as a man who is a doctor, by an exercise of the moral authority he has acquired in relation to the man who is his patient and to his family, and not by virtue of his medical expertise.

Even when he could succeed, a doctor may and sometimes should allow his medical judgment to defer to a patient's estimate of the higher importance of the worth and the relations for which his life was lived. In doing so the doctor acts the more as a man than as a medical expert, acknowledging the preeminence of the human relations in which he stands with these and all other men, rather than solely in his capacity as a scientist or as a healer.

In this age of scientific medicine and of the authority figure in a white coat, it is salutary to remind ourselves of some of the measures which, until not so long ago, no one needed to use to save his life. Fr. Kelly lists the following examples: "Leaving one's home to go to a more healthful climate; the maiden's repugnance to being treated by a (male) physician or surgeon; the amputation of a limb; other major operations, especially those involving the opening of the abdomen; and all very costly treatments." Thomas J. O'Donnell, S.J., has roundly criticized these out-of-date cases and his fellow moralists for not keeping up with advancements in medical practice.[14] Still we should notice the humane wisdom contained in some of these illustrations, a sensitivity to human factors that is too likely to be evacuated in this age of technology. We should notice the good moral reasons that could be adduced for formerly deeming only elective certain of the medical practices that have become established practices with the advancement of the science and art of medicine. . . .

Not every means for prolonging life, once it is successful and made available—even "customary" medical practice—becomes thereby ordinary and mandatory upon both patient and doctor. There are always broader human factors to be taken into account, and these always in Christian medical ethics kept the saving of life from being made an absolute and inflexible norm, a hardship inhumanly applied. Medical progress may be described as a process of constantly creating ordinary means out of extraordinary ones, but also as a process of constantly creating more and more extraordinary means that need not be used and perhaps ought not to be chosen.

As amputation of an arm or leg became ordinary, the saving of men who suffered quadruple amputation by accident or in war came into view. This as well as a number of other ways of saving life, such as organ transplantation, may be such that they can never become proper specifications of the requirement that we always should save life, or desire to live by all ordinary means. After all, the moralists' main reason for holding amputations to be only elective surgery was the "serious inconvenience of living with a mutilated body," not the pain or the risk of infection endured for only a short time. Looked at in this light, terminal wards and the present-day practice of geriatrics increasingly testify to the fact that "progress" in the science and art of medicine can also be described as the mounting use of means that are irremediably extraordinary. This also can be the result of the mistaken notion that men and medicine are required to save life by every physically effective means.

Not only morally relevant features of practices but also morally relevant features of patients themselves can render merely elective remedies morally required. For example, if a person need not save his life by using exquisite or painful procedures so far as he alone is concerned, perhaps he ought to do so if he bears some special relation to the common good. It may be that the next peace congress greatly depends on him. Then extraordinary means of extending his life for yet a while longer are, for that patient, "ordinary." To gain time to put in order one's fiduciary relations with God and man—to give and receive forgiveness—may also warrant extraordinary efforts to prolong life. Thus also, it is arguable that the one hundred heart transplants performed in 1968 were warranted because these were investigative operations having in view the common good to come. As therapy they were dispensable. The transplants were elective, however, through the consent of patients and surgeons to become coadventurers in the cause of medical progress. The experimental nature of these operations should, then, have been made very clear to recipients and donors alike.

Before concluding this section on the broader, nonmedical grounds for the possible rightness of electing not to oppose death, there are two final points that need to be mentioned. A physician may, we have said, either (1) on medical grounds only care for patients who have been seized by their particular process of dying, or (2) make room for the dispensability of extraordinary life-sustaining treatments because he as a man acknowledges that there may be sufficient moral and human reasons for this decision. If he does either of these things, he has a special problem in relation to the family of a patient who is unconscious or otherwise incompetent to consent or ask that either course of action be taken. He cannot and would not proceed without the agreement of the close relatives of such a patient. His problem, however, is that the family of seriously or irreversibly ill patients and of the dying have, in this situation, an enormous load of guilt. The guilt need not be for anything overtly done in the past. It is only that every one of us has the guilt of failing to enrich the life of an ill or dying loved one as much as we might have done.

Such is the human condition, that all are responsible for all—and in face of the death of a loved one, we are guilty of many a sin of omission. Out of their guilt, members of the family are likely—at long last—to require that everything possible be done for the hopelessly ill and the dying loved one. This may mean the prolongation of dying or the continuation of extraordinary life-sustaining measures beyond reasonable moral justification. At the same time, guilt-ridden people in their grief may be unable to bear the additional burden of a decision to discontinue useless treatment, and they are often relieved if this decision is not wholly placed on them. This means that the physician must exercise the authority he has acquired as a physician and as a man in relation to the relatives and take the lead in suggesting what should be done. In doing this, the doctor acts more as a man than as a medical expert, acknowledging the preeminence of the human relations in which he with these and all other men stand. For this reason, the medical imperative and the moral imperative or permission are, while distinguishable, not separable in the person or in the vocation of the man who is a physician.

Second, while in caring for patients a moral judgment concerning mandatory and elective treatment may be based on broader grounds than a strictly medical judgment, still a physician has in relation to disease a strictly medical imperative that is more encompassing than the patient-doctor relation itself. His is the ethics of a scientific mission in regard to disease itself. He is bound by a medical imperative that is more extensive than the human and moral considerations that may warrant elective death on the part of the man who is the patient of his care. It is not contrary to the common good or to the care now needed for a doctor to admit that a patient is incurable, or that he is now dying, and to cease trying to effect his cure or prolong his dying. But, while as a doctor he should act in accord with the incurability of the patient and as a human being should act in accord with the humanity of the patient, "it would be contrary to the common good [for him] to cease trying to find a remedy for the disease itself." [15] Here the medical imperative governing a doctor's profession and specifying the requirement that he never cease trying to find the cure or relief which future patients need proves more extensive in its turn and preeminent over the humane moral judgment that can clearly warrant the choiceworthiness of death for other than medical reasons in many a particular instance. The question of questions is whether both judgments (with appropriate actions) can dwell together in the same person and calling. Or must one be bartered against the other, and in practice the one weaken the other resolve?

The medical imperative to continue to try to find a remedy for incurable diseases, while admitting that a patient is incurable and while ceasing to try to effect his cure, may involve the creation of a consensual community between doctors and incurable patients in which they both become joint adventurers in the common cause of curing these diseases. No advantage should be taken of the desperation of dying men, of course; but they also should be accorded the nobility and opportunity of personally nontherapeutic service of mankind, if this is the true account of trials made upon them to save life from that disease. An understanding partnership between a physician-investigator and the dying or the incurably ill would be one way, and perhaps a satisfying way, of not dying alone.

Notes

1. Belding H. Scribner, "Ethical Problems of Using Artificial Organs to Sustain Human Life," in Harold M. Schmeck, Jr., *The Semi-Artificial Man: A Dawning Revolution in Medicine* (New York: Walker, 1965).

2. E. H. Rynearson, "You Are Standing at Bedside of Patient Dying of Untreatable Cancer," C.A., 9 (May–June 1959), 85–87.

3. Gerald Kelly, "The Duty of Using Artificial Means of Preserving Life," *Theological Studies,* 11 (June 1950), 215–16. I presume that the above debate is about the dying cancer patient or a quite advanced incurable cancer. There are, of course, stages of cancer for which treatment holds out the hope of, say, ten years of relatively normal life. The diabetes of such a patient should certainly be treated. While it may be that the disease has seized him from which he one day will die, he is not yet dying of it.

4. Kieran Nolan, "The Problem of Care for the Dying," in Charles E. Curran, ed., *Absolutes in Moral Theology?* (Washington, D.C., and Cleveland: Corpus Books, 1968), p. 253.

5. *Ibid.,* p. 256.

6. *Ibid.,* p. 260.

7. David Daube, "Transplantation: Acceptability of Procedures and Their Required Legal Sanctions," in G. E. W. Wolstenholme and Maeve O'Connor, *Ethics in Medical Progress* (Boston: Little Brown, 1966), pp. 190–91.

8. John R. Cavanagh, "Bene Mori: The Right of a Patient to Die with Dignity," *Linacre Quarterly,* May 1963 (unpaginated reprint).

9. H. P. Wasserman, "Problematic Aspects of the Phenomenon of Death," *World Medical Journal,* 14 (1967), 148–49.

10. Charles D. Aring, "Intimations of Mortality: An Appreciation of Death and Dying," *Annals of Internal Medicine,* 69, no. 1 (July 1968), 149.

11. *Ibid.,* pp. 141, 137, 138, 144–45, 151.

12. Symposium on "The Culture of Unbelief," held in Rome under the sponsorship of the Vatican Secretariat for Nonbelievers and the University of California at Berkeley.

13. Kelly, "The Duty of Using Artificial Means of Preserving Life," p. 214.

14. Kelly, "The Duty of Using Artificial Means of Preserving Life," pp. 204–5; Thomas J. O'Donnell, S.J., *Morals in Medicine* (Westminister, Md.: Newman, 1960), pp. 63–67.

15. Kelly, "The Duty of Preserving Life," *Theological Studies,* 12 (December 1951), p. 555.

Many physicians have styles of care that emphasize "heroic" measures, but they may often stop short of orders for resuscitation. Many families desire that every "heroic" measure be attempted—to assuage guilt, etc.—short of resuscitation. It is usually assumed that a decision *not* to use such measures in the dying patient would more or less be followed by orders *not* to resuscitate in the event of sudden cessation of vital functions. But the patient ordinarily is little involved in such decision making, and hospital policies may be nonexistent or poorly articulated and loosely implemented. Thus, orders not to resuscitate may be dependent on the presence or absence of key head nurses to whom the communication has been made.

The selection that follows reports the development of procedures leading to orders not to resuscitate and of a policy statement in one hospital concerning the order not to resuscitate. The selection points out an instance of patients' rights and informed consent involving the complex relationships between the psychological attitudes involved (including those of the family), the rights and obligations of the physician, and the impact of medical and hospital policy and practice.

Mitchell T. Rabkin
Gerald Gillerman
Nancy R. Rice

ORDERS NOT TO RESUSCITATE *

Medical opinions on the inappropriateness of cardiopulmonary resuscitation of certain patients are now openly discussed, as acknowledged by the New Jersey Supreme Court in its recent Quinlan decision. As early as 1974 the A.M.A. proposed that decisions not to resuscitate be formally entered in patients' progress notes and communicated to all attending staff. There has been little open discussion, however, of the process by which a decision not to resuscitate is formulated. Within a single institution, practices may vary among physicians in part from the lack of a clearly articulated hospital policy.

An apparent need for hospital definitions of the process by which decisions not to resuscitate should be made led to the development of the following statement, which is proposed as a policy statement for hospitals concerned with regulating the process whereby Orders Not to Resuscitate may be considered and then implemented. . . .

Having witnessed impressive medical developments over the past 25 years, the health-care community is now confronted with complex ques-

* From the *New England Journal of Medicine*, 295 (August 12, 1976), 364–66. Reprinted by permission.

tions arising from interplay of two such developments, technologic advances and the increased emphasis on the patient's role in decisions concerning his own health care. There is a growing concern that it may be inappropriate to apply technologic capabilities to the fullest extent in all cases and without limitation. Moreover, increased awareness of the rights of patients to be treated in accordance with their own decisions and expectations means that the use of heroic measures to sustain life can be justified only by adherence to the dictates of both sound medical practice and the patient's right to elect or decline the benefits of medical technology.

Both as a standard of medical care and as a statement of philosophy, it is the general policy of hospitals to act affirmatively to preserve the life of all patients, including persons who suffer from irreversible terminal illness. It is essential that all hospital staff understand this policy and act accordingly.

As a matter of policy hospitals also respect the competent patient's informed acceptance or rejection of treatment, including cardiopulmonary resuscitation, and recognize that in certain cases the unwanted use of heroic measures on a patient irreversibly and irreparably terminally ill might be both medically unsound and so contrary to the patient's wishes or expectations as not to be justified.

To ensure adherence to each of these policies, we have prepared this statement to guide a hospital in the process of decision making regarding the use of cardiopulmonary resuscitation.

Notwithstanding the hospital's pro-life policy, the right of a patient to decline available medical procedures must be respected. For example, if a competent patient who is not irreversibly and irreparably ill issues instructions that under stated circumstances, he is opposed to the use of certain procedures, the following guidelines should be observed. The physician should explore thoroughly with the patient the types of circumstances that might arise, and warn that the consequences of a generalized prohibition may be to allow an unintended termination of life. If after a careful disclosure the patient persists in some form of order declining use of certain medical procedures when otherwise applicable, the physician is legally required to respect such instructions. Such situations are not unknown to hospitals that have treated Jehovah's Witnesses and other persons with fixed opinions unlikely to be affected by unforeseen medical exigencies. If the physician finds the medical program as ordered by the patient so inconsistent with his own medical judgment as to be incompatible with his continuing as the responsible physician, he may attempt to transfer the care of the patient to another physician more sympathetic to the patient's desires.

The specific issue of the appropriateness of cardiopulmonary resuscitation arises frequently with the irreversibly, irreparably ill patient whose death is imminent. We refer to the medical circumstance in which the disease is "irreversible" in the sense that no known therapeutic measures can be effective in reversing the course of illness; the physiologic status of the patient is "irreparable" in the sense that the course of illness has progressed beyond the capacity of existing knowledge and technic to stem the process; and when death is "imminent" in the sense that in the ordinary course of events, death probably will occur within a period not exceeding two weeks.

When it appears that a patient is irreversibly and irreparably ill, and that death is imminent, the question of the appropriateness of cardiopulmonary resuscitation in the event of sudden cessation of vital functions may be considered by the patient's physician, if not already raised by the patient, to avoid an unnecessary abuse of the patient's presumed reliance on the physician and hospital for continued life-supporting care. The initial medical judgment on such question should be made by the primarily responsible physician for the patient after discussion with an ad hoc committee consisting not only of the other physicians attending the patient and the nurses and others directly active in the care of the patient, but at least one other senior staff physician not previously involved in the patient's care. The inquiry should focus on whether the patient's death is so certain and so imminent that resuscitation in the event of sudden cessation of vital functions would serve no purpose. Although the unanimous opinion of the ad hoc committee in support of the decision of the responsible physician is not necessarily required (for some may be uncertain), a strongly held dissenting view not negated by other staff members should generally dissuade the responsible physician from his or her initial judgment on the appropriateness of resuscitation efforts.

Even if a medical judgment is reached that a patient is faced with such an illness and imminence of death that resuscitation is medically inappropriate, the decision to withhold resuscitation (Orders Not to Resuscitate, "ONTR") will become effective only upon the informed choice of a competent patient or, with an incompetent patient, by strict adherence to the guidelines discussed below, and then only to the extent that all appropriate family members are in agreement with the views of the involved staff. In this context, "appropriate" means at least the family members who would be consulted for permission to perform a postmortem examination if the patient died.

"Competence" in this context is not to be restricted to the legal and medical tests to determine competence to stand trial or to form a criminal intent. For the purpose of making an informed choice of medical treatment, "competence" is understood to rest on the test of whether the patient understands the relevant risks and alternatives, and whether the resulting decision reflects a deliberate choice by the patient. Caution should be exercised that a patient does not unwittingly "consent" to an ONTR, as a result of temporary distortion (for example, from pain, medication or metabolic abnormality) in his ability to choose among available alternatives.

It is recognized that it may be inappropriate to introduce the subject of withholding cardiopulmonary resuscitation efforts to certain competent patients when, in the physician's judgment, the patient will probably be unable to cope with it psychologically. In such event, Orders Not to Resuscitate may not be directed because of the absence of an informed choice. Appropriate family members should be so informed, and the physician should explain the course that will thus follow in the event of sudden cessation of the patient's vital functions. This discussion with the family should be noted by the physician in the medical record. If, however, the physician is able to discuss the essential elements of the case with a competent patient without violating the principles of reasonable and humane medical practice, a valid consent may follow.

If the competent patient thus chooses the ONTR alternative, this is his choice, and it may not be overridden by contrary views of family members. Nevertheless, it is important to inform the family members of the patient's decision (with the patient's permission and in accordance with his directions) so that the failure to resuscitate or to take other heroic measures is not unanticipated. In any event, the decision should be documented by the responsible physician and at least one witness. Such decisions shall remain in effect if the patient subsequently becomes incompetent and if the clinical circumstances for Orders Not to Resuscitate otherwise remain in existence.

Minors who are not emancipated by state law will be deemed incompetent to make a decision not to resuscitate. Such persons, however, will be kept informed if such a communication is appropriate, and have the right to reject a decision not to resuscitate, despite their presumed incompetence.

If a patient is incompetent, he should not be denied the benefits of the evaluation process described above. The physician and the ad hoc committee will consider initially whether the conditions of irreversibility, irreparability, and imminence of death are satisfied in their opinion. The basis for a final decision for Orders Not to Resuscitate must be concern from the patient's point of view, and not that of some other person who might present what he regards as sufficient reasons for not resuscitating the patient. It is only the clinical interest of the patient that must be considered; consideration of other factors would violate the fundamental policy of the hospital. An additional condition for the issuance of Orders Not to Resuscitate for an incompetent patient is approval of at least the same family members who are required to consent to postmortem examination. Failure to obtain and record family approval of Orders Not to Resuscitate may expose those involved to charges of negligent or unlawful conduct. Thus, the failure to obtain such approval would foreclose further consideration of Orders Not to Resuscitate in cases in which the patient is incompetent.

To prevent any uncertainty or confusion over the status of a patient's treatment, the decision for Orders Not to Resuscitate and its accompanying consent by the competent patient or the appropriate family members should be recorded promptly in the medical chart. In addition to the formal consent, the written and dated record must include the following: a summary of the staff discussion and decision; the disclosures to the patient, which must include the elements of informed consent, the patient's response, the responsible physician's documentation of the patient's competence, the patient's decision to inform appropriate family members and the resulting discussion with them that may then follow. Each hospital must specify what it deems to be the elements of informed consent and the formats in which consent must be witnessed and documented. Whether or not the patient's signature must be required invariably should also be decided; the signature removes ambiguity, but the physical act of signing may be deemed unpalatable by certain patients and therefore unacceptable to them as a necessary or appropriate formalization of the meaningful discussion and their resulting verbal consent.

It is the responsibility of the physician to convey the meaning of the Orders Not to Resuscitate to all medical, nursing and other staff as appropriate, and, simultaneously, to insist upon being notified immediately if the patient's condition should change so that the orders seem no longer applicable. If the circumstances described to such a patient do not change, a subsequent resuscitation would constitute treatment without consent.

After the issuing of Orders Not to Resuscitate, the patient's course, including continued evaluation of competence and consent, must be reviewed by the responsible physician at least daily, or at more frequent intervals, if appropriate, and documentation made in the medical chart to determine the continued applicability of such orders. If the patient's condition alters in such a way that the orders are no longer deemed applicable, the Orders Not to Resuscitate must be revoked, and the revocation communicated without delay.

Nothing in the entire procedure leading to Orders Not to Resuscitate, nor the ONTR itself, should indicate to the medical and nursing staff or to the patient and family any intention to diminish the appropriate medical and nursing attention to be received by the patient. It is the responsibility of the physician in charge to be certain that no diminution of necessary and appropriate measures for the patient's care and comfort follows from this decision.

When the incompetent patient is sufficiently alert to appreciate at least some aspects of the care he is receiving (the benefit of doubt must always assign to the patient the likelihood of at least partial alertness or receptivity to verbal stimuli), and especially with a child, whose "incompetence" by legal definition may not be supported by clinical observation, every effort must be made to provide the comfort and reassurance appropriate to the patient's state of consciousness and emotional condition regardless of the designation of incompetence.

In every case in which Orders Not to Resuscitate are issued, the hospital shall make available to the greatest extent practicable resources to provide counseling, reassurance, consolation and other emotional support as appropriate, for the patient's family and for all involved hospital staff, as well as for the patient.

Occasionally, a proposal for Orders Not to Resuscitate may be initiated by family members. It is essential to recognize that a family member's instructions not to resuscitate are not to be viewed as the choice of the patient. Thus, the attending physician and the ad hoc committee must not simply concur in the Orders Not to Resuscitate suggested by the family, but such concurrences shall be forthcoming only upon the timing and conditions described above.

Some courts have not hesitated to enforce the overruling by doctors of a patient's refusal of treatment of life-saving procedures. This confrontation comes to the fore (frequently in emergency situations) in the case of Jehovah's Witnesses, who believe that there is a Biblical injunction against accepting blood transfusions—even if the doctor deems it essential to the saving of life. In the next selection Charles H. Montange discusses both the uncertain status of legal precedents and the wide variety of judicial formulations that relate to control by the patient. As noted in the Introduction, dying in the hospital (rather than at home) introduces, in a significant way, the standards of the health provider. Montange argues for standards of informed consent other than those of the health provider (including the scope of disclosure), even when the patient is suffering from terminal illness. The patient's right to select treatment may be severely limited when it is based only on information deemed worthy of disclosure according to a medical community standard. Such issues as the concealment of information that might cause the patient to forego treatment and the standard of the reasonable person are raised.

Charles H. Montange

INFORMED CONSENT AND THE DYING PATIENT *

People afflicted with terminal illness rarely die at home. The success of medicine has shifted the locus of dying to public and private health-care

* Reprinted by permission of The Yale Law Journal Company and Fred B. Rothman & Company. From *The Yale Law Journal,* 83, no. 8 (July 1974), 1632–64.

institutions, thus transferring control over treatment away from the patient and his family to the health-care provider and the state. This has been a tacit accommodation to the way health sciences treat the dying, rather than an explicit legal choice.

The terminally ill patient may nevertheless wish to forego treatment offered by the health-care institution for a number of reasons: religious beliefs, pain and suffering, exhaustion of financial resources, acquiescence to death on the loss of control over most bodily functions. The patient's wish may conflict with the interests of the health-care providers who are committed to prolongation of life through medical technology, or with what seem to be the interests of the state, asserted through laws against suicide and homicide. The application of these laws is fraught with difficulty in cases of "passive euthanasia," the withholding of life-sustaining medical treatment; nonetheless, some courts have not hesitated to enforce the overruling by doctors of a patient's refusal of treatment. The proper legal outcome, however, is far from settled.

The doctrine of informed consent offers an established basis for court resolution of the issue. Since Judge Cardozo's opinion in *Schloendorff* v. *Society of New York Hospital,* courts have, in nonterminal cases, regularly premised the doctrine on the basic principle that "[e]very human being of adult years and sound mind has a right to determine what shall be done with his own body . . . ." This axiom has been restated recently in the leading case of *Natanson* v. *Kline* [1] as follows:

> Anglo-American law starts with the premise of thorough-going self-determination. It follows that each man is considered to be master of his own body, and he may, if he be of sound mind, expressly prohibit the performance of life-saving surgery, or other medical treatment. A doctor might well believe that an operation or form of treatment is desirable or necessary but the law does not permit him to substitute his own judgment for that of the patient by any form of artifice or deception. [2]

While purporting to apply the basic principle, however, courts in different jurisdictions have developed a wide variety of formulations that inhibit realization of ultimate control by the patient. When a court focuses on the doctor's therapeutic privilege to withhold information or bases its determination of the doctor's liability on the disclosure standards observed by the local medical community, the patient's self-determination may be too easily overlooked.

This Note argues that, in accordance with the postulate of self-determination, someone other than the health-care provider should set the standard and scope of disclosure. Courts should scrutinize with care any accretions to the doctrine of informed consent that diminish the information a patient receives or that circumscribe his entitlement to consent before treatment. The stress some courts place on interests countervailing the *Schloendorff* axiom may represent an implicit questioning of the validity of that principle. However, this Note contends that probing the underpinnings of the principle will reveal even more fundamental interests which require results consistent with the axiom in those cases in which the courts engage in some variety of balancing.

Viewed in this light, the doctrine of informed consent requires that any competent patient should retain control over decisions about treatment, even if he is suffering from a terminal illness. . . .

I. INFORMED CONSENT

The doctrine of informed consent emerged from medical malpractice cases involving rendition of some treatment to which the patient had not consented. Treatment necessarily involves a touching of the patient's body. If performed without a valid consent, it has been viewed as an intentional interference with the person—a battery. Expert testimony as to the standard medical community practice is not required in a battery action, since liability is not based on any standard of care but rather on an unlawful touching. For situations in which the doctor performs a treatment for which no consent whatsoever has been obtained, battery is the appropriate theory for recovery in many jurisdictions.

However, in situations in which the patient consents to a treatment but an undisclosed risk materializes, courts have been reluctant to find that the physician has committed an intentional tort. In such cases, physicians have generally been allowed to interpose the defense that disclosure of the risk in question was not customary in the local medical community. This encouraged some courts to view insufficient disclosure of risks and alternatives as a failure to exercise due care. A due-care standard is doctrinally more consistent with negligence than with battery; therefore a trend has developed to view failure to obtain an informed consent as a tort of negligence.

A. Information and Consent

Whether battery or negligence is the theory, informed consent involves the two vital elements its name implies: the patient must be given information on the risks involved in the treatment, and he must assent to the treatment. The fiduciary relationship between the doctor and patient obligates the doctor to assure the presence of both elements before undertaking a procedure.

However, risks which are everyday knowledge need not be mentioned to the patient, and disclosure of "material" risks is sufficient. Furthermore, physicians will be held responsible for revealing only such risks as are known to reasonably prudent comparable practitioners. However, courts adopting a negligence theory for informed consent differ greatly over what constitutes a material risk.

The view accepted by the majority of American jurisdictions bases the duty to disclose on a community standard; it requires only such disclosure of risks as is consistent with the practice of the local medical community. Expert medical testimony is required to show a breach of local medical standards. The majority rule results from a view of the fiduciary relationship between physician and patient that perceives the doctor's duty to disclose as subservient to his general duty "to do what is best" for the patient. The latter duty is a function of the local medical community standard which must be established by expert testimony. Since the obligation to disclose is seen as part of, or subservient to, the more general duty, the standard of disclosure is described as a question of medical judgment. Thus no disclosure is required unless expert testimony indicates that otherwise the relevant standard of medical care would be breached.

This view, however, threatens to emasculate the individual self-determination which the doctrine of informed consent was meant to protect. The patient's right to select treatment is severely limited when it is based only on information deemed worthy of disclosure according to a medical community standard set by those under the obligation to inform. Thus the medical community standard test runs contrary to vesting ultimate determination of treatment questions in the patient and diminishes rather than assures his self-determination. Furthermore, it is open to abuse. It may be used as a device either to conceal information which might cause the patient to forego treatment, or to avoid possible confrontations with patients and their families which might be emotionally difficult for the patient or doctor.

In recent years, courts in several jurisdictions have recognized these objections and have abolished the medical-community standard, adopting new tests for disclosure. Seeking to retain some limits on physician liability, the new tests utilize a reasonable-man standard. However, they apply the standard to differing elements of the case. One scheme applies the reasonable-man test to materiality of the information withheld. Another applies the test to causation and appears to leave materiality to a more subjective standard. Yet another formulation weighs both materiality and causation according to an objective test.

The Rhode Island Supreme Court in *Wilkinson* v. *Vesey* [3] concluded that the patient must be given all material information necessary for a decision. The character of material information could not be determined by a "local medical group" which has no knowledge of the individual or the unique situation involved. The court reasoned that the decision as to materiality is a human judgment which does not require expert medical testimony, but may be determined by the jury. Disclosure should extend to all facts which a reasonable man would regard as material in light of the severity of the risk and the likelihood of its occurrence—the more severe or likely the risk, the more probable that it is material.

Wilkinson also discussed causation. To recover in a malpractice action for lack of informed consent, the patient must show not only that the physician failed to disclose a material fact, but also that he, the patient, would have refused consent had he been informed of the fact, and that he has been injured as a result of the concealment. The focus is on what the particular patient would have done, thus wisely making the causation test more subjective than the materiality requirement.

However, *Wilkinson* unduly restricted recovery to cases in which the patient would have refused treatment altogether. The rule should be broader. If the patient shows that, had he been warned, he would have delayed consent in order to attend to personal or business matters, he should recover for damages which he can prove resulted from the concealment. Such a modified rule would be consistent with the requirement of causation for tort liability, while increasing the scope of protection consistently with the reasons for informed consent.

The California Supreme Court in *Cobbs* v. *Grant*[4] also began with the familiar postulate of self-determination over one's body as the basis for requiring that the physician disclose to his patient "all information relevant to a meaningful decisional process."[5] This court, rejecting the community-standard rule as "overbroad" and " nebulous," opted for a standard more protective of patient's rights. *Cobbs* required that known risks of death or serious bodily harm be disclosed. The test for adequate disclosure is the patient's need for information, a need which encompasses "whatever is material to the decision."[6] . . .

B. Underpinnings of the Doctrine

Judicial deviation from the basic principle of informed consent—self-determination over one's own body—perhaps results from a failure to probe the underpinnings of that axiom. The principle implies that there exist categories of decisions which an individual must be permitted to make, even if others believe the individual decides irrationally or incorrectly. It indicates that an implicit weighing of the interests of competing decision makers has already taken place and that the balance has been resolved in favor of individual choice. Courts and commentators may analyze the class of decisions reserved to the individual to rest on John Stuart Mill's concept of freedom of choice over matters which have a direct adverse effect on no one but the decision maker. Alternatively, courts may come increasingly to view informed consent as a manifestation of constitutionally protected privacy, especially after *Roe* v. *Wade*. However, courts have explored the connection between informed consent and constitutional doctrine most in the context of freedom of religion. Competent, informed patients have been held entitled to refuse treatment solely because of religious beliefs, even if the treatment is necessary to preserve their lives. Constitutional rights may thus indeed lie at the foundation of informed-consent doctrine, but the issue remains far from settled.

The doctrine's underpinnings, however, may also be explained in terms more commonly applied to tort doctrine in general. To the extent that tort law seeks to achieve an efficient allocation of resources, it aspires to place the responsibility for particular decisions upon the individuals who can best avoid costs arising from that decision making. This cost avoidance includes an effort to reduce the number and severity of incorrect decisions, and an attempt to reduce the costs of gathering and considering information in making decisions. Decision making for purposes of informed consent may be evaluated in terms of cost avoidance. The physician is primarily an expert in diagnosis and treatment who can determine at less expense than the patient the desirability of a particular treatment from a medical point of view. However, the physician is not equipped to evaluate a treatment in terms of a patient's nonmedical needs. The cost to the physician of discovering all the patient's psychological, social, and business needs and obligations is simply too great. Only the patient knows sufficiently his own value preferences, capacity for pain and suffering, future business and social plans, and religious beliefs to evaluate the desirability of a particular treatment so it will maximize the patient's satisfaction. Moreover, a system which overtly ignored the individual values of patients might encourage them to avoid or delay consulting physicians for fear that their values would be disregarded. This would risk deterioration of health standards at considerable cost to society as individuals neglected to seek medical advice.

This analysis suggests that the most efficient decision-making method for medical treatment places responsibility on the physician to make sufficient medical disclosures to his patients. On the basis of both the medical information and his own values, the patient would then be responsible for evaluating alternative procedures proposed by the physician and for making the ultimate decision as to the most appropriate treatment. The physician would be liable for insufficient disclosure, but the patient would bear the risks of the treatment or nontreatment which he selected after receiving adequate information. As the previous discussion indicated, recent informed-consent cases have moved in this direction of an economically efficient allocation of decision-making authority.

II. IMPLICATIONS FOR EUTHANASIA

Society engages in a denial of death. This denial of death entails two attitudes which must be squarely confronted and overcome in order to achieve reasoned discussion of voluntary euthanasia. First, the denial has encouraged the view that society attaches unqualified paramount value to human life, or, put another way, that society engages in thoroughgoing protection of life. In actuality such protection is an illusion, for society has tended to prevent only direct takings of life, while permitting the indirect, but statistically certain, deaths. For example, the recent reduction of speed limits on highways during the energy shortage made clear that the higher speeds tolerated for years have resulted in a substantially higher death toll. Death of a human being should be of equal concern whether direct or indirect. Direct takings, however, would confront the denial by shattering the illusion, whereas the illusion may be maintained when the takings are indirect. Voluntary euthanasia is sufficiently open and direct that it constitutes an explicit challenge to the illusion.

Second, denial of death has made many unable to appreciate that a dying person may accept the prospect of death "with equanimity and without mental disturbance."[7] This in turn prompts the attitude that a decision to die by a terminal patient is a manifestation of mental incompetency; hence that a terminal patient cannot competently consent to any form of euthanasia.

Once one begins to see through these attitudes, the question becomes not, "Why make an exception permitting a death?" but rather, "What exceptions should be made?" This latter question may be addressed in part through the doctrine of informed consent.

The patient's right to an informed consent makes no sense without a right to an informed refusal. The right to refuse should be extended to the dying patient, for his decision on proffered treatment is no different from that involved in any other medical situation. The individual continues to know best his own value preferences, capacity for pain and suffering, and uncompleted business and social obligations. He remains the optimal cost avoider.

The problem of euthanasia can be viewed as a continuum of situations requiring implementation of the patient's right to be the decision maker. At one end of the continuum is the nonterminal patient confronted with risks and alternatives in selecting treatment. Next is the terminal patient deciding whether to submit to life-sustaining therapy. Further along the continuum comes the terminal patient requesting the discontinuance of a life-sustaining treatment. Finally there is the terminal patient requesting that his life be shortened by rendition of a death-inducing agent.

The doctrine of informed consent requires that the competent, nonterminal patient in a nonemergency situation be given a chance to consent or refuse. The situation is no different for the terminal patient advised by his doctor to undergo a particular treatment. He should likewise have a choice, since the decision involved is analytically the same as in the first case.

However, the case of the competent terminal patient requesting discontinuance of life-sustaining treatment presents several problems. Arguably, once a patient submits to a life-sustaining treatment, the physician has an obligation not only to him but also to society to maintain him, at a minimum, in his present condition. In addition, a patient is sometimes viewed as submitting to the physician's "professional standards" or "school of practice" when he requests treatment. According to this view, the physician may thereafter treat the patient according to his school, which may mean that termination of treatment before death will not be permitted.

This argument forces the patient to choose between extreme alternatives. The patient is compelled either to forego treatment altogether or, once treatment commences, to submit completely to the physician's decisions. This failure to honor the patient's decision to terminate treatment converts the initial consent into a contract of adhesion from which the patient is permitted no escape even though new facts might be brought to his attention after his initial consent.

The primary duty of the physician should not be only to act in the best interests of the patient as defined by some school of practice, but rather to act in the best interests of the patient as the patient himself views those best interests. Self-determination, the basis of informed consent, implies that a competent patient must have the right to redefine his best interests for the duration of a medical procedure. Hence, the patient should be able to withdraw his consent at any time and discontinue the treatment. . . .

III. CLOSING COMPETENCY LOOPHOLES

Even in those jurisdictions which have eliminated the medical community standard as the test for adequacy of disclosure, physicians may still escape liability for failure to disclose material information. This is true for two reasons. First, the patient may be deemed incompetent, in which case information need be provided not to the patient but only to the family. Second, the physician might feel the patient would be "upset" by the information and therefore withhold the relevant facts on grounds of therapeutic privilege.

These grounds for failing to provide information may be abused, creating a loophole through which the implications of informed consent may be avoided. Because of his lack of expertise in comparison to the physician, the patient must rely heavily upon the doctor for information concerning the quality and nature of the treatment. It has been suggested that physicians in fact attempt to manipulate or enhance patient uncertainty in order to preserve power over the patient in the doctor-patient relationship. Such control over the patient, being contrary to interests in self-determination sought to be protected by informed consent, must be restrained. Consequently, the courts should be particularly alert to prevent manipulation of the patient. This concern may be expressed by the formulation of adequate legal safeguards to control determinations of competency and the use of therapeutic privilege.

Unfortunately, some courts tend to confuse competency to consent with competency to receive certain "upsetting" information. Further, even when the concepts are kept separate, adequate legal tests protective of patient interests have not been forthcoming. This Note will examine separately the two notions, and offer approaches designed to maintain and safeguard patient self-determination.

A. Competency to Consent

Courts generally except from the requirement of informed consent persons who are not competent. Information need not be tendered nor consent obtained from an incompetent patient, though an informed consent must be obtained from the patient's guardian. The definition of competency is critical. It must be formulated consistently with the objective of informed consent—to secure for the patient the right to forego treatment even if the medical profession or society would feel the reasons to be irrational. At the outset, it should be noted that competency may be defined in different ways for different purposes. Therefore, the discussion following will elaborate a concept of competency applicable specifically for informed consent to medical treatment.

Judicial opinions dealing with informed consent generally do not articulate tests for competency. Apparently courts are usually content to rely on physicians' unguided judgments as to what constitutes competency to consent. However, some courts have been successful in establishing a legal test for competency which both serves the interests of informed consent and avoids confusion with therapeutic privilege.

The Supreme Court of Washington set forth such a test of competency in *Grannum* v. *Berard*. Competency is presumed; to overcome this presumption, clear, cogent, and convincing evidence is necessary. The test of competency is the same as that used to determine the capacity of an individual to execute an agreement. Thus, the question is whether the person at the time of making the agreement possessed sufficient reason to understand the nature, terms, and effect of the agreement. This test focuses on the patient's capacity to comprehend his situation, risks, and alternatives. It does not import an examination of whether the patient's choice is rational or dispassionately conceived, but allows a patient to make decisions which may seem to others to be unreasonable.

B. Therapeutic Privilege: The Patient's Competency to Receive Certain Information

Many courts have permitted doctors to exercise a therapeutic privilege to withhold information which they believe might seriously upset or depress patients. Concealment is thus permitted even from an apparently competent patient. In *Nishi* v. *Hartwell,* a recent Hawaiian case, information was concealed from a competent patient on grounds of therapeutic privilege, and was also concealed from the patient's wife. The court held that no disclosure to the family was necessary, since the patient was competent, even when information was concealed from the patient to avoid "upsetting" him.

This decision fails to consider the interest of the patient and his family in receiving information so they might prepare for contingencies. Furthermore, it fails to provide protection against manipulating the consent of the patient by selective provision of information. Finally, although the Hawaii court avoided this analysis, the invocation of therapeutic privilege implies a judgment that the patient is incompetent to receive certain material information which might be distressing. It is contradictory at the same time to view him as competent to consent. Meaningful consent requires disclosure of material information. If a patient is not competent to receive all material information, then he is not competent to give a valid consent. In such a case consent should be sought from an informed family or guardian.

Canterbury v. *Spence* [8] recognized that the "physician's privilege to withhold information for therapeutic reasons must be carefully circumscribed . . . for otherwise it might devour the disclosure rule itself." [9] *Canterbury* unfortunately places only an outer limit on the privilege, but it does suggest that disclosure to a close relative is necessary if the privilege is exercised. The opinion represents a movement toward viewing invocation of therapeutic privilege as equivalent to an assertion that the patient is incompetent.

Doctors would be caught between Scylla and Charybdis if they were restricted in the use of therapeutic privilege but yet were held liable for making frightening disclosures to competent patients. Unfortunately there are indications in some jurisdictions that physicians will be held liable in damages for mental anguish caused by disclosures. Any tendency of the law in the direction of holding doctors liable for any honest disclosures must be closely scrutinized, for it may impede the flow of material information to the patient.

In place of permissive judicial approaches allowing therapeutic privilege and of intimations that physicians may be liable for frightening disclosures, the law should concentrate on developing a duty to inform patients carefully of material information, even if it is distressing. Requiring a tactful disclosure would provide the patient with the information necessary to make an informed decision while avoiding excessive discomfort in the patient. The interest in self-determination of a competent patient is not served by distorted information. Furthermore, there is evidence that patients desire a full disclosure, even of distressing information. Courts should permit only one exception to this rule of full tactful disclosure. A physician should exercise a therapeutic privilege to withhold information from a competent patient when the patient expressly waives his right to a disclosure. However, in order to avoid abuse, courts should insist that the waiver be express and unequivocal, and not a doctor's inference from subjective impressions of the competent patient's behavior.

C. Competency and the Dying Patient

It might be argued that a decision by a terminal patient to refuse treatment provides prima facie evidence of mental incompetency or is itself so irrational that it should be disregarded. However, given the patient's implicit choice between prolonged dying or more rapid death, a decision to die may be quite reasonable even if other individuals or groups in our society judge it unacceptable for themselves. If a terminal patient were to decide to die for what others would deem irrational reasons, the decision should still be honored; informed consent protects all decisions by competent patients, rational or irrational. This proposition was recognized in *In re Yetter,* a Pennsylvania lower court case which held a schizophrenic sufficiently competent to refuse life-saving surgery even though the patient's grounds for refusal were considered by some as irrational.

Some commentators have argued that terminal patients may be particularly vulnerable to the influence of family members, drugs, pain, or financial factors.[10] These contentions basically pose the problem of coercion of the terminal patient's decision. Coercion may take the form of subtle pressure from other individuals, unconscious motivations, or simple failures to comprehend information in the form in which it is conveyed. The concern is that coercion of the terminal patient's decision will increase the number and frequency of incorrect decisions by the patient—decisions which are irreversible[11]—imposing societal costs greater than the costs if the responsibility were placed on the individual's family, physicians and the state. If that were the case, it might be argued that the state should override the patient's expressed will. However, the state should avoid coercing an individual to protect him from coercion if some less drastic way of vindicating the state's interests is available. The state can structure its approach so that only patients who are relatively uncoerced may make the ultimate decision as to treatment, striving to assure that the patient makes the decision with genuine understanding of information material to the decision. Furthermore, even if the issue is a close one, interests in privacy argue that society opt for an approach encouraging self-determination; voluntary euthanasia is not espoused simply to alleviate pain, but rather to preserve to the terminal patient his last meaningful freedom, that of control over the time of his death. If the terminal patient is competent according to the *Grannum* test, then he has the same right to self-determination through informed consent as his brethren with more comforting prospects for longevity.

There is evidence that nondisclosure to dying patients is an accepted practice among doctors. Apparently, a strong feeling exists that a dying patient would be shocked, depressed, or otherwise adversely affected if he were acquainted with the facts, or that he usually knows he is dying anyway. On the other hand, from the patient's point of view, a majority of Americans want to be able to tell their doctor to let them die if they suffer from an incurable condition. Furthermore, dignity of the patient, informed consent, and the opportunity to arrange one's affairs dictate that the patient should be told of his condition.

By either ignoring the dying patient's wishes as irrational or failing to inform the patient of his condition in the first place, the issue of competency has often been used by the medical profession to make its own decisions as to what treatment to give terminal patients. Thus, courts should carefully consider the competency test. Therapeutic privilege should not expand into a presumption of incompetency, with the result of denying to the patient the right to render an informed consent or to make his own decision about euthanasia. . . .

CONCLUSION

The individual's right to self-determination over his own body is frequently asserted as the axiomatic foundation of informed consent. Recent informed-consent cases abolishing the medical community standard rule for disclosure have returned to a position of greater consistency with the *Schloendorff* axiom. It is fundamental to the doctrine that a right to consent presupposes a right to refuse. Hence, if courts take informed consent seriously, they must recognize the right of a competent terminal patient to forego treatment.

Countervailing concerns about the psychological impact of refusals of treatment upon society are not strong enough to overcome the law's commitment to decision making by the individual with respect to his own medical treatment. Society's interests in minimizing incorrect decisions may be met by proper tests for competency and by measures to assure sufficient comprehension of relevant material information. The outcome remains the same: recognition of the patient's right to refuse, whether the patient is terminal or not. Through application of developing tort doctrine, the courts alone might achieve this result. However, legislation which dispels the fear of possible criminal liability in cases of voluntary euthanasia is desirable.

Lawmakers should mitigate the uncertainties and generate adequate legal measures to permit a dignified death.

Notes

1. 186 Kan. 393, 350 P.2d 1093, *rehearing denied,* 187 Kan. 186, 354 P.2d 670 (1960).
2. *Ibid.* at 406–07, 350 P.2d at 1104.
3. 110 R.I. 606, 295 A.2d 676 (1972).
4. 8 Cal. 3d 229, 502 P.2d 1, 104 Cal. Rptr. 505 (1972).
5. *Ibid.* at 242, 502 P.2d at 9–10, 104 Cal. Rptr. at 513 (1972).
6. *Ibid.* at 245, 502 P.2d at 11, 104 Cal. Rptr. at 515 (1972).
7. E. Kübler-Ross, *On Death and Dying* (New York: The Macmillan Company, 1969), pp. 112–37.
8. 150 U.S. App. D.C., 263, 464 F.2d 772, *cert. denied,* 409 U.S. 1064 (1972).
9. *Ibid.* at 280, 464 F.2d at 789. This recognition is not surprising since claims of therapeutic privilege to conceal information achieve the same results as assertions of a community standard against disclosure.
10. *See, e.g.,* Kamisar, in the chapter on Euthanasia below in this text.
11. Kamisar argues that voluntary euthanasia should not be permitted because "the consequence of error is so irreparable." Kamisar's point is apparently that the patient may be nonterminal. That the refusal of treatment in a nonterminal situation may result in harm is, however, a part of the price the doctrine of informed consent must pay in order to assure self-determination. The way to reduce possible error is to maximize the supply of accurate information to the decisionmaker (here, the competent patient), not to deprive him of choice.

For Hegland, the individual's right to determine what shall be done with his own body and the sanctity of life come into direct conflict. He interprets the common law and the first amendment as *not* giving the individual the right to reject life-saving treatment in the emergency situation. His thesis is that the use of such treatment on the person of an objecting adult patient is proper. He argues that a valid public interest in the life of the individual exists, and he defends his views by reference to "analogous" areas such as euthanasia, poisonous snake rituals, and the prevention of suicide. Hegland argues that the individual does not have a legally enforceable right to choose death. Limitations of medical discretion are noted—especially in the case of the patient who has not sought aid, as compared to the one who has.

Kenney F. Hegland

UNAUTHORIZED RENDITION OF LIFESAVING MEDICAL TREATMENT *

Anglo-American law starts with the premise of thorough-going self-determination. It follows that each man is considered to be master of his own body, and he may, if he be of sound mind, expressly prohibit the performance of lifesaving surgery. . . .[1]

Do our humane laws make it the duty of a physician to leave the bedside of a dying man, because he demands it, and, if he remains and relieves him by physical touch, hold him guilty of assault? [2]

An adult hospital patient refuses to consent to lifesaving medical treatment, such as a blood transfusion: The individual's right to determine what shall be done with his own body and the sanctity of life come into direct conflict. Should a court order that the treatment be given, or should it respect the individual's commands and let him die? The few courts which have faced this problem are divided as to the proper course.

In September 1963 the mother of a seven-month-old baby entered the Georgetown College Hospital.[3] Massive internal bleeding, caused by a ruptured ulcer, necessitated an immediate transfusion. Due to religious conviction,[4] both the patient and her husband refused to authorize the transfusion. Hospital officials sought a court order authorizing the transfusion. After a district judge had refused the order, Circuit Judge Wright was contacted and after conferring with the patient, her husband, and attending physicians, signed an order authorizing the administration of "such transfusions as are in the opinion of the physicians in attendance necessary to save . . . [her] life."[5] Transfusions were given and the patient recovered.[6]

Application of the President of Georgetown College, Inc.[7] is one of several cases in which a court has authorized lifesaving treatment on the adult patient who has refused to consent.[8] The Illinois Supreme Court, however, has recently held that where the refusal of treatment was due to religious conviction, such action constituted an unconstitutional infringement of religious liberty.[9]

The thesis of this Comment is that the rendition of emergency lifesaving medical treatment on the person of the objecting adult patient is proper. It will be seen that neither the common law nor the "free exercise" clause of the First Amendment of the United States Constitution gives the individual a right to reject lifesaving treatment. The law's traditional view

* Copyright © 1965, California Law Review, Inc. Reprinted by permission of the publisher and Fred B. Rothman.

of the sanctity of human life and the importance of the individual's life to the welfare of society deny the individual a right to, in effect, consent to his own death. It will be shown that denial of the right to reject lifesaving treatment will not result in wholesale substitution of medical opinion for that of the individual. It will also be argued that a prior court order is not necessary in such a situation and the physician should be allowed to save the patient's life without one.

RIGHT TO REFUSE MEDICAL TREATMENT

In most circumstances the individual is afforded the right to reject medical treatment. Both the common law and the first amendment afford protection of the individual's right to determine what shall be done with his own body. However, an examination of these two sources of protection indicates that they do not give the individual the right to reject lifesaving treatment in the emergency situation.

Common-Law Protection: Unauthorized Medical Treatment as Battery

Common law recognizes the right to refuse medical treatment at least in the nonemergency situation. Tort liability is imposed on the physician who renders treatment without his patient's authorization,[10] or, having once obtained it, goes beyond it by rendering treatment different from,[11] or more extensive than, that authorized.[12] The plaintiff suing for an intentional, as opposed to a negligent, tort need only show that the treatment was given without authorization; he need not rely on the expert witnesses generally required in a malpractice action. Since the heart of the battery action is the absence of legal consent, it is no defense that the unauthorized treatment was given with a high degree of skill or that it actually benefitted the patient.

The common law does not, however, afford an absolute right to reject medical treatment, at least under certain circumstances. An exception to the requirement of prior consent is recognized in the emergency situation where the patient is in a condition, such as unconsciousness, which renders him incapable of either giving or withholding his consent.[13] The physician is then privileged to give the emergency aid. The privilege is supported on two grounds. First, it is assumed that the patient, if capable, would consent to the treatment, and hence its rendition does not conflict with his right to determine what shall be done with his own body. Second, although the particular patient might reject the treatment were he able to do so, the lives of other patients in like circumstances would be lost if the physician were held to act at his peril, i.e., if the physician were held liable for battery if it developed that the patient would have refused consent. Thus, without yet reaching the question of whether there is ever a right to reject lifesaving treatment, it appears proper in many emergencies to ignore the patient's refusal. Certainly the physician may ignore the refusal to consent of an insane or delirious patient.

Where the patient is neither insane nor delirious, it would be proper in many cases to render the treatment over the patient's commands when failure to do so would mean the patient's death. Assuming that the individual has, in effect, a right to choose death, the law should require a high degree of certainty that he really desires to exercise this prerogative before giving it operative significance. In many emergency situations, such certainty is not possible.

Assume that an individual's leg has been crushed in an automobile accident. Without immediate amputation he will die of blood poisoning. Stating that he would rather die than live with one leg, the patient refuses to consent. Just as it is assumed that an unconscious patient, if capable, would consent to emergency treatment, it seems justified to assume that this refusal of lifesaving aid is due to weakness, confusion, and pain rather than deliberation.

Such an assumption could, of course, be overcome if the refusal had been confirmed by a course of conduct antedating the emergency. For example, refusal by a Jehovah's Witness to consent to a blood transfusion is probably an expression of true preference. Yet, in a case like *Georgetown,* where the patient is suddenly seized by a condition requiring a transfusion, his refusal may be due to his physically weakened condition.[14] Even here there may be insufficient certainty to allow the patient to die.

In many cases involving the refusal of lifesaving aid, the physician should, therefore, be allowed to proceed, either by prior judicial order or by holding him privileged in a subsequent battery action, because of the inherent difficulties in distinguishing the rash refusal from that representing true choice. Whether the refusal was in fact rash should not be determinative, for to require the physician to act at his peril would tend to deter all action, thus costing the lives of those whose refusal was due to confusion and weakened physical conditions.

This rationale, however, cannot be applied where it is clear that the patient's true desire is to refuse consent. For example, physicians inform a pregnant woman that blood transfusions will be necessary to save her life after the delivery of her child. While in perfect health, before any loss of blood, she refuses to consent. Here the issue is clearly raised: Does the individual have a legally protected right to reject lifesaving treatment? The few cases which have faced the issue in the battery context have given no clear answer. Does the Constitution afford such a right?

Constitutional Protection: Freedom of Religion

If the refusal of required treatment is due to religious belief, to ignore it might violate the free exercise of religion clause of the First Amendment to the United States Constitution. Yet reliance on the First Amendment raises rather than answers the question because that amendment has not been held to give absolute freedom to religious practice.

In the early case of *Reynolds* v. *United States*,[15] the private secretary of Brigham Young appealed his conviction for bigamy, arguing that the statute was unconstitutional as applied to him because his religion required its violation. The United States Supreme Court, affirming, held that whereas freedom of conscience was absolute, the right to free exercise of religion could not justify acts against the public well-being.

In the cases since *Reynolds,* the question has been whether a religious practice is sufficiently detrimental to the public good to justify its curtailment: Courts have held that the practice must present an immediate threat to a valid public interest. Whether a religiously motivated refusal of lifesaving medical treatment is constitutionally protected turns on whether there is a valid public interest in the individual's life. In many analagous areas of the law, courts have recognized this interest.

PUBLIC INTEREST IN THE LIFE OF THE INDIVIDUAL

Refusal of lifesaving treatment does not constitute an immediate and direct threat to the well-being of others; however, several areas of the law recognize the propriety of curtailing activities which do not directly endanger others. Certain activities, because they adversely affect the participants and thus indirectly affect the welfare of society, have fallen under legal proscription. Polygamy, for example, does not present an immediate and direct threat to the welfare of other individuals, but this practice may be made criminal even for those whose religion dictates it. It is likewise arguable that much of modern narcotics legislation is designed primarily to protect users. The use of narcotics presents primarily an indirect threat to society by harming the individual user.

Similarly, this Comment argues that refusal of lifesaving treatment constitutes an activity which should be curtailed despite the fact that it does not endanger others. Such a refusal is tantamount to consenting to death. In the analogous areas of euthanasia, the "snake cases" and suicide, the law has uniformly denied operative significance to the individual's consent to his own death and consequently it should be expected that the same result will follow in the case of the refusal of lifesaving treatment.

Euthanasia

It is no defense to homicide prosecution that the decedent desired to die. In effect, the individual cannot consent to his own death at the hands of a second party. The primary concern of the law in condemning "mercy killing" is apparently not with the difficult proof problems in the prosecution of homicide that the defense of consent would generate; hence, the case of taking life cannot be distinguished from that of saving it by un-authorized treatment. First, there is society's interest in the life of the individual. If this is the reason why the individual has no right to consent to his own death in the euthanasia situation, then he would have no right to prohibit lifesaving medical treatment. Second, there is the fear that any exception to the sanctity of life cannot but cheapen it. The same fear would lead to hesitation before condemning any act which saves life, *e.g.,* the rendition of lifesaving aid. If the individual has the right to command his own death, the form of the command should not be determinative: that is, whether it commands another individual to do something, as in the case of euthanasia, or whether it commands him not to do something, as in the case of the refusal of required medical treatment.

Poisonous Snake Rituals

The "snake cases"[16] provide additional precedent for the proposition that the state may act to prevent the individual from consenting to his own death. A small religious sect, known as the Holiness Church, believes that the true test of faith is the handling of poisonous snakes: the true believer will not be harmed. Several state legislatures made this practice criminal. Several state courts, upholding the constitutionality of the statutes, iterated the traditional language about the safety of onlookers, but a close reading of the cases indicates that the concern was with the individuals who handled the snakes.[17]

It is difficult to find a meaningful distinction between an individual who handles a poisonous snake and one who refuses required medical treatment. A distinction between misfeasance and nonfeasance is nonsense; each individual is making basically the same decision. Walking into a burning house is tantamount to refusing to walk out. In terms of the danger to others presented by the two acts, there is little distinction. The ceremonies of the Holiness Church create a slight public danger in that the poisonous snake might escape. If minor considerations are determinative, then it could be argued that the hospital patient, in refusing lifesaving treatment, creates a danger to others by bringing otherwise unneeded physicians to his bedside and by generally interrupting the smooth operation of the hospital.

A stronger argument for curtailing religious practice can be made in the case of the hospital patient than in the case of the snake handler. First, the extent of social harm presented by the practice is greater because death from the refusal of lifesaving treatment is as certain as medical knowledge can be, whereas death from the handling of snakes is a mere possibility. Second, the extent that religious practice must be curtailed is less in the case of the hospital patient. Handling snakes is essential to the ritual of the Holiness Church; the proscription of a given form of medical treatment is generally just one of many proscriptions found in religious doctrines. In addition, while the members of the Holiness Church are forever barred from practicing the dictates of their religion, the members of a sect which prohibits a given form of treatment are free to follow their religious dictates in all but the most limited of situations: the life-and-death situation. As to the manner of curtailment, criminal sanctions are imposed on the individual who handles snakes due to his religion, while in the case of the individual who refuses a form of medical treatment due to his religion, no such sanctions are imposed. When a patient refuses lifesaving treatment, the propriety of his decision is not at issue: The only question is whether a physician's act in violation of that decision is proper.

Analogy to Prevention of Suicide

It is obviously proper for a physician to save his patient's life by unauthorized treatment if the physician in doing so is in the same position as the individual who has prevented a suicide. It is not a legal wrong to prevent suicide. To hold the physician liable and the rescuer from suicide privileged, a distinction must be found either in their respective actions or in the actions of the person saved.

There are two possible ways to distinguish the acts of the suicide from that of the patient who refuses lifesaving treatment: first, by the misfeasance-nonfeasance analysis, and second, in terms of the motivation of the person saved. Neither, however, appear to justify intervention in one case but not in the other.

The misfeasance-nonfeasance analysis would be misapplied in this context because the concern is not with whether the individual is "guilty" of his own death but rather with the preservation of his life. The misfeasance-nonfeasance analysis is employed to determine an individual's culpability in relation to a given result which society has condemned, and not to reassess the social disutility of that result. For example, a defendant drowns another by pushing him in a lake. He is guilty of homicide. A second defendant refuses to take affirmative action which would effectuate an easy rescue. He is guilty of nothing. In both cases, however, the man is dead, and the loss to society is equally great. Similarly, the result of the suicide's "misfeasance" and the patient's "nonfeasance" is the same.

The second ground for a possible distinction between the suicide and the hospital patient lies in their respective motivations. The suicide wishes to die, whereas the patient who declines treatment for religious reasons, wishes to live, but prefers death to a breach of religious commandment. The act of the patient does not "seem" like suicide. It may well be that society's condemnation of suicide is directed at the motivation behind the act and not at the act itself because, as one author explains:

> Suicide shows contempt for society. It is rude. . . . This most individualistic of all actions disturbs society profoundly. Seeing a man who

appears not to care for the things which it prizes, society is compelled to question all it has thought desirable. The things which make its own life worth living, the suicide boldly jettisons. Society is troubled, and its natural and nervous reaction is to condemn the suicide. Thus it bolsters up again its own values.[18]

This may be good psychology, but to use motivation as a basis of legal distinction in this context would be absurd. Take, for example, two hospital patients both in dire need of blood transfusions. One rejects them because of a desire to die, the other because of religious conviction. Should the law allow the patient wishing to live but preferring death to breach of religious faith, to die, while forcing the one wishing to die, to live? To ask the question is to answer it.

In *Reynolds* v. *United States*,[19] the Court stated in a dictum that it is within the power of government to prevent a religious suicide.[20] The dictum makes sense. If the nonreligious suicide may be prevented, so may the religious suicide. If judicial response were to vary in the two situations, it would be the sheerest of hypocrisies: Life may be saved, not because it is valuable, but rather because suicide is "rude."

Failure to find a meaningful distinction between the refusal of life-saving treatment and suicide, either in their respective motivations or in the misfeasance-nonfeasance analysis, leads to the conclusion that, based on the quality of their respective conduct, neither the patient nor the suicide can demand legal protection from lifesaving touching. Consequently, if the physician who renders unauthorized treatment is to be held liable while the individual who prevents suicide is held privileged, a distinction must be found in the respective acts of the rescuers. It may be that the latter would be held privileged because he was justified in assuming that the would-be suicide was acting rashly. However, it is apparent that not all suicide attempts are rash. If the rescuer knew that the would-be suicide was not acting rashly, would he commit a legal wrong if he prevented the suicide? If he would not be, then neither would the physician.

Is There a Right to Choose Death?

To hold that a court order which allows the physician to proceed with lifesaving treatment over the religious objections of the patient is an unconstitutional infringement of religious liberty, or to hold that the physician who has rendered the treatment is liable for battery, is to hold that the individual has a legally enforceable right to choose death. Because of society's interest in the life of the individual, because of the law's traditional view of the sanctity of human life, and because life can be saved without too great a curtailment of the religious liberty of those patients who refuse treatment on religious grounds, the law should not give its protection to the individual's decision to choose death.

Society has an interest in the life of the individual. In the *Georgetown* case, the patient was the mother of a seven-month-old child and it is apparent that others than herself would have suffered had she died.[21] Once it is admitted that there is sufficient interest in the life of a particular patient to deny him a legal right to refuse lifesaving treatment, then the decision must be the same for all patients. That is, the criterion of the "social worth" of the patient would lead the courts into insolvable problems. Any distinction based on "social worth" in this area is repugnant to the basic ideal of equality: If the mother of several children is to be saved, then so must the childless individual.

It would be out of line with the law's traditional affirmation of life were it to label the saving of life as either unconstitutional or as a civil wrong. To bring the issue into focus, take the case of a Buddhist monk's attempt to burn himself. Does the individual commit battery if he prevents the attempted suicide? Does a court unconstitutionally deny the free exercise of religion if it acts to prevent the suicide? There seems but one answer.

To deny the individual a legally enforceable right to reject lifesaving treatment for religious reasons does not greatly curtail his religious freedom, where objection to treatment is on this ground. First, no criminal sanctions are imposed on him. Second, he is allowed to practice the dictates of his religion in all but the most limited of circumstances: the life-and-death situation. Third, neither he nor his religion, at least in the case of the Jehovah's Witnesses, will deem him to have sinned. He did not voluntarily breach religious dictates. . . .

CONCLUSION

The *Georgetown* case, in ordering that lifesaving treatment may be given to the objecting adult patient, seems to be in accord with the traditional legal view of the sanctity of human life and the interest society has in the life of the individual. To hold otherwise is to hold that the individual has a legally enforceable right, in effect, to choose death, and that the saving of human life, under these circumstances, is a legal wrong.

As medical science becomes more sophisticated, one can expect more such cases to arise, and hence it is essential that the courts clarify the respective rights of the patient and his physician. Today, a life may depend on the individual judge's opinion as to the propriety of judicial intervention into this area.

Notes

1. *Natanson* v. *Kline,* 186 Kan. 393, 406–07, 350 P.2d 1093, 1104 (1960) (dictum), cited with approval in *Woods* v. *Brumlop,* 71 N.M. 221, 227, 377 P.2d 520, 524 (1962) (dictum).

2. *Meyer* v. *Knights of Pythias,* 178 N.Y. 63, 67, 70 N.E. 111, 112 (1904) (dictum).

3. *Application of President of Georgetown College, Inc.,* 331 F.2d 1000 (D.C. Cir.), *cert. denied,* 377 U.S. 978 (1964).

4. Mrs. Jones and her husband are members of the religious sect known as Jehovah's Witnesses. Objection to blood transfusions, which are equated with the drinking of blood, is based on the Biblical text. See Acts 15:28–29.

5. 331 F.2d at 1002 n.4.

6. Her petition for rehearing en banc was denied (apparently on the grounds of mootness). 331 F.2d at 1010.

7. 331 F.2d 1000 (D.C. Cir.), *cert. denied,* 377 U.S. 978 (1964).

8. These cases are not reported. See Watchtower Bible and Tract Soc'y of New York, Inc., "Do Hospital Patients Have Rights?" *Awake!* Sept. 8, 1964, p. 21.

9. *In re* Estate of Brooks, 32 Ill. 2d 361, 205 N.E.2d 435 (1965); *accord, Erickson* v. *Dilgard,* 44 Misc. 2d 27, 252 N.Y.S.2d 705 (Sup. Ct. 1962).

10. *Gill* v. *Selling,* 125 Ore. 587, 267 Pac. 812 (1928) (operation on wrong patient).

11. *Mohr* v. *Williams,* 95 Minn. 261, 104 N.W. 12 (1905) (operation on left ear instead of right as agreed to by the patient).

12. *Tabor* v. *Scobee,* 254 S.W.2d 474 (Ky. 1952) (during operation for appendicitis, diseased fallopian tubes removed).

13. The classic case is *Jackovach* v. *Yocum,* 212 Iowa 914, 237 N.W. 444 (1931), where a boy of seventeen jumped from a freight train, sustaining severe head and arm injuries. Attending physicians, while the boy was anesthetized, amputated the arm due to their fear of gangrene. The efforts to reach the boy's parents had failed. The court held the physicians were privileged because of the emergency situation.

14. In the *Georgetown* case, Judge Wright found the patient *in extremis* and "hardly compos mentis" when he arrived at the hospital, 331 F.2d at 1008.

15. 98 U.S. 145 (1878).

16. *Hill* v. *State,* 38 Ala. App. 623, 88 So. 2d 880 (Ct. App. 1956), *cert. denied,* 38 Ala. 697, 88 So. 2d 887 (1956); *Lawson* v. *Commonwealth,* 291 Ky. 473, 164 S.W.2d 972 (Ct. App. 1942); *State* v. *Massey,* 229 N.C. 734, 51 S.E.2d 179 (1949), *appeal dismissed sub nom. Dunn* v. *North Carolina,* 336 U.S. 942 (1949); *Harden* v. *State,* 188 Tenn. 17, 216 S.W.2d 708 (1948).

17. For example, in one case the court stated that the legislative purpose in outlawing such activities was to protect people "participating in or attending religious services," and later, after finding that the precautions taken to protect the audience were inadequate, stated that "of course, such precautions do not at all protect those who are actually handling these poisonous snakes." *Harden* v. *State,* 188 Tenn. 17, 24, 216 S.W.2d 708, 710 (1948).

18. Feeden, *Suicide* (1938), 42, as quoted in Williams, *The Sanctity of Life and the Criminal Law* (1957), 267.

19. 98 U.S. 145 (1878).

20. *Ibid.* at 166.

21. Judge Wright argued that the "state, as *parens patriae,* will not allow a parent to abandon a child, and so it should not allow this most ultimate of voluntary

abandonments. The patient had a responsibility to the community to care for her infant. Thus the people had an interest in preserving the life of this mother." 331 F.2d at 1008.

In the next selection Norman L. Cantor analyzes a variety of public and private interests at stake in a patient's decision to decline lifesaving medical treatment. Public interests include preservation of society, sanctity of life, upholding of public morals, protection of the individual against himself, and protection of third parties. Unlike Hegland, Cantor concludes that an independent adult's decision must be recognized on the basis of constitutional rights of personal privacy. According to Cantor, deference to the patient's refusal of treatment "reflects sensitivity towards personal interests in bodily integrity and self-determination, not callousness towards life."

Norman L. Cantor

A PATIENT'S DECISION TO DECLINE LIFE-SAVING MEDICAL TREATMENT: BODILY INTEGRITY VERSUS THE PRESERVATION OF LIFE *

The scene is a local community hospital. The patient is a 25-year-old man or woman suffering from a perforated ulcer, potentially fatal but curable by a simple operation. The patient is unmarried, childless, and fully coherent. With the threat of death looming, physicians request that the patient consent to surgery and an accompanying blood transfusion. The patient refuses because: (a) religious convictions forbid either the surgery or the blood transfusion; (b) the patient wants to die because of shame and anxiety over recent financial or romantic setbacks; (c) the patient wants to die because he or she is also the victim of a terminal illness which will inevitably entail considerable pain and gradual bodily degeneration; or (d) the patient is refusing treatment as a symbolic protest against a governmental policy, such as Viet Nam, and will only submit to surgery when that policy is officially changed. The hospital administrator, acting on the principle that a hospital's paramount mission is to preserve life, seeks a judicial order appointing himself temporary guardian for purposes of consenting to the necessary life-saving medical treatment.

Can or should a judge grant the relief requested? Does refusal to

* From *Rutgers Law Review*, 26, no. 2 (Winter 1973), 228–64. Reprinted by permission.

intervene entail acceptance of a "right to die" in the context of suicide and euthanasia? Does it matter whether the patient is motivated by reasons of conscience or simply by the will to die? Does it matter that the patient has dependents who will be disadvantaged by his or her death? The strong temptation is to respond positively to the opportunity to preserve life. Judges have been anguished by the knowledge that failure to order treatment would likely mean the patient's death, particularly where the patient did not really wish to die but was only following religious dictates. Religious freedom, bodily integrity, or individual self-determination appear as evanescent or ephemeral principles in the face of an immediate threat to life. Yet both religious freedom and control of one's body are cherished values in our society and both are of constitutional dimension when threatened by governmental invasion. . . .

ANALYSIS OF INTERESTS

A variety of public interests have been arrayed both by courts and commentators in support of judicial intervention to order life-saving medical treatment for a reluctant patient. These interests run the gamut from a noble reference to the sanctity of life to a banal concern for the economic burden left by a patient who dies after refusing treatment. Most of these interests have been described briefly in the prior discussion of case law on point. A few have not. All deserve careful scrutiny.

Preservation of Society

One writer has argued that the "importance of the individual's life to the welfare of society" precludes allowing a patient to spurn life-saving treatment.[1] This is an appealing notion, but it cannot withstand critical examination. Certainly, a society and its duly constituted institutions have a strong and legitimate interest in their own preservation. Any significant diminution in population might be a matter of real concern, but no one has ever suggested that the volume of persons declining medical treatment constitutes a threat to the maintenance of population levels. Nor is the refusal of treatment an act likely to be widely imitated or duplicated if openly allowed; it is unlike narcotics addiction in that respect. In short, society's existence is by no means threatened by patients' refusals of treatment.

The state also has a legitimate interest in promoting a thriving and productive population. Compulsory education laws are one manifestation of such an interest, yielding both economic and political benefits to society as a whole. In this context, the state might assert an interest in the productivity of an individual—talents, skills, taxpaying potential, military service potential—justifying compelled treatment to keep the individual alive. It is submitted, however, that this concern with productivity cannot override the competing interests in bodily integrity or religious liberty. In the first place, the marginal social utility involved is generally outweighed by the direct and immediate invasion of the patient's personal privacy, both because of the small numbers involved and the attenuated impact on the economy. Secondly, in each instance of refusal, the societal interest would vary according to the individual patient's attributes. In terms of productivity, for example, an industrialist or nuclear physicist has more "social worth" than a vagrant. The problem here is obvious. It is both unseemly and unrealistic to measure the social worth of each patient who declines medical treatment. One solution would be to assume the high value of every patient. But this approach exalts the interest of government, the state, or society over individual self-determination. It is also a fictive approach, since in reality the vast majority of us do not contribute so much to the social fabric as to enable the state to claim a paramount interest in our preservation.

Sanctity of Life

The state has an indisputable interest in the preservation of life. The criminal law and police power are focused on the protection of public safety. But this use of governmental authority is grounded on the assumption that citizens invariably want to enjoy bodily safety and uninterrupted life. Where a competent individual choses to decline life-saving treatment, the normal congruity of interest between individual welfare and state protection against death is disrupted. Entirely new interests, self-determination and privacy from state intrusions, are asserted. The assumption that the citizen demands self-preservation can no longer be operative.

Some writers have nonetheless argued that preservation of a resisting patient's life is relevant to the lives and safety of the general public. The theory is that by denying the patient an opportunity to choose death, a court promotes general respect for life. If a court acquiesced in a patient's rejection of treatment and consequent death, the value of life would be degraded since "any exception to the sanctity of life cannot but cheapen it."[2]

This argument cannot be taken lightly. Sanctity of life is not just a vague theological precept. It is the foundation of a free society. Indeed, libertarians recently campaigned against capital punishment on a similar theory that destruction of life (even the life of a convicted malefactor) degrades the value of life and undermines a society's regard for its sanctity. The countervailing consideration, of course, is the dignity tied up with bodily control and self-determination.

> Control by men over their circumstances of action is, along with knowledge of their circumstances, an indispensable part of their personal integrity. Knowledge and control are what make the difference between puppets and people.[3]

It is true that noninterference in an individual's decision to refuse treatment may mean that the patient dies for a reason which may appear silly or inconsequential to most observers. But the rejection of life-saving medical treatment normally represents a principled invocation of personal or religious convictions, not a deprecation of life. Restraint by courts would be impelled by profound respect for the individual's bodily integrity and religious freedom, not by disregard or disdain for the sanctity of life. Human dignity is enhanced by permitting the individual to determine for himself what beliefs are worth dying for. Through the ages, a multitude of noble causes, religious and secular, have been regarded as worthy of self-sacrifice. Certainly, most governments and societies, our own included, do not consider the sanctity of life to be the supreme value. Nations still insist on the prerogative to engage in mass killing for furtherance of the "national interest," "wars of liberation," or the "defense of democracy." Bodily control, self-determination, and religious freedom are beneficial both to the individual and to the society whose atmosphere and tone are determined by the human values which it respects.

Public Morals

As the debate over so-called victimless crimes illustrates, the use of law to reinforce a dominant morality without tangible benefit to public health, safety, and welfare is fraught with difficulties. This is particularly true where the moral underpinnings of laws no longer enjoy a wide community consensus. Many laws aimed primarily at morality nonetheless have been enacted, and we must acknowledge that all law is infused with some moral view.

These factors are relevant here because the rejection of life-saving treatment is a form of suicide—in that it is a voluntary act undertaken with knowledge that death will likely result. Suicide, in turn, has traditionally been anathema in a Judaeo-Christian culture. In the religious sphere, the revulsion toward suicide is grounded primarily on the sixth commandment and the belief that only a divinity can control the withdrawal of life. Antipathy toward suicide, however, extends well beyond the theological realm, and public attitudes have sometimes mirrored religious ones. The English common law attached both criminal and civil penalties to suicide or attempted suicide. Suicide was viewed as an offense against nature, violating instincts of self-preservation, as well as an offense against God, the society, and the king. The common revulsion of western culture toward self-imposed death has, then, an ethical or moral base as well as a religious one. Self-destruction is considered to be contrary to man's natural inclinations, a deprivation of a person's productive capacity, an evil example to others, and even a rude expression of contempt for society. "Public morals," specifically the "immorality" of self-destruction, cannot provide a legitimate basis for intervention in the patient's decision, however. Contemporary condemnation of suicide as "immoral" is largely clerical in nature, and public attitudes toward suicide have markedly changed. While embarrassment about the subject persists, the individual is no longer generally regarded as a sinner or crazed demon. Changes in law have accompanied changes in public opinion. In the vast majority of states, attempted suicide is no longer covered by the criminal law. To the extent that anti-suicide laws remain on the books, they are directed toward authorizing officials to take temporary custody of the individual to prevent the immediate infliction of harm and to render psychological assistance. Suicide is no longer considered, either legally or popularly, as inherently immoral. A morality grounded on an individual's service to the state would be threatened by a patient's conduct in refusing treatment. However, that moral scheme is not widely accepted within a democratic society which stresses maximum individual liberty compatible with the comfort and welfare of others.

Protection of the Individual against Himself

Normally, the state's police power is exercised for the general public's health, safety, or welfare. This is so even in the case of certain ostensibly individual invasions, such as compulsory immunizations or blood tests. There are a few areas of law, however, where the state apparently undertakes to protect the individual against his own imprudence.

The "snake cases," involving statutory prohibition of the public handling of snakes, provide one commonly cited example of government paternalism. A number of courts have sustained the validity of such statutes against claims by fundamentalist religious sects that the prohibitions interfere with their expression of religious faith. These cases do not, however, stand for the proposition that government can readily interfere with an individual's course of conduct in order to prevent the individual from harming himself. For these statutes undoubtedly protect observers and peripheral participants, as well as the snake handlers themselves. No court has addressed the issue of whether a legislature could protect the handler alone.

The motorcycle helmet cases are more apposite. Scores of state cases have considered challenges to statutes requiring motorcyclists to wear protective helmets. Motorcyclists claim that their individual liberty and privacy are infringed without a corresponding protection of legitimate public interests. The majority of courts have avoided the basic issue of whether state concern for the welfare of the cyclist can justify such requirements; they have made strained findings that all highway travelers are protected because cyclists struck by stones or limbs might lose control of their vehicles and injure others. Thus, the public health, safety, and welfare is being promoted. A number of courts have proceeded beyond this fictive argument to address whether the state may protect an individual from himself. The results are inconclusive. Several cases have urged that the police power encompasses authority to protect individuals despite their reluctance to be safeguarded. A few cases have ruled that the helmet statutes constitute unconstitutional infringement of liberty, since they have only a tenuous relation to public safety or welfare. It is submitted that without a clearer judicial consensus, and without Supreme Court guidance, the motorcycle helmet cases provide no resolution of whether the state can generally protect individuals against themselves. Certainly, they do not determine the outcome where a patient resists compelled treatment and invokes religious freedom or a right to bodily integrity as his protection. Indeed, constitutional standards may differ where liberty (substantive due process) is invoked as opposed to religious freedom or bodily privacy.

There is, however, an area of paternalistic state conduct which has universally been upheld despite its ostensible interference with individual freedom of choice. A plethora of pure food and drug laws, licensure schemes, and regulations controlling noxious substances exist which incidentally prevent consumers from injuring themselves. Even where the restrictions apply to sellers or distributors, the objective is to prevent the buyer from subjecting himself to risks which the government deems unadvisable. Some observers have articulated concern about the legal implications of this interference with individual self-determination, but these protective health measures nonetheless proliferate. They are generally salutary and are seldom challenged. Yet they may occasionally prevent consumer access to an enjoyable food (for example, swordfish, cyclamate-containing beverages) or to an experimental drug which might be highly beneficial. The individual is effectively precluded from selecting his own risks. Because such protective laws remain judicially inviolate, the question arises whether they provide an effective precedent for governmental prevention of individual risk taking which might be extended to the life-saving medical treatment problem.

Most protective legislation is clearly warranted because it guards against abuses which individual consumers are generally helpless to detect or control. For example, most consumers cannot determine the minimum competency of a physician, the iodine content of a food, or the spoilage of meat without regulatory controls. Furthermore consumers alone may be impotent to eliminate the dangerous products of an entire industry (for example, flammable fabrics or unsafe cars). The regulated items also have such wide potential distribution that the public safety and welfare is actually promoted by the protective legislation. These observations about regulatory schemes, however, in no way apply to refusal of medical treatment, since judicial intervention to compel treatment is a very different matter than common regulatory controls. Although both forms of governmental action interfere with individual choice, the regulatory schemes are generally impelled by conditions which preclude real individual choice. The elimination of dangerous products also constitutes, in most instances, a lesser deprivation than interference with religious liberty or bodily integrity. Thus, while precedents may be cited for governmental efforts to preclude individual risk taking, none sanctions judicial intervention to protect a patient against his own decision to decline treatment. Clearly, there are limitations on attempts to guarantee the individual's safety, for otherwise an individual's personal habits, including eating and sleeping, would be potentially subject to governmental dictates. The rights to freedom of religion and personal privacy circumscribe paternalistic impulses in the context of compelled medical treatment.

Protection of Third Parties

The patient's important interests in religious freedom or bodily integrity could be overridden if refusal of medical treatment were shown to inflict legally cognizable harm on persons other than the patient. Various third-party injuries have been suggested by courts and commentators discussing compelled treatment. They all warrant consideration.

1. *Surviving Adults.* The death of a relative or close friend may provoke grief, despair, or other emotional harm in the surviving person. This phenomenon will undoubtedly be present in cases of compelled treatment, and may be urged as a ground for judicial intervention. It is submitted, however, that this factor cannot justify a court in overriding a patient's determination. A variety of conduct by an individual may inflict emotional harm upon his loved ones. The dissolution of a marriage by separation or divorce, or simply abusive conduct toward loved ones, can cause emotional wounds, yet no court would contemplate a judicial order to force an adult to be considerate or kind to adult relatives. A similar independence of conduct must be accorded to the patient who may be asserting religious or personal principles in his refusal of treatment. The emotional consequences to survivors will likely be temporary, should be tempered by respect for the patient's principled decision, and, in any event, do not outweigh the patient's interests at stake.

2. *Fellow Patients.* One source has argued that a patient's rejection of live-saving treatment will distract physicians, provoke turmoil in the hospital staff, and generally disrupt hospital procedure to the detriment of other patients. This argument is speculative and seems rather farfetched. If the patient's choice is honored, precisely the converse of the predicted result should follow. That is, by declining treatment, medical care may well be reduced to the administration of analgesics, freeing staff to attend to other functions. Once a policy of judicial nonintervention is established and publicized, the hospital staff will not expend futile effort in seeking court

orders. Although there may be occasions when the rejection of therapy engenders medical complications which necessitate diverting hospital staff to the patient, this situation is more likely to be the exception than the rule and cannot operate as a general justification for judicial interference with patients' decisions.

3. *Physicians.*   Several courts have noted the interests of physicians in compelling life-saving treatment. One concern is that the physician, if required to respect the patient's choice to decline treatment, must act against his best professional judgment. It is difficult for a physician, trained and dedicated to preservation of life, to allow a salvageable patient to die. In addition, by withholding therapy, the physician may theoretically risk subsequent civil or criminal liability, particularly if the physician were found to have honored an incompetent patient's choice.

While a physician's interest in proper practice of medicine is both valid and legally cognizable, the above concerns do not justify judicial intervention to compel life-saving treatment. Unfettered exercise of medical judgment has never been a sacrosanct value. The doctrine of informed consent is grounded on the premise that a physician's judgment is subservient to the patient's right to self-determination. Further, other situations exist where a physician's professional judgment is legally restricted or precluded. Laws governing contraception, narcotics, experimental drugs, and compulsory reporting demonstrate that professional judgment is not always a paramount consideration. The assertion of constitutional interests in bodily integrity and free exercise of religion in the context of refusal of care deserve no less deference, even in derogation of a physician's best judgment. While it may be harrowing for a physician to determine whether a patient is voluntarily and competently declining life-saving treatment, difficult medical decisions must inevitably be made. This is so, for example, whenever a patient is certified as mentally ill for purposes of civil commitment or when a patient ostensibly consents to medical operations which entail substantial risks.

4. *Surviving Minors.*   As previously noted, both courts and commentators have supported judicial intervention to compel medical treatment where the patient is the parent of a minor child, based on an extension of the parens patriae doctrine. Since the state can generally act to safeguard a child's welfare, it can act to prevent "ultimate abandonment" of a child by the parent's self-destruction. By keeping the parent alive, the child presumably benefits emotionally, by continued love and reassurance from the parent, and economically, by continued financial support.

The argument that a court should act to preserve the emotional well-being of children is an appealing one. The legitimacy of the state's interest can be sustained on either of two grounds: there may be altruistic concern with providing each child with a healthful environment, or, development of stable children may be viewed as promoting the political and social well-being of the country. Of course, the loss of a parent will not always produce emotional harm in a child. Not all parents are loving and supportive of their children. It is conceivable that in some instances the surviving child would benefit emotionally from a court's acquiescence in the parent's decision to decline life-saving treatment. But judicial inquiry, on a case-by-case basis, into the complex emotional relationships among parents and children might well be too time-consuming and unpleasant to be undertaken. Assuming that the death of a parent will likely provoke some emotional harm to a surviving child, the question becomes whether that harm justifies exercise of the state's parens patriae authority to compel a patient to undergo unwanted treatment.

There are numerous situations where a child may be left alone by a parent with consequent emotional upheaval in the child. Death of a parent from natural causes, service in the armed forces, divorce, or even extended travel might cause some emotional wounds. Yet these unintended inflictions of emotional harm are never the source of state intervention; to suggest such intervention would undoubtedly provoke indignant cries of interference with personal liberty. Indeed, an infinite variety of parental conduct could be regulated if prevention of the infliction of emotional harm upon children were accepted as an unlimited basis for interference with parental conduct not intended to harm the child. The state could, under such a theory, compel medical checkups or dictate diets in order to preserve the health of parents.

Some interference with parental conduct is not only justified, but necessary, as the existence of "neglect" statutes demonstrates. Nevertheless, the loss of one of two parents because of the parent's adherence to religious or personal convictions in declining treatment is, arguably, too remote from the state's interest in a child's emotional well-being to support judicial intervention. Perhaps a legislature could make a contrary judgment and dictate intervention, but a court operating without such authorization must hesitate to intervene on the basis of protecting children's psychic well-being.

A second, less speculative basis exists for judicial intervention to preserve parents' lives—the economic interest of the state in avoiding the burden of supporting surviving children. In many contexts, protection of the public fisc has served as a justification for state conduct or regulations which otherwise would be considered to infringe upon fundamental personal rights. This has been the case with compulsory sterilization laws, motorcycle helmet laws, and certain welfare regulations having an indirect impact on parents' behavior. In *Wisconsin* v. *Yoder*,[4] the Supreme Court treated avoidance of "public wards" as a legitimate state interest to be balanced against competing individual rights. It must be conceded, then, that some judicial concern with the financial plight of a patient's survivors is both understandable and proper.

The economic issue is placed in even sharper perspective if the refusal of medical treatment threatens permanent disability but not death; for example, where rejection of a blood transfusion results in insufficient oxygen to the brain and consequent neurological damage. The ensuing permanent disability could result in the patient, as well as the surviving family, becoming public economic burdens. In such an instance, the economic impact would be direct and probably substantial. Judicial intervention to avoid that impact would likely be sustained even in the face of constitutional challenges bottomed on privacy and religious freedom. Similar considerations would probably support judicial intervention where the patient by declining treatment would die and leave an impecunious family to be sustained by the public.

Despite this concession, an important caveat should be considered before a court intervenes to compel treatment on an "avoidance of public wards" theory. The economic factors justifying intervention are not present in every case of a parent's refusal of treatment. The surviving spouse, accumulated savings, or other sources may be available to avoid penury even if the patient dies. Thus, the problem would have to be approached on a case-by-case basis and the economic circumstances sifted in each instance. This type of judicial inquiry is neither difficult nor unseemly; courts commonly examine financial status with regard to support payments, bankruptcy, and enforcement of judgments, to cite a few examples. However, tying the question of judicial intervention to financial circumstances of the patient may prove distasteful to the judiciary. The effect is to tell the patient that his convictions will not be respected because he does not have enough money. It is at least arguable that this de facto wealth discrimination would violate the equal-protection clause. In any event, it appears rather mercenary to hinge exercise of rights of privacy and free exercise upon wealth. Perhaps the public should be expected to absorb the economic burden when the refusal of medical treatment leaves indigent survivors. Courts might well take this approach. In light of the relatively small number of people who can be expected to spurn medical treatment when they know their family will be left impecunious, the overall economic burden shifted to the public can be expected to be slight. Judges who rely on the public ward theory to compel life-saving medical treatment will likely be impelled not by real concern for the public coffers, but by their personal distaste for the patient's decision. . . .

CONCLUSION

As to an independent adult who genuinely objects to treatment, the patient's decision to refuse life-saving treatment must be respected by the judiciary no matter what the reason for refusal. Respect for bodily integrity, as dictated by constitutional rights of personal privacy, mandates this result in light of the inadequacy or inapplicability of asserted governmental interests in compelling treatment. Even where familial circumstances would constitutionally permit judicial intervention, a judge should normally respect the patient's decision. Intervention to protect survivors' emotional or economic interests, with concomitant government avoidance of fiscal burdens, would too often reflect judicial distaste for a decision to accept death rather than recognition of compelling state interests sufficient to override a patient's decision.

Acceptance of a patient's right to decline life-saving treatment will mean emotional strain for both physicians and judges. On occasion, it will even be difficult to determine whether the patient's decision is the product of a sound mind. Yet deference to the patient's refusal of treatment reflects sensitivity toward personal interests in bodily integrity and self-determination, not callousness toward life.

Notes

1. "Unauthorized Rendition of Lifesaving Medical Treatment," *California Law Review*, 53 (August 1965), p. 862.
2. "Unauthorized Rendition," *supra*, p. 867.
3. Fletcher, *Morals and Medicine* (1954), p. 66.
4. 406 U.S. 205 (1972).

SUGGESTED READINGS FOR CHAPTER 3

Books and Articles

ANNAS, GEORGE J., *The Rights of Hospital Patients: The Basic ACLU Guide to a Hospital Patient's Rights.* An American Civil Liberties Union Handbook. New York: Avon Books, 1975.

ALFIDI, R. J. "Informed Consent: A Study of Patient Reaction." *Journal of the American Medical Association,* 216 (1971), 1325–29.

BRANSON, ROY, "Is Acceptance a Denial of Death? Another Look at Kübler-Ross." *Christian Century,* May 7, 1975, 464–68.

BRIM, ORVILLE G., JR., FREEMAN, HOWARD E., LEVINE, SOL, and SCOTCH, NORMAN A., eds., *The Dying Patient.* New York: Russell Sage Foundation, 1970.

CASSELL, ERIC J. *The Healer's Art: A New Approach to the Doctor–Patient Relationship.* Philadelphia: J. B. Lippincott Company, 1976.

ETZIONY, M. B., comp. *The Physician's Creed: An Anthology of Medical Prayers, Oaths, and Codes of Ethics Written and Recited by Medical Practitioners through the Ages.* Springfield, Ill.: Charles C Thomas, 1973.

GOROVITZ, SAMUEL, ET AL. "Moral Problems in the Physician-Patient Relationship." *Moral Problems in Medicine.* Englewood Cliffs, N.J.: Prentice-Hall, 1976. Chap. 2, pp. 54–241.

GROUP FOR THE ADVANCEMENT OF PSYCHIATRY. *The Right to Die: Decision and Decision Makers.* Proceedings of a Symposium, vol. VIII, symposium no. 12, November 1973. New York, 1973.

KASS, LEON R. "Death as an Event: A Commentary on Robert Morison." *Science,* 173 (1971), 698–702.

KASTENBAUM, ROBERT, and AISENBERG, RUTH. *A Psychology of Death.* New York: Springer-Verlag, 1972.

KÜBLER-ROSS, ELISABETH. *On Death and Dying.* New York: The Macmillan Company, 1969.

MASSACHUSETTS GENERAL HOSPITAL, CLINICAL CARE COMMITTEE. "Optimum Care for Hopelessly Ill Patients." *New England Journal of Medicine,* 295 (1976), 362–64.

MORISON, ROBERT S. "Death: Process or Event?" *Science,* 173 (1971), 694–98.

PARIS, JOHN J. "Compulsory Medical Treatment and Religious Freedom: Whose Law Shall Prevail?" *University of San Francisco Law Review,* 10 (1975), 1–35.

POTTER, RALPH B., JR. "The Paradoxical Preservation of a Principle." *Villanova Law Review,* 13 (1968), 784–92.

SHNEIDMAN, EDWIN S., ed. *Death: Current Perspectives.* Palo Alto, Calif.: Mayfield Publishing Co., 1976.

"Standards for Cardiopulmonary Resuscitation (CPR) and Emergency Cardiac Care (ECC)." *Journal of the American Medical Association,* 227

(1974), 831–70. Issued as no. 7, supplement, February 18, 1974. National Conference Steering Committee: American Heart Association, Committee on Cardiopulmonary Resuscitation and Emergency Cardiac Care, and National Academy of Sciences—National Research Council, Division of Medical Sciences, Committee on Emergency Medical Services. Reprints available from American Heart Association.

VEATCH, ROBERT M. *Death, Dying, and the Biological Revolution.* New Haven: Yale University Press, 1976.

VERNICK, JOHN, and KARON, MYRON. "Who's Afraid of Death on a Leukemia Ward?" *American Journal of Diseases of Children,* 109 (1965), 393–97.

WEISMAN, AVERY D. *On Dying and Denying: A Psychiatric Study of Terminality.* Foreword by Herman Feifel. New York: Behavioral Publications, Inc., 1972.

WILLIAMS, ROBERT H., ed. *To Live and to Die: When, Why, and How.* New York: Springer-Verlag, 1973.

Bibliographies

SOLLITTO, SHARMON, and VEATCH, ROBERT M., comps. *Bibliography of Society, Ethics, and the Life Sciences.* Hastings-on-Hudson, N.Y.: Institute of Society, Ethics, and the Life Sciences. Issued annually, since 1973. See "Death and Dying: II. Care of the Dying Patient" and other entries under "Death and Dying."

VERNICK, JOEL J. *Selected Bibliography on Death and Dying.* Washington, D.C.: National Institutes of Health; U.S. Government Printing Office. n.d.

WALTERS, LEROY, ed. *Bibliography of Bioethics.* Detroit: Gale Research Co. Issued annually since 1975. See "Patients' Rights," "Treatment Refusal," "Prolongation of Life," "Terminal Care."

Encyclopedia of Bioethics Articles

DEATH AND DYING: ETHICS: Systematic Perspective—SISSELA BOK

DEATH AND DYING: ETHICS: Right to Refuse Treatment—ALEXANDER M. CAPRON

DEATH AND DYING: ETHICS: Rights of the Terminally Ill—GEORGE J. ANNAS

HEALTH CARE: Humanization and Dehumanization of Health Care—JAN HOWARD

INFORMED CONSENT: Consent in the Therapeutic Relationship: Clinical Aspects—ERIC CASSELL

INFORMED CONSENT: Consent in the Therapeutic Relationship: Ethical and Legal Aspects—JAY KATZ

PATERNALISM—TOM L. BEAUCHAMP

PATIENTS' RIGHTS MOVEMENT—GEORGE J. ANNAS

TRUTH-TELLING: Attitudes of Patients and Health-Care Professionals—ROBERT M. VEATCH

TRUTH-TELLING: Ethical Aspects—SISSELA BOK

4

EUTHANASIA AND NATURAL DEATH

INTRODUCTION

We saw in Chapter 3 that the scope of patients' rights to refuse treatment has recently been extended in many legal jurisdictions. (In 1976 a "Natural Death Act," included in the present chapter, was passed into law in California. It grants patients the right to refuse certain forms of life-saving therapies, where death is virtually certain to result. This bill and the repeal of suicide laws in the past two decades—as discussed in Chapter 2—have been greeted enthusiastically by some and disparaged by others because they seem to manifest a new social attitude toward the intentional taking of life, and even new attitudes toward allowing to die.) (To proponents of such bills this attitude favors human dignity and individual freedom over the coercive strictures of law.) To its antagonists the new attitude represents an increasing moral permissiveness and an indifference toward human death—an attitude so serious that it threatens our belief in the sanctity of life. Controversy emerged once again in the seventies over proposed *euthanasia* legislation (as well as over some controversial practices commonly used by some doctors to end life).

Euthanasia, insofar as it is voluntarily consented to, is construed by many as a form of suicide (specifically as "assisted suicide"). Yet, for reasons to be mentioned, euthanasia has not met with the same legislative success as suicide. Recent advances in biomedicine, however, have introduced an array of methods for the prolongation of life that make the issue of euthanasia an even more pressing one, and numerous so-called "death with dignity" bills are now being considered by state legislatures.

Arguments for and against Euthanasia

The literature on euthanasia reveals three pervasive arguments for euthanasia and four against. These arguments attempt to resolve two fundamental questions: (1) Under what conditions, if any, is euthanasia morally justified? (2) Should euthanasia be legalized, so that there is a right to "die with dignity"? Arguments favoring its moral legitimacy (and/or legalization) include the following:

1. *An Argument from Individual Liberty.*   Many people argue that a primary moral principle, which ought to be incorporated into law wherever possible, is the right of free choice. They argue that state coercion is never permissible unless an individual's actions produce harm to others. Since the sufferer's choice to accelerate death does not harm others, it is a permissible exercise of individual liberty and ought not to be subject to the compulsion of law. (This right of free choice seems to be what is often meant by the phrase "the *right* to die.")

2. *An Argument from Loss of Human Dignity.*   As we have seen, medical technology has increased, and will continue to increase, our capacity to prolong lives. Sometimes dying persons see themselves gradually stripped of their former character and of all the activities they formerly enjoyed. Such patients are not only subjected to intense and abiding pain, they are often aware of their own deterioration, as well as of the burden they have become to others. To some it seems uncivilized and incompassionate, under these conditions, not to allow them to choose their own death.

3. *An Argument from the Reduction of Suffering.*   Some kinds of suffering are so intense and others so protracted as to be unendurable. This suffering can be borne by patient and family alike. As in argument 2 it seems to some immoral under such circumstances not to allow a patient (and in some cases his family) to elect his own death. Euthanasia is here said to be justified on grounds of prevention of cruelty.

Arguments against the moral legitimacy (and/or the legalization) of euthanasia include the following:

1. *An Argument from the Sanctity of Human Life.*   Anti-euthanasiasts often appeal to the principle that human life is inviolable, and for this reason ought not to be taken under any circumstances. The reasons for this appeal to the sacredness of human life vary. Some are religiously based; others are rooted in the conviction that the sanctity of life principle is the pillar of social order. And still others spring from reflection on various ancient and modern periods in human history when human lives were disposed of at the whim of the state or family.

2. *The Wedge Argument.*   Some appeal to the danger of deteriorating standards. If we once permit the taking of human life by consent of

patients as a permissible practice, this will erode other strictures against the taking of life. Such euthanasia proposals are said to be the "thin end of a wedge" leading to euthanasia without consent, infanticide, and so on. Euthanasia proposals must be resisted in the beginning, it is argued, or we will ultimately be unable to draw the line ending practices that take human life; for it is not so distant a move from the incurably ill to the socially deviant.

3. *Arguments from Probable Abuse.*   This argument appeals to the likelihood of abuse by doctors, members of the family, and other interested parties. The claim is that provision of wide discretion to medical practitioners concerning the methods of terminating life introduces a risk of abuse so serious that it outweighs any possible benefits of euthanasia. There are serious problems concerning whether the conditions under which a patient gives his consent are appropriate, especially when one considers possible family and financial pressures.

4. *Arguments from Wrong Diagnoses and New Treatments.*   Another argument is encapsulated in the saying, "Where there's life there's hope." It is well known that doctors often misdiagnose maladies. This is not so serious when the diagnoses are correctable, but in cases of euthanasia if the information given is wrong, or if a new treatment appears shortly after death, the case is not correctable. And there are many cases on record of "hopelessly incurable" patients who recovered.

These seven arguments appear in various forms in several of the articles in this chapter. They are not the only arguments for and against euthanasia, but they do seem to be the most popular ones.

The Nature and Types of Euthanasia

Many moral and legal differences in arguments concerning euthanasia may be the result of different conceptions or definitions of euthanasia. Certainly it is an elusive and difficult concept, marked by a number of changes of meaning in recent history. In its original meaning the term "euthanasia" derived from the Greek for "good death," a notion so broad as to be almost useless. Until rather recently the term basically was used for the act of painlessly and mercifully putting to death incurably ill persons. But with recent advances in biomedical equipment, which make it possible to sustain life much beyond what formerly was the natural point of death, the meaning has shifted for most users of the term. It now refers not only to the active and intentional putting to death of the incurably ill, but has spread also to the withdrawing or withholding of artificial means used merely to prolong life (some also appeal to "extraordinary" means). Accordingly, "euthanasia" is now generally understood as the action of bringing about a seriously suffering person's death by at least one other person, where the motive for ending the life is merciful and the means chosen is as painless as possible.[1]

Perhaps because of the recently extended scope of the concept of euthanasia, a distinction is commonly drawn between *active* and *passive* euthanasia. Active or positive euthanasia results when death is directly and intentionally caused by another person (as, for example, when a lethal injection of a drug is administered), while passive or negative euthanasia occurs when death results because others refrain from actions that might prolong life (usually though not necessarily by withholding or withdrawing artificial supports). Often in literature on euthanasia this distinction is intentionally associated with the distinction between killing and letting die. Another widely used distinction is that between *voluntary* and *involuntary* euthanasia. "Voluntary" here refers to choice by the patient, and hence the distinction is that between euthanasia with patient consent and euthanasia without patient consent (e.g., where someone is in a comatose and vegetative condition). These two distinctions, if accepted, generate four different types of euthanasia, which may be diagrammed as follows:

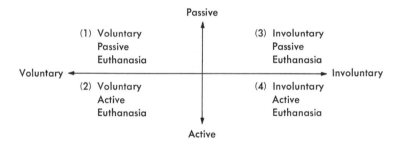

Active or positive euthanasia is illegal in all states in the United States, but physicians may lawfully remove life-prolonging therapy in a variety of cases. The American Medical Association generally supports this position, as do many religious bodies. However, it is a debated question whether cessation of therapy under such conditions is or is not truly a form of euthanasia, and also whether its being *passive* provides grounds to morally *justify* one's failure to act. Similarly there is much debate concerning what does and what does not constitute an active causing of death (e.g., whether the actual shutting down of a respirator is active). Also debated is the issue of which means entail merely "letting die." For example, would hastening "natural death" by removing a respirator or ceasing dialysis treatment be *merely* passive withdrawal? The situation seems as controversy-ridden in current legal thinking as in current ethical theory. This chapter is largely a reflection of the unsettled state of the debate over euthanasia.

Note

1. This definition is not intended to state necessary and sufficient conditions of the term. Such a formulation would be much more detailed.

Initiating a debate with Glanville Williams, Yale Kamisar argues against laws that would permit voluntary euthanasia. He concedes that voluntary euthanasia may sometimes be acceptable on ethical grounds but finds other reasons against legalization. He advances three important arguments, all of which are based on euthanasia's giving rise to undesirable consequences: (1) it is difficult to determine whether consent is voluntary, and for this reason there exists a danger that euthanasia laws might be exploited; (2) the medical decision that a person is incurably or irreversibly ill could be mistaken, either because the doctor's diagnosis may be in error or because it is wrongly believed that no therapy or cure will be available within the patient's life expectancy; (3) the wedge argument can be formulated to show that there is danger of the legalization of *involuntary* euthanasia.

Yale Kamisar

EUTHANASIA LEGISLATION:
SOME NONRELIGIOUS OBJECTIONS *

A book by Glanville Williams, *The Sanctity of Life and the Criminal Law,*[1] once again brought to the fore the controversial topic of euthanasia, more popularly known as "mercy-killing." In keeping with the trend of the euthanasia movement over the past generation, Williams concentrates his efforts for reform on the *voluntary* type of euthanasia, for example the cancer victim begging for death, as opposed to the *involuntary* variety— that is, the case of the congenital idiot, the permanently insane or the senile. . . .

The existing law on euthanasia is hardly perfect. But if it is not too good, neither, as I have suggested, is it much worse than the rest of the criminal law. At any rate, the imperfections of existing law are not cured by Williams's proposal. Indeed, I believe adoption of his views would add more difficulties than it would remove.

Williams strongly suggests that "euthanasia can be condemned only according to a religious opinion."[2] He tends to view the opposing camps as Roman Catholics versus Liberals. Although this has a certain initial

* From Minnesota Law Review, 42, no. 6 (May 1958). Reprinted by permission of Minnesota Law Review Foundation.

appeal to me, a non-Catholic and self-styled liberal, I deny that this is the only way the battle lines can, or should, be drawn. I leave the religious arguments to the theologians. I share the view that "those who hold the faith may follow its precepts without requiring those who do not hold it to act as if they did."[3] But I do find substantial utilitarian obstacles on the high road to euthanasia. I am not enamoured of the *status quo* on mercy-killing. But while I am not prepared to defend it against all comers, I am prepared to defend it against the proposals for change which have come forth to date.

As an ultimate philosophical proposition, the case for voluntary euthanasia is strong. Whatever may be said for and against suicide generally, the appeal of death is immeasurably greater when it is sought not for a poor reason or just any reason, but for "good cause," so to speak; when it is invoked not on behalf of a "socially useful" person, but on behalf of, for example, the pain-racked "hopelessly incurable" cancer victim. If a person is *in fact* (1) presently incurable, (2) beyond the aid of any respite which may come along in his life expectancy, suffering (3) intolerable and (4) unmitigable pain and of a (5) fixed and (6) rational desire to die, I would hate to have to argue that the hand of death should be stayed. But abstract propositions and carefully formed hypotheticals are one thing; specific proposals designed to cover everyday situations are something else again.

In essence, Williams's specific proposal is that death be authorized for a person in the above situation "by giving the medical practitioner a wide discretion and trusting to his good sense."[4] This, I submit, raises too great a risk of abuse and mistake to warrant a change in the existing law. That a proposal entails risk of mistake is hardly a conclusive reason against it. But neither is it irrelevant. Under any euthanasia programme the consequences of mistake, of course, are always fatal. As I shall endeavour to show, the incidence of mistake of one kind or another is likely to be quite appreciable. If this indeed be the case, unless the need for the authorized conduct is compelling enough to override it, I take it the risk of mistake *is* a conclusive reason against such authorization. I submit, too, that the possible radiations from the proposed legislation—for example, involuntary euthanasia of idiots and imbeciles (the typical "mercy-killings" reported by the press)—and the emergence of the legal precedent that there are lives not "worth living," give additional cause for reflection.

I see the issue, then, as the need for voluntary euthanasia versus (1) the incidence of mistake and abuse; and (2) the danger that legal machinery initially designed to kill those who are a nuisance to themselves may some day engulf those who are a nuisance to others. . . .

THE "CHOICE"

Under current proposals to establish legal machinery, elaborate or otherwise, for the administration of a quick and easy death, it is not enough that those authorized to pass on the question decide that the patient, in effect, is "better off dead." The patient must concur in this opinion. Much of the appeal in the current proposal lies in this so-called "voluntary" attribute.

But is the adult patient really in a position to concur? Is he truly able to make euthanasia a "voluntary" act? There is a good deal to be said, is there not, for Dr. Frohman's pithy comment that the "voluntary" plan is supposed to be carried out "only if the victim is both sane and crazed by pain."[5]

By hypothesis, voluntary euthanasia is not to be resorted to until narcotics have long since been administered and the patient has developed a tolerance to them. *When,* then, does the patient make the choice? While heavily drugged? Or is narcotic relief to be withdrawn for the time of decision? But if heavy dosage no longer deadens pain, indeed, no longer makes it bearable, how overwhelming is it when whatever relief narcotics offer is taken away too?

"Hypersensitivity to pain after analgesia has worn off is nearly always noted."[6] Moreover, "the mental side-effects of narcotics, unfortunately for anyone wishing to suspend them temporarily without unduly tormenting the patient, appear to outlast the analgesic effect" and "by many hours."[7] The situation is further complicated by the fact that "a person in terminal stages of cancer who had been given morphine steadily for a matter of weeks would certainly be dependent upon it physically and would probably be addicted to it and react with the addict's response."[8]

The narcotics problem aside, Dr. Benjamin Miller, who probably has personally experienced more pain than any other commentator on the euthanasia scene, observes:

> Anyone who has been severely ill knows how distorted his judgment became during the worst moments of the illness. Pain and the toxic effect of disease, or the violent reaction to certain surgical procedures may change our capacity for rational and courageous thought.[9]

Undoubtedly, some euthanasia candidates will have their lucid moments. How they are to be distinguished from fellow-sufferers who do not, or how these instances are to be distinguished from others when the patient is exercising an irrational judgment, is not an easy matter. Particularly is this so under Williams's proposal, where no specially qualified persons, psychiatrically trained or otherwise, are to assist in the process.

Assuming, for purposes of argument, that the occasion when a euthanasia candidate possesses a sufficiently clear mind can be ascertained and that a request for euthanasia is then made, there remain other problems. The mind of the pain-racked may occasionally be clear, but is it not also likely to be uncertain and variable? This point was pressed hard by the great physician, Lord Horder, in the House of Lords debates:

During the morning depression he [the patient] will be found to favour the application under this Bill, later in the day he will think quite differently, or will have forgotten all about it. The mental clarity with which noble Lords who present this Bill are able to think and to speak must not be thought to have any counterpart in the alternating moods and confused judgments of the sick man.[10]

The concept of "voluntary" in voluntary euthanasia would have a great deal more substance to it if, as is the case with voluntary admission statutes for the mentally ill, the patient retained the right to reverse the process within a specified number of days after he gives written notice of his desire to do so—but unfortunately this cannot be. The choice here, of course, is an irrevocable one.

The likelihood of confusion, distortion, or vacillation would appear to be serious drawbacks to any voluntary plan. Moreover, Williams's proposal is particularly vulnerable in this regard, since as he admits, by eliminating the fairly elaborate procedure of the American and British Societies' plans, he also eliminates a time period which would furnish substantial evidence of the patient's settled intention to avail himself of euthanasia.[11] But if Williams does not always choose to slug it out, he can box neatly and parry gingerly:

> [T]he problem can be exaggerated. Every law has to face difficulties in application, and these difficulties are not a conclusive argument against a law if it has a beneficial operation. The measure here proposed is designed to meet the situation where the patient's consent to euthanasia is clear and incontrovertible. The physician, conscious of the need to protect himself against malicious accusations, can devise his own safeguards appropriate to the circumstances; he would normally be well advised to get the patient's consent in writing, just as is now the practice before operations. Sometimes the patient's consent will be particularly clear because he will have expressed a desire for ultimate euthanasia while he is still clear-headed and before he comes to be racked by pain; if the expression of desire is never revoked, but rather is reaffirmed under the pain, there is the best possible proof of full consent. If, on the other hand, there is no such settled frame of mind, and if the physician chooses to administer euthanasia when the patient's mind is in a variable state, he will be walking in the margin of the law and may find himself unprotected.[12]

If consent is given at a time when the patient's condition has so degenerated that he has become a fit candidate for euthanasia, when, if ever, will it be "clear and incontrovertible"? Is the suggested alternative of consent in advance a satisfactory solution? Can such a consent be deemed an informed one? Is this much different from holding a man to a prior statement of intent that if such and such an employment opportunity would present itself he would accept it, or if such and such a young woman were to come along he would marry her? Need one marshal authority for the proposition that many an "iffy" inclination is disregarded when the actual facts are at hand?

Professor Williams states that where a pre-pain desire for "ultimate euthanasia" is "reaffirmed" under pain, "there is the best possible proof of full consent." Perhaps. But what if it is alternately renounced and reaffirmed under pain? What if it is neither affirmed nor renounced? What if it is only renounced? Will a physician be free to go ahead on the ground that the prior desire was "rational," but the present desire "irrational"? Under Williams's plan, will not the physician frequently "be walking in the margin of the law"—just as he is now? Do we really accomplish much more under this proposal than to put the euthanasia principle on the books?

Even if the patient's choice could be said to be "clear and incontrovertible," do not other difficulties remain? Is this the kind of choice, assuming that it can be made in a fixed and rational manner, that we want to offer a gravely ill person? Will we not sweep up, in the process, some who are not really tired of life, but think others are tired of them; some who do not really want to die, but who feel they should not live on, because to do so when there looms the legal alternative of euthanasia is to do a selfish or a cowardly act? Will not some feel an obligation to have themselves "eliminated" in order that funds allocated for their terminal care might be better used by their families or, financial worries aside, in order to relieve their families of the emotional strain involved?

It would not be surprising for the gravely ill person to seek to inquire of those close to him whether he should avail himself of the legal alternative of euthanasia. Certainly, he is likely to wonder about their attitude in the matter. It is quite possible, is it not, that he will not exactly be gratified by any inclination on their part—however noble their motives may be in fact—that he resort to the new procedure? At this stage, the patient-family relationship may well be a good deal less than it ought to be.

And what of the relatives? If their views will not always influence the patient, will they not at least influence the attending physician? Will a physician assume the risks to his reputation, if not his pocketbook, by administering the *coup de grâce* over the objection—however irrational— of a close relative. Do not the relatives, then, also have a "choice"? Is not the decision on their part to do nothing and say nothing *itself* a "choice"? In many families there will be some, will there not, who will consider a stand against euthanasia the only proof of love, devotion, and gratitude for past events? What of the stress and strife if close relatives differ over the desirability of euthanatizing the patient?

At such a time, members of the family are not likely to be in the best state of mind, either, to make this kind of decision. Financial stress and conscious or unconscious competition for the family's estate aside,

The chronic illness and persistent pain in terminal carcinoma may place strong and excessive stresses upon the family's emotional ties with the patient. The family members who have strong emotional attachment to start with are most likely to take the patient's fears, pains, and fate personally. Panic often strikes them. Whatever guilt feelings they may have toward the patient emerge to plague them.

If the patient is maintained at home, many frustrations and physical demands may be imposed on the family by the advanced illness. There may develop extreme weakness, incontinence, and bad odors. The pressure of caring for the individual under these circumstances is likely to arouse a resentment and, in turn, guilt feelings on the part of those who have to do the nursing.[13]

Nor should it be overlooked that while Professor Williams would remove the various procedural steps and personnel contemplated in the British and American Bills and bank his all on the "good sense" of the general practitioner, no man is immune to the fear, anxieties and frustrations engendered by the apparently helpless, hopeless patient. Not even the general practitioner. . . .

THE "HOPELESSLY INCURABLE" PATIENT AND THE FALLIBLE DOCTOR

Professor Williams notes as "standard argument" the plea that "no sufferer from an apparently fatal illness should be deprived of his life because there is always the possibility that the diagnosis is wrong, or else that some remarkable cure will be discovered in time."[14] . . .

Until the Euthanasia Societies of Great Britain and America had been organized and a party decision reached, shall we say, to advocate euthanasia only for incurables on their request, Dr. Abraham L. Wolbarst, one of the most ardent supporters of the movement, was less troubled about putting away "insane or defective people [who] have suffered mental incapacity and tortures of the mind for many years" than he was about the "incurables."[15] He recognized the "difficulty involved in the decision as to incurability" as one of the "doubtful aspects of euthanasia": "Doctors are only human beings, with few if any supermen among them. They make honest mistakes, like other men, because of the limitations of the human mind."[16]

He noted further that "it goes without saying that, in recently developed cases with a possibility of cure, euthanasia should not even be considered," that "the law might establish a limit of, say, ten years in which there is a chance of the patient's recovery."[17]

Dr. Benjamin Miller is another who is unlikely to harbour an ulterior theological motive. His interest is more personal. He himself was left to die the death of a "hopeless" tuberculosis victim, only to discover that he was suffering from a rare malady which affects the lungs in much the same manner but seldom kills. Five years and sixteen hospitalizations later, Dr. Miller dramatized his point by recalling the last diagnostic clinic of the brilliant Richard Cabot, on the occasion of his official retirement:

> He was given the case records [complete medical histories and results of careful examinations] of two patients and asked to diagnose their illnesses. . . . The patients had died and only the hospital pathologist knew the exact diagnosis beyond doubt, for he had seen the descriptions of the postmortem findings. Dr. Cabot, usually very accurate in his diagnosis, that day missed both.
>
> The chief pathologist who had selected the cases was a wise person. He had purposely chosen two of the most deceptive to remind the medical students and young physicians that even at the end of a long and rich experience one of the greatest diagnosticians of our time was still not infallible.[18]

Richard Cabot was the John W. Davis, the John Lord O'Brian, of his profession. When one reads the account of his last clinic, one cannot help but think of how fallible the *average* general practitioner must be, how fallible the *young doctor just starting practice* must be—and this, of course, is all that some small communities have in the way of medical care—how fallible the *worst* practitioner, young or old, must be. If the range of skill and judgment among licensed physicians approaches the wide gap between the very best and the very worst members of the bar—and I have no reason to think it does not—then the minimally competent physician is hardly the man to be given the responsibility for ending another's life. Yet, under Williams's proposal at least, the marginal physician, as well as his more distinguished brethren, would have legal authorization to make just such decisions. Under Williams's proposal, euthanatizing a patient or two would all be part of the routine day's work. . . .

Faulty diagnosis is only one ground for error. Even if the diagnosis is correct, a second ground for error lies in the possibility that some measure of relief, if not a full cure, may come to the fore within the life expectancy of the patient. Since Glanville Williams does not deign this objection to euthanasia worth more than a passing reference,[19] it is necessary to turn elsewhere to ascertain how it has been met. One answer is: "It must be little comfort to a man slowly coming apart from multiple sclerosis to think that fifteen years from now, death might not be his only hope."[20]

To state the problem this way is of course, to avoid it entirely. How do we know that fifteen *days* or fifteen *hours* from now, "death might not be [the incurable's] only hope"?

A second answer is: "[N]o cure for cancer which might be found 'tomorrow' would be of any value to a man or woman 'so far advanced in cancerous toxemia as to be an applicant for euthanasia.' "[21]

As I shall endeavour to show, this approach is a good deal easier to formulate than it is to apply. For one thing, it presumes that we know today *what* cures will be found tomorrow. For another, it overlooks that if such cases can be said to exist, the patient is likely to be *so far* advanced in cancerous toxemia as to be no longer capable of understanding the step he is taking and hence *beyond* the stage when euthanasia ought to be administered.

Thirty-six years ago, Dr. Haven Emerson, then President of the American Public Health Association, made the point that "no one can say today what will be incurable tomorrow. No one can predict what disease will be fatal or permanently incurable until medicine becomes stationary and sterile."[22] . . .

VOLUNTARY VERSUS INVOLUNTARY EUTHANASIA

Ever since the 1870s, when what was probably the first euthanasia debate of the modern era took place, most proponents of the movement—at least when they are pressed—have taken considerable pains to restrict the question to the plight of the unbearably suffering incurable who *voluntarily seeks* death, while most of their opponents have striven equally hard to frame the issue in terms which would encompass certain involuntary situations as well, e.g. the "congenital idiots," the "permanently insane," and the senile.

Glanville Williams reflects the outward mood of many euthanasiasts when he scores those who insist on considering the question from a broader angle:

> The [British Society's] bill [debated in the House of Lords in 1936 and 1950] excluded any question of compulsory euthanasia, even for hopelessly defective infants. Unfortunately, a legislative proposal is not assured of success merely because it is worded in a studiously moderate and restrictive form. The method of attack, by those who dislike the proposal, is to use the "thin end of the wedge" argument. . . . There is no proposal for reform on any topic, however conciliatory and moderate, that cannot be opposed by this dialectic.[23]

Why was the bill "worded in a studiously moderate and restrictive form"? If it were done as a matter of principle, if it were done in recognition of the ethico-moral-legal "wall of separation" which stands between voluntary and compulsory "mercy-killings," much can be said for the euthanasiasts' lament about the methods employed by the opposition. But if it were done as a matter of political expediency—with great hopes and expectations of pushing through a second and somewhat less restrictive bill as soon as the first one had sufficiently "educated" public opinion and next a third, still less restrictive bill—what standing do the euthanasiasts then have to attack the methods of the opposition? No cry of righteous indignation could ring more hollow, I would think, than the protest from those utilizing the "wedge" principle themselves that their opponents are making the wedge objection. . . .

The boldness and daring which characterize most of Glanville Williams's book dim perceptibly when he comes to involuntary euthanasia proposals. As to the senile, he states:

> At present the problem has certainly not reached the degree of seriousness that would warrant an effort being made to change traditional attitudes towards the sanctity of life of the aged. Only the grimmest necessity could bring about a change that, however cautious in its approach, would probably cause apprehension and deep distress to many people, and inflict a traumatic injury upon the accepted code of behaviour built up by two thousand years of the Christian religion. It may be, however, that as the problem becomes more acute it will itself cause a reversal of generally accepted values.[24]

To me, this passage is the most startling one in the book. On page 310 Williams invokes "traditional attitudes towards the sanctity of life" and "the accepted code of behaviour built up by two thousand years of the Christian religion" to check the extension of euthanasia to the senile, but for 309 pages he had been merrily rolling along debunking both. Substitute "cancer victim" for "the aged" and Williams's passage is essentially the argument of many of his *opponents* on the voluntary euthanasia question.

The unsupported comment that "the problem [of senility] has certainly not reached the degree of seriousness" to warrant euthanasia is also rather puzzling, particularly coming as it does after an observation by Williams on the immediately preceding page that "it is increasingly common for men and women to reach an age of 'second childishness and mere oblivion,' with a loss of almost all adult faculties except that of digestion."[25]

How "serious" does a problem have to be to warrant a change in these "traditional attitudes"? If, as the statement seems to indicate, "seriousness" of the problem is to be determined numerically, the problem of the cancer victim does not appear to be as substantial as the problem of the senile. For example, taking just the 95,837 first admissions to "public prolonged-care hospitals" for mental diseases in the United States in 1955, 23,561— or one-fourth—were cerebral arteriosclerosis or senile brain disease cases. I am not at all sure that there are twenty thousand cancer victims per year who die *unbearably painful* deaths. Even if there were, I cannot believe that among their ranks are some twenty thousand per year who, when still in a rational state, so long for a quick and easy death that they would avail themselves of legal machinery for euthanasia.

If the problem of the incurable cancer victim has reached "the degree of seriousness that would warrant an effort being made to change traditional attitudes towards the sanctity of life," as Williams obviously thinks it has, then so has the problem of senility. In any event, the senility problem will undoubtedly soon reach even Williams's requisite degree of seriousness:

> A decision concerning the senile may have to be taken within the next twenty years. The number of old people are increasing by leaps and bounds. Pneumonia, "the old man's friend," is now checked by antibiotics. The effects of hardship, exposure, starvation and accident are now minimized. Where is this leading us? . . . What of the drooling, helpless, disoriented old man or the doubly incontinent old woman lying log-like in bed? Is it here that the real need for euthanasia exists?[26]

If, as Williams indicates, "seriousness" of the problem is a major criterion for euthanatizing a category of unfortunates, the sum total of mentally deficient persons would appear to warrant high priority, indeed.

When Williams turns to the plight of the "hopelessly defective infants," his characteristic vim and vigour are, as in the senility discussion, conspicuously absent:

> While the Euthanasia Society of England has never advocated this, the Euthanasia Society of America did include it in its original programme. The proposal certainly escapes the chief objection to the similar proposal for senile dementia: it does not create a sense of insecurity in society, because infants cannot, like adults, feel anticipatory dread of being done to death if their condition should worsen. Moreover, the proposal receives some support on eugenic grounds, and more importantly on humanitarian grounds—both on account of the parents, to whom the child will be a burden all their lives, and on account of the handicapped child itself. (It is not, however, proposed that any child should be destroyed against the wishes of its parents.) Finally, the legalization of euthanasia for handicapped children would bring the law into closer relation to its practical administration, because juries do not regard parental mercy-killing as murder. For these various reasons the proposal to legalize humanitarian infanticide is put forward from time to time by individuals. They remain in a very small minority, and the proposal may at present be dismissed as politically insignificant.[27]

It is understandable for a reformer to limit his present proposals for change to those with a real prospect of success. But it is hardly reassuring for Williams to cite the fact that only "a very small minority" has urged euthanasia for "hopelessly defective infants" as the *only* reason for not pressing for such legislation now. If, as Williams sees it, the only advantage voluntary euthanasia has over the involuntary variety lies in the organized movements on its behalf, that advantage can readily be wiped out.

In any event, I do not think that such "a very small minority" has advocated "humanitarian infanticide." Until the organization of the British and American societies led to a concentration on the voluntary type, and until the by-products of the Nazi euthanasia programme somewhat embarrassed, if only temporarily, most proponents of involuntary euthanasia, about as many writers urged one type as another. Indeed, some euthanasiasts have taken considerable pains to demonstrate the superiority of defective infant euthanasia over incurably ill euthanasia.

As for dismissing euthanasia of defective infants as "politically insignificant," the only poll that I know of which measured the public response to both types of euthanasia revealed that *45 percent favoured euthanasia for defective infants under certain conditions while only 37.3 percent approved euthanasia for the incurably and painfully ill under any conditions.*[28] Furthermore, of those who favoured the mercy-killing cure for incurable adults, some 40 percent would require only family permission or medical board approval, but not the patient's permission.

Nor do I think it irrelevant that while public resistance caused Hitler to yield on the adult euthanasia front, the killing of malformed and idiot children continued unhindered to the end of the war, the definition of "children" expanding all the while. Is it the embarrassing experience of the Nazi euthanasia programme which has rendered destruction of defective infants presently "politically insignificant"? If so, is it any more of a jump from the incurably and painfully ill to the unorthodox political thinker than it is from the hopelessly defective infant to the same "unsavoury character"? Or is it not so much that the euthanasiasts are troubled by the Nazi experience as it is that they are troubled that the public is troubled by the Nazi experience?

I read Williams's comments on defective infants for the proposition that there are some very good reasons for euthanatizing defective infants, but the time is not yet ripe. When will it be? When will the proposal become politically significant? After a voluntary euthanasia law is on the books and public opinion is sufficiently "educated"?

Williams's reasons for not extending euthanasia—once we legalize it in the narrow "voluntary" area—to the senile and the defective are much less forceful and much less persuasive than his arguments for legalizing voluntary euthanasia in the first place. I regard this as another reason for not legalizing voluntary euthanasia in the first place.

Notes

1. First published in the United States in 1957, by arrangement with the Columbia Law School. Page references in the notes following relate to the British edition (Faber & Faber, 1958).
2. Williams, p. 278.
3. Wechsler and Michael, "A Rationale of the Law of Homicide," 37 *Columbia Law Review* (1937).
4. Williams, p. 302.

5. Frohman, "Vexing Problems in Forensic Medicine: A Physician's View," 31 *New York University Law Review* 1215, 1222 (1956).

6. Goodman and Gilman, *The Pharmacological Basis of Therapeutics,* 2d ed. (1955), p. 235.

7. Sharpe, "Medication as a Threat to Testamentary Capacity," 35 *North Carolina Law Review* 380, 392 (1975), and medical authorities cited therein.

8. Sharpe, *op. cit.,* 384.

9. "Why I Oppose Mercy Killings," *Woman's Home Companion* (June 1950), pp. 38, 103.

10. *House of Lords Debates,* 103, 5th series (1936), cols. 466, 492–93.

11. Williams, pp. 306–7.

12. *Ibid.,* p. 307.

13. Zarling, "Psychological Aspects of Pain in Terminal Malignancies," *Management of Pain in Cancer* (Schiffrin edition, 1956), pp. 211–12.

14. *Williams,* p. 283.

15. Wolbarst, "Legalize Euthanasia!," *The Forum* 94 (1935), 330, 332. But see Wolbarst, "The Doctor Looks at Euthanasia," *Medical Record,* 149 (1939), 354.

16. Wolbarst, "Legalize Euthanasia!," *loc. cit.*

17. *Ibid.,* 332.

18. *Op. cit.* (n. 9 above), p. 39.

19. See Williams, p. 283.

20. "Pro & Con: Shall We Legalize 'Mercy Killing'?," *Reader's Digest* (November 1938), pp. 94, 96.

21. James, "Euthanasia—Right or Wrong?" *Survey Graphic* (May 1948), pp. 241, 243; Wolbarst, "The Doctor Looks at Euthanasia," *Medical Record,* 149 (1939), 354, 355.

22. Emerson, "Who Is Incurable? A Query and a Reply," *New York Times* (October 22, 1933), sec. 8, p. 5, col. 1.

23. Williams, pp. 297–98.

24. Williams, p. 310.

25. *Ibid.*

26. Banks, "Euthanasia," *Bulletin of the New York Academy of Medicine,* 26 (1950), 297, 305.

27. Williams, pp. 311–12.

28. The Fortune Quarterly Survey: IX, *Fortune Magazine* (July 1937), pp. 96, 106.

Glanville Williams, in a direct reply to Kamisar, argues for the legalization of voluntary euthanasia. He argues both that it is *cruel* to refuse a suffering and incurably ill person's voluntary request for "merciful release" and that individual liberty is seriously and unwarrantably stifled by present anti-euthanasia laws. Williams does not in general deny that some of Kamisar's arguments have moral force, but he believes that the possible detrimental consequences of introducing pro-euthanasia legislation are insufficient to warrant continued legal prohibition of voluntary euthanasia. He finds the wedge argument seriously deficient and minimizes the potential dangers mentioned by Kamisar. Williams thus believes that there is a moral right to voluntary euthanasia and that there ought to be a legal right.

Glanville Williams

EUTHANASIA LEGISLATION: A REJOINDER TO THE NONRELIGIOUS OBJECTIONS *

I welcome Professor Kamisar's reply to my argument for voluntary euthanasia, because it is on the whole a careful, scholarly work, keeping to knowable facts and accepted human values. It is, therefore, the sort of reply that can be rationally considered and dealt with. In this short rejoinder I shall accept most of Professor Kamisar's valuable notes, and merely submit that they do not bear out his conclusion.

The argument in favour of voluntary euthanasia in the terminal stages of painful diseases is a quite simple one, and is an application of two values that are widely recognized. The first value is the prevention of cruelty. Much as men differ in their ethical assessments, all agree that cruelty is an evil—the only difference of opinion residing in what is meant by cruelty. Those who plead for the legalization of euthanasia think that it is cruel to allow a human being to linger for months in the last stages of agony, weakness and decay, and to refuse him his demand for merciful release. There is also a second cruelty involved—not perhaps quite so compelling, but still worth consideration: the agony of the relatives in seeing their loved one in his desperate plight. Opponents of euthanasia are apt to take a cynical view of the desires of relatives, and this may sometimes be justified. But it cannot be denied that a wife who has to nurse her husband through the last stages of some terrible disease may herself be so deeply affected by the experience that her health is ruined, either mentally or physically. Whether the situation can be eased for such a person by voluntary euthanasia I do not know; probably it depends very much upon the individuals concerned, which is as much as to say that no solution in terms of a general regulatory law can be satisfactory. The conclusion should be in favour of individual discretion.

The second value involved is that of liberty. The criminal law should not be invoked to repress conduct unless this is demonstrably necessary on

* From the *New England Journal of Medicine,* 292, no. 2 (January 1975), no. 1 (1958), 1–12 (slightly edited). By permission of Minnesota Law Review Foundation.

social grounds. What social interest is there in preventing the sufferer from choosing to accelerate his death by a few months? What positive value does his life still possess for society, that he is to be retained in it by the terrors of the criminal law?

And, of course, the liberty involved is that of the doctor as well as that of the patient. It is the doctor's responsibility to do all he can to prolong worth-while life, or, in the last resort, to ease his patient's passage. If the doctor honestly and sincerely believes that the best service he can perform for his suffering patient is to accede to his request for euthanasia, it is a grave thing that the law should forbid him to do so.

This is the short and simple case for voluntary euthanasia, and, as Kamisar admits, it cannot be attacked directly on utilitarian grounds. Such an attack can only be by finding possible evils of an indirect nature. These evils, in the view of Professor Kamisar, are (1) the difficulty of ascertaining consent, and arising out of that the danger of abuse; (2) the risk of an incorrect diagnosis; (3) the risk of administering euthanasia to a person who could later have been cured by developments in medical knowledge; (4) the "wedge" argument.

Before considering these matters, one preliminary comment may be made. In some parts of his essay Kamisar hints at recognition of the fact that a practice of mercy-killing exists among the most reputable of medical practitioners. Some of the evidence for this will be found in my book.[1] In the first debate in the House of Lords, Lord Dawson admitted the fact, and claimed that it did away with the need for legislation. In other words, the attitude of conservatives is this: let medical men do mercy-killing, but let it continue to be called murder, and be treated as such if the legal machinery is by some unlucky mischance made to work; let us, in other words, take no steps to translate the new morality into the concepts of the law. I find this attitude equally incomprehensible in a doctor, as Lord Dawson was, and in a lawyer, as Professor Kamisar is. Still more baffling does it become when Professor Kamisar seems to claim as a virtue of the system that the jury can give a merciful acquittal in breach of their oaths. The result is that the law frightens some doctors from interposing, while not frightening others—although subjecting the braver group to the risk of prosecution and possible loss of liberty and livelihood. Apparently, in Kamisar's view, it is a good thing if the law is broken in a proper case, because that relieves suffering, but also a good thing that the law is there as a threat in order to prevent too much mercy being administered; thus, whichever result the law has, is perfectly right and proper. It is hard to understand on what moral principle this type of ethical ambivalence is to be maintained. If Kamisar does approve of doctors administering euthanasia in some clear cases, and of juries acquitting them if they are prosecuted for murder, how does he maintain that it is an insuperable objection to euthanasia that diagnosis may be wrong and medical knowledge subsequently extended?

However, the references to merciful acquittals disappear after the early part of the essay, and thenceforward the argument develops as a straight attack on euthanasia. So although at the beginning Kamisar says that he would hate to have to argue against mercy-killing in a clear case, in fact he does proceed to argue against it with some zest. . . .

Kamisar's first objection, under the heading "The Choice," is that there can be no such thing as truly voluntary euthanasia in painful and killing diseases. He seeks to impale the advocates of euthanasia on an old dilemma. Either the victim is not yet suffering pain, in which case his consent is merely an uninformed and anticipatory one—and he cannot bind himself by contract to be killed in the future—or he is crazed by pain and stupefied by drugs, in which case he is not of sound mind. I have dealt with this problem in my book; Kamisar has quoted generously from it, and I leave the reader to decide. As I understand Kamisar's position, he does not really persist in the objection. With the laconic "perhaps," he seems to grant me, though unwillingly, that there are cases where one can be sure of the patient's consent. But having thus abandned his own point, he then goes off to a different horror, that the patient may give his consent only in order to relieve his relatives of the trouble of looking after him.

On this new issue, I will return Kamisar the compliment and say: "Perhaps." We are certainly in an area where no solution is going to make things quite easy and happy for everybody, and all sorts of embarrassments may be conjectured. But these embarrassments are not avoided by keeping to the present law: we suffer from them already. If a patient, suffering pain in a terminal illness, wishes for euthanasia partly because of his pain and partly because he sees his beloved ones breaking under the strain of caring for him, I do not see how this decision on his part, agonizing though it may be, is necessarily a matter of discredit either to the patient himself or to his relatives. The fact is that, whether we are considering the patient or his relatives, there are limits to human endurance.

Kamisar's next objection rests on the possibility of mistaken diagnosis. . . . I agree with him that, before deciding on euthanasia in any particular case, the risk of mistaken diagnosis would have to be considered. Everything that is said in the essay would, therefore, be most relevant when the two doctors whom I propose in my suggested measure come to consult on the question of euthanasia; and the possibility of mistake might most forcefully be brought before the patient himself. But have these medical questions any true relevance to the legal discussion?

Kamisar, I take it, notwithstanding his wide reading in medical literature, is by training a lawyer. He has consulted much medical opinion in order to find arguments against changing the law. I ought not to object to this, since I have consulted the same opinion for the opposite purpose. But what we may well ask ourselves is this: is it not a trifle bizarre that we should be doing so at all? Our profession is the law, not medicine. How does it come about that lawyers have to examine medical literature to assess the advantages and disadvantages of a medical practice?

If the import of this question is not immediately clear, let me return to my imaginary State of Ruritania. Many years ago, in Ruritania as elsewhere, surgical operations were attended with great risk. Lister had not discovered antisepsis, and surgeons killed as often as they cured. In this state of things, the legislature of Ruritania passed a law declaring all surgical operations to be unlawful in principle, but providing that each specific type of operation might be legalized by a statute specially passed for the purpose. The result is that, in Ruritania, as expert medical opinion sees the possibility of some new medical advance, a pressure group has to be formed in order to obtain legislative approval for it. Since there is little public interest in these technical questions, and since, moreover, surgical operations are thought in general to be inimical to the established religion, the pressure group has to work for many years before it gets a hearing. When at last a proposal for legalization is seriously mooted, the lawyers and politicians get to work upon it, considering what possible dangers are inherent in the new operation. Lawyers and politicians are careful people, and they are perhaps more prone to see the dangers than the advantages in a new departure. Naturally they find allies among some of the more timid or traditional or less knowledgeable members of the medical profession, as well as among the priesthood and the faithful. Thus it is small wonder that whereas appendicectomy has been practised in civilized countries since the beginning of the present century, a proposal to legalize it has still not passed the legislative assembly of Ruritania.

It must be confessed that on this particular matter the legal prohibition has not been an unmixed evil for the Ruritanians. During the great popularity of the appendix operation in much of the civilized world during the 'twenties and 'thirties of this century, large numbers of these organs were removed without adequate cause, and the citizens of Ruritania have been spared this inconvenience. On the other hand, many citizens of that country have died of appendicitis, who would have been saved if they had lived elsewhere. And whereas in other countries the medical profession has now learned enough to be able to perform this operation with wisdom and restraint, in Ruritania it is still not being performed at all. Moreover, the law has destroyed scientific inventiveness in that country in the forbidden fields.

Now, in the United States and England we have no such absurd general law on the subject of surgical operations as they have in Ruritania. In principle, medical men are left free to exercise their best judgment, and the result has been a brilliant advance in knowledge and technique. But there are just two—or possibly three—"operations" which are subject to the Ruritanian principle. These are abortion, euthanasia, and possibly sterilization of convenience. In these fields we, too, must have pressure groups, with lawyers and politicians warning us of the possibility of inexpert practitioners and mistaken diagnosis, and canvassing medical opinion on the risk of an operation not yielding the expected results in terms of human happiness and the health of the body politic. In these fields we, too, are forbidden to experiment to see if the foretold dangers actually come to pass. Instead of that, we are required to make a social judgment on the probabilities of good and evil before the medical profession is allowed to start on its empirical tests.

This anomaly is perhaps more obvious with abortion than it is with euthanasia. Indeed, I am prepared for ridicule when I describe euthanasia as a medical operation. Regarded as surgery it is unique, since its object is not to save or prolong life but the reverse. But euthanasia has another object which it shares with many surgical operations—the saving of pain. And it is now widely recognized, as Lord Dawson said in the debate in the House of Lords, that the saving of pain is a legitimate aim of medical practice. The question whether euthanasia will effect a net saving of pain and distress is, perhaps, one that we can attempt to answer only by trying it. But it is obscurantist to forbid the experiment on the ground that until it is performed we cannot certainly know its results. Such an attitude, in any other field of medical endeavour, would have inhibited progress.

The argument based on mistaken diagnosis leads into the argument based on the possibility of dramatic medical discoveries. Of course, a new medical discovery which gives the opportunity of remission or cure will almost at once put an end to mercy-killings in the particular group of cases for which the discovery is made. On the other hand, the discovery cannot affect patients who have already died from their disease. The argument based on mistaken diagnosis is therefore concerned only with those patients who have been mercifully killed just before the discovery becomes available for use. The argument is that such persons may turn out to have been "mercy-killed" unnecessarily, because if the physician had waited a bit longer they would have been cured. Because of this risk for this tiny fraction of the total number of patients, patients who are dying in pain must be left to do so, year after year, against their entreaty to have it ended.

Just how real is the risk? When a new medical discovery is claimed, some time commonly elapses before it becomes tested sufficiently to justify large-scale production of the drug, or training in the techniques involved. This is a warning period when euthanasia in the particular class of case would probably be halted anyway. Thus it is quite probable that when the new discovery becomes available, the euthanasia process would not in fact show any mistakes in this regard.

Kamisar says that in my book I "did not deign this objection to euthanasia more than a passing reference." I still do not think it is worth any more than that.

He advances the familiar but hardly convincing arguments that the quantitative need for euthanasia is not large. As one reason for this argument, he suggests that not many patients would wish to benefit from euthanasia, even if it were allowed. I am not impressed by the argument. It may be true, but it is irrelevant. So long as there are *any* persons dying in weakness and grief who are refused their request for a speeding of their end, the argument for legalizing euthanasia remains. Next, he suggests that there is no great need for euthanasia because of the advances made with pain-killing drugs. . . . In my book, recognizing that medical science does manage to save many dying patients from the extreme of physical pain, I pointed out that it often fails to save them from an artificial, twilight existence, with nausea, giddiness, and extreme restlessness, as well as the long hours of consciousness of a hopeless condition. A dear friend of mine, who died of cancer of the bowel, spent his last months in just this state, under the influence of morphine, which deadened pain, but vomiting incessantly, day in and day out. The question that we have to face is whether the unintelligent brutality of such an existence is to be imposed on one who wishes to end it. . . .

The last part of the essay is devoted to the ancient "wedge" argument which I have already examined in my book. It is the trump card of the traditionalist, because no proposal for reform, however strong the arguments in its favour, is immune from the wedge objection. In fact, the stronger the arguments in favour of a reform, the more likely it is that the traditionalist will take the wedge objection—it is then the only one he has. C. M. Cornford put the argument in its proper place when he said that the wedge objection means this: that you should not act justly today, for fear that you may be asked to act still more justly tomorrow.

We heard a great deal of this type of argument in England in the nineteenth century, when it was used to resist almost every social and economic change. In the present century we have had less of it, but it is still accorded an exaggerated importance in some contexts. When lecturing on the law of torts in an American university a few years ago, I suggested that just as compulsory liability insurance for automobiles had spread practically throughout the civilized world, so we should in time see the law of tort superseded in this field by a system of state insurance for traffic accidents, administered independently of proof of fault. The suggestion was immediately met by one student with a horrified reference to "creeping socialism." That is the standard objection made by many people to any proposal for a new department of state activity. The implication is that you must resist every proposal, however admirable in itself, because otherwise you will never be able to draw the line. On the particular question of socialism, the fear is belied by the experience of a number of countries which have extended state control of the economy without going the whole way to socialistic state regimentation.

Kamisar's particular bogey, the racial laws of Nazi Germany, is an effective one in the democratic countries. Any reference to the Nazis is a powerful weapon to prevent change in the traditional taboo on sterilization as well as euthanasia. The case of sterilization is particularly interesting on this; I dealt with it at length in my book, though Kamisar does not mention its bearing on the argument. When proposals are made for promoting voluntary sterilization on eugenic and other grounds, they are immediately condemned by most people as the thin end of a wedge leading to involuntary sterilization; and then they point to the practices of the Nazis. Yet a more persuasive argument pointing in the other direction can easily be found. Several American states have sterilization laws, which for the most part were originally drafted in very wide terms to cover desexualization as well as sterilization, and authorizing involuntary as well as voluntary operations. This legislation goes back long before the Nazis; the earliest statute was in Indiana in 1907. What has been its practical effect? In several American states it has hardly been used. A few have used it, but in practice they have progressively restricted it until now it is virtually confined to voluntary sterilization. This is so, at least, in North Carolina, as Mrs. Woodside's study strikingly shows. In my book I summed up the position as follows:

> The American experience is of great interest because it shows how remote from reality in a democratic community is the fear—frequently voiced by Americans themselves—that voluntary sterilization may be the "thin end of the wedge," leading to a large-scale violation of human rights as happened in Nazi Germany. In fact, the American experience is the precise opposite—starting with compulsory sterilization, administrative practice has come to put the operation on a voluntary footing.

But it is insufficient to answer the "wedge" objection in general terms; we must consider the particular fears to which it gives rise. Kamisar professes to fear certain other measures that the Euthanasia Societies may bring up if their present measure is conceded to them. Surely these other measures, if any, will be debated on their merits? Does he seriously fear that anyone in the United States or in Great Britain is going to propose the extermination of people of a minority race or religion? Let us put aside such ridiculous fancies and discuss practical politics.

Kamisar is quite right in thinking that a body of opinion would favour the legalization of the involuntary euthanasia of hopelessly defective infants, and some day a proposal of this kind may be put forward. The proposal would have distinct limits, just as the proposal for voluntary euthanasia of incurable sufferers has limits. I do not think that any responsible body of opinion would now propose the euthanasia of insane adults, for the perfectly clear reason that any such practice would greatly increase the sense of insecurity felt by the borderline insane and by the large number of insane persons who have sufficient understanding on this particular matter.

Kamisar expresses distress at a concluding remark in my book in which I advert to the possibility of old people becoming an overwhelming burden on mankind. I share his feeling that there are profoundly disturbing possibilities here; and if I had been merely a propagandist, intent upon securing agreement for a specific measure of law reform, I should have done wisely to have omitted all reference to this subject. Since, however, I am merely an academic writer, trying to bring such intelligence as I have to bear on moral and social issues, I deemed the topic too important and threatening to leave without a word. I think I have made it clear, in the passages cited, that I am not for one moment proposing any euthanasia of the aged in present society; such an idea would shock me as much as it shocks Kamisar and would shock everybody else. Still, the fact that we may one day have to face is that medical science is more successful in preserving the body than in preserving the mind. It is not impossible that, in the foreseeable future, medical men will be able to preserve the mindless body until the age, say, of a thousand, while the mind itself will have lasted only a tenth of that time. What will mankind do then? It is hardly possible to imagine that we shall establish huge hospital-mausolea where the aged are kept in a kind of living death. Even if it is desired to do this, the cost of the undertaking may make it impossible.

This is not an immediately practical problem, and we need not yet face it. The problem of maintaining persons afflicted with senile dementia is well within our economic resources as the matter stands at present. Perhaps some barrier will be found to medical advance which will prevent the problem becoming more acute. Perhaps, as time goes on, and as the alternatives become more clearly realized, men will become more resigned to human control over the mode of termination of life. Or the solution may be that after the individual has reached a certain age, or a certain degree of decay, medical science will hold its hand, and allow him to be carried off by natural causes. But what if these natural causes are themselves painful? Would it not then be kinder to substitute human agency?

In general, it is enough to say that we do not have to know the solutions to these problems. The only doubtful moral question upon which we have to make an immediate decision in relation to involuntary euthanasia is whether we owe a moral duty to terminate the life of an insane person who is suffering from a painful and incurable disease. Such a person is left unprovided for under the legislative proposal formulated in my book. The objection to any system of involuntary euthanasia of the insane is that it may cause a sense of insecurity. It is because I think that the risk of this fear is a serious one that a proposal for the reform of the law must exclude its application to the insane.

Note

1. *The Sanctity of Life and Criminal Law* (1958), pp. 299 ff.; American edition (1957), pp. 334–39.

We have now explored some of the major arguments for and against the legalization of euthanasia. In those arguments an appeal was sometimes made to the rather traditional distinction between active and passive euthanasia, as discussed in the Introduction to this chapter. In the following article, James Rachels argues that this distinction is both morally and conceptually troublesome. Rachels believes that there is no moral significance in the distinction itself, and he thinks its use leads to confused moral reasoning. He challenges the distinction because: (1) it leads to less humane decisions than might otherwise be reached; (2) it leads to moral decisions on morally irrelevant grounds; and (3) it is a distinction that rests on the distinction between killing and letting die, and the bare difference between these two acts is of no moral importance. Rachels does not specifically advocate euthanasia, but he does seriously advocate rethinking the conceptual and moral bases on which we either accept or oppose euthanasia.

James Rachels

ACTIVE AND PASSIVE EUTHANASIA *

The distinction between active and passive euthanasia is thought to be crucial for medical ethics. The idea is that it is permissible, at least in some cases, to withhold treatment and allow a patient to die, but it is never permissible to take any direct action designed to kill the patient. This doctrine seems to be accepted by most doctors, and it is endorsed in a statement adopted by the House of Delegates of the American Medical Association on December 4, 1973:

* From the *New England Journal of Medicine*, 292, no. 2 (January 1975), 78–80. Reprinted by permission from the *New England Journal of Medicine*.

The intentional termination of the life of one human being by another —mercy killing—is contrary to that for which the medical profession stands and is contrary to the policy of the American Medical Association.

The cessation of the employment of extraordinary means to prolong the life of the body when there is irrefutable evidence that biological death is imminent is the decision of the patient and/or his immediate family. The advice and judgment of the physician should be freely available to the patient and/or his immediate family.

However, a strong case can be made against this doctrine. In what follows I will set out some of the relevant arguments, and urge doctors to reconsider their views on this matter.

To begin with a familiar type of situation, a patient who is dying of incurable cancer of the throat is in terrible pain, which can no longer be satisfactorily alleviated. He is certain to die within a few days, even if present treatment is continued, but he does not want to go on living for those days since the pain is unbearable. So he asks the doctor for an end to it, and his family joins in the request.

Suppose the doctor agrees to withhold treatment, as the conventional doctrine says he may. The justification for his doing so is that the patient is in terrible agony, and since he is going to die anyway, it would be wrong to prolong his suffering needlessly. But now notice this. If one simply withholds treatment, it may take the patient longer to die, and so he may suffer more than he would if more direct action were taken and a lethal injection given. This fact provides strong reason for thinking that, once the initial decision not to prolong his agony has been made, active euthanasia is actually preferable to passive euthanasia, rather than the reverse. To say otherwise is to endorse the option that leads to more suffering rather than less, and is contrary to the humanitarian impulse that prompts the decision not to prolong his life in the first place.

Part of my point is that the process of being "allowed to die" can be relatively slow and painful, whereas being given a lethal injection is relatively quick and painless. Let me give a different sort of example. In the United States about one in 600 babies is born with Down's syndrome. Most of these babies are otherwise healthy—that is, with only the usual pediatric care, they will proceed to an otherwise normal infancy. Some, however, are born with congenital defects such as intestinal obstructions that require operations if they are to live. Sometimes, the parents and the doctor will decide not to operate, and let the infant die. Anthony Shaw describes what happens then:

> . . . When surgery is denied [the doctor] must try to keep the infant from suffering while natural forces sap the baby's life away. As a surgeon whose natural inclination is to use the scalpel to fight off death, standing by and watching a salvageable baby die is the most emotionally exhausting experience I know. It is easy at a conference, in a theoretical discussion,

to decide that such infants should be allowed to die. It is altogether different to stand by in the nursery and watch as dehydration and infection wither a tiny being over hours and days. This is a terrible ordeal for me and the hospital staff—much more so than for the parents who never set foot in the nursery.[1]

I can understand why some people are opposed to all euthanasia, and insist that such infants must be allowed to live. I think I can also understand why other people favor destroying these babies quickly and painlessly. But why should anyone favor letting "dehydration and infection wither a tiny being over hours and days?" The doctrine that says that a baby may be allowed to dehydrate and wither, but may not be given an injection that would end its life without suffering, seems so patently cruel as to require no further refutation. The strong language is not intended to offend, but only to put the point in the clearest possible way.

My second argument is that the conventional doctrine leads to decisions concerning life and death made on irrelevant grounds.

Consider again the case of the infants with Down's syndrome who need operations for congenital defects unrelated to the syndrome to live. Sometimes, there is no operation, and the baby dies, but when there is no such defect, the baby lives on. Now, an operation such as that to remove an intestinal obstruction is not prohibitively difficult. The reason why such operations are not performed in these cases is, clearly, that the child has Down's syndrome and the parents and doctor judge that because of that fact it is better for the child to die.

But notice that this situation is absurd, no matter what view one takes of the lives and potentials of such babies. If the life of such an infant is worth preserving, what does it matter if it needs a simple operation? Or, if one thinks it better that such a baby should not live on, what difference does it make that it happens to have an unobstructed intestinal tract? In either case, the matter of life and death is being decided on irrelevant grounds. It is the Down's syndrome, and not the intestines, that is the issue. The matter should be decided, if at all, on that basis, and not be allowed to depend on the essentially irrelevant question of whether the intestinal tract is blocked.

What makes this situation possible, of course, is the idea that when there is an intestinal blockage, one can "let the baby die," but when there is no such defect there is nothing that can be done, for one must not "kill" it. The fact that this idea leads to such results as deciding life or death on irrelevant grounds is another good reason why the doctrine should be rejected.

One reason why so many people think that there is an important moral difference between active and passive euthanasia is that they think killing someone is morally worse than letting someone die. But is it? Is killing, in itself, worse than letting die? To investigate this issue, two cases may be considered that are exactly alike except that one involves killing whereas the other involves letting someone die. Then, it can be asked whether this difference makes any difference to the moral assessments. It is important that the cases be exactly alike, except for this one difference, since otherwise one cannot be confident that it is this difference and not some other that accounts for any variation in the assessments of the two cases. So, let us consider this pair of cases:

In the first, Smith stands to gain a large inheritance if anything should happen to his six-year-old cousin. One evening while the child is taking his bath, Smith sneaks into the bathroom and drowns the child, and then arranges things so that it will look like an accident.

In the second, Jones also stands to gain if anything should happen to his six-year-old cousin. Like Smith, Jones sneaks in planning to drown the child in his bath. However, just as he enters the bathroom Jones sees the child slip and hit his head, and fall face down in the water. Jones is delighted; he stands by, ready to push the child's head back under if it is necessary, but it is not necessary. With only a little thrashing about, the child drowns all by himself, "accidentally," as Jones watches and does nothing.

Now Smith killed the child, whereas Jones "merely" let the child die. That is the only difference between them. Did either man behave better, from a moral point of view? If the difference between killing and letting die were in itself a morally important matter, one should say that Jones's behavior was less reprehensible than Smith's. But does one really want to say that? I think not. In the first place, both men acted from the same motive, personal gain, and both had exactly the same end in view when they acted. It may be inferred from Smith's conduct that he is a bad man, although that judgment may be withdrawn or modified if certain further facts are learned about him—for example, that he is mentally deranged. But would not the very same thing be inferred about Jones from his conduct? And would not the same further considerations also be relevant to any modification of this judgment? Moreover, suppose Jones pleaded, in his own defense, "After all, I didn't do anything except just stand there and watch the child drown. I didn't kill him; I only let him die." Again, if letting die were in itself less bad than killing, this defense should have at least some weight. But it does not. Such a "defense" can only be regarded as a grotesque perversion of moral reasoning. Morally speaking, it is no defense at all.

Now, it may be pointed out, quite properly, that the cases of euthanasia with which doctors are concerned are not like this at all. They do not involve personal gain or the destruction of normal healthy children. Doctors are concerned only with cases in which the patient's life is of no further use to him, or in which the patient's life has become or will soon become a terrible burden. However, the point is the same in these cases: the bare difference between killing and letting die does not, in itself, make a moral difference. If a doctor lets a patient die, for humane reasons, he is in the same moral position as if he had given the patient a lethal injection for humane reasons. If his decision was wrong—if, for example, the patient's illness was in fact curable—the decision would be equally regrettable no matter which method was used to carry it out. And if the doctor's decision was the right one, the method used is not in itself important.

The AMA policy statement isolates the crucial issue very well; the crucial issue is "the intentional termination of the life of one human being by another." But after identifying this issue, and forbidding "mercy killing," the statement goes on to deny that the cessation of treatment is the intentional termination of a life. This is where the mistake comes in, for what is the cessation of treatment, in these circumstances, if it is not "the intentional termination of the life of one human being by another?" Of course it is exactly that, and if it were not, there would be no point to it.

Many people will find this judgment hard to accept. One reason, I think, is that it is very easy to conflate the question of whether killing is, in itself, worse than letting die, with the very different question of whether most actual cases of killing are more reprehensible than most actual cases of letting die. Most actual cases of killing are clearly terrible (think, for example, of all the murders reported in the newspapers), and one hears of such cases every day. On the other hand, one hardly ever hears of a case of letting die, except for the actions of doctors who are motivated by humanitarian reasons. So one learns to think of killing in a much worse light than of letting die. But this does not mean that there is something about killing that makes it in itself worse than letting die, for it is not the bare difference between killing and letting die that makes the difference in these cases. Rather, the other factors—the murderer's motive of personal gain, for example, contrasted with the doctor's humanitarian motivation—account for different reactions to the different cases.

I have argued that killing is not in itself any worse than letting die; if my contention is right, it follows that active euthanasia is not any worse than passive euthanasia. What arguments can be given on the other side? The most common, I believe, is the following:

> The important difference between active and passive euthanasia is that, in passive euthanasia, the doctor does not do anything to bring about the patient's death. The doctor does nothing, and the patient dies of whatever ills already afflict him. In active euthanasia, however, the doctor does something to bring about the patient's death: he kills him. The doctor who gives the patient with cancer a lethal injection has himself caused his patient's death; whereas if he merely ceases treatment, the cancer is the cause of the death.

A number of points need to be made here. The first is that it is not exactly correct to say that in passive euthanasia the doctor does nothing, for he does do one thing that is very important: he lets the patient die. "Letting someone die" is certainly different, in some respects, from other types of action—mainly in that it is a kind of action that one may perform by way of not performing certain other actions. For example, one may let a patient die by way of not giving medication, just as one may insult someone by way of not shaking his hand. But for any purpose of moral assessment, it is a type of action nonetheless. The decision to let a patient die is subject to moral appraisal in the same way that a decision to kill him would be subject to moral appraisal: it may be assessed as wise or unwise, compassionate or sadistic, right or wrong. If a doctor deliberately let a patient die who was suffering from a routinely curable illness, the doctor would certainly be to blame for what he had done, just as he would be to blame if he had needlessly killed the patient. Charges against him would then be appropriate. If so, it would be no defense at all for him to insist that he didn't "do anything." He would have done something very serious indeed, for he let his patient die.

Fixing the cause of death may be very important from a legal point of view, for it may determine whether criminal charges are brought against the doctor. But I do not think that this notion can be used to show a moral difference between active and passive euthanasia. The reason why it is considered bad to be the cause of someone's death is that death is regarded as a great evil—and so it is. However, if it has been decided that euthanasia—even passive euthanasia—is desirable in a given case, it has also been decided that in this instance death is no greater an evil than the patient's continued existence. And if this is true, the usual reason for not wanting to be the cause of someone's death simply does not apply.

Finally, doctors may think that all of this is only of academic interest—the sort of thing that philosophers may worry about but that has no practical bearing on their own work. After all, doctors must be concerned about the legal consequences of what they do, and active euthanasia is clearly forbidden by the law. But even so, doctors should also be concerned with the fact that the law is forcing upon them a moral doctrine that may well be indefensible, and has a considerable effect on their practices. Of course, most doctors are not now in the position of being coerced in this matter, for they do not regard themselves as merely going along with what the law requires. Rather, in statements such as the A.M.A. policy statement that I have quoted, they are endorsing this doctrine as a central point of medical ethics. In that statement, active euthanasia is condemned not merely as illegal but as "contrary to that for which the medical profession stands," whereas passive euthanasia is approved. However, the preceding considerations suggest that there is really no moral difference between the two, considered in themselves (there may be important moral differences in some cases in their *consequences*, but, as I pointed out, these differences may make active euthanasia, and not passive euthanasia, the morally preferable option). So, whereas doctors may have to discriminate between active and passive euthanasia to satisfy the law, they should not do any more than that. In particular, they should not give the distinction any added authority and weight by writing it into official statements of medical ethics.

Note

1. A. Shaw, "Doctor, Do We Have a Choice?" *The New York Times Magazine*, January 30, 1972, p. 54.

Whereas Rachels completely rejects both the distinction between active and passive euthanasia and the A.M.A. position on euthanasia, Tom L. Beauchamp attempts to reinstate some of the importance of the distinction. Beauchamp agrees with Rachels that most of the traditional ways of morally justifying euthanasia (active or passive) are unsatisfactory and that the bare difference between killing and letting die is morally insignificant. But Beauchamp thinks it does not follow that the distinction between active and passive euthanasia should not play any significant role in our thinking about euthanasia. Using a form of utilitarianism, he argues that the best consequences for society *might* result by permitting passive euthanasia, while rejecting active euthanasia —a point of substantial, though not total, agreement with the ethical position of the American Medical Association (which does seem to endorse a limited form of passive euthanasia). Beauchamp concludes that society is presently faced with a dilemma over whether to retain or to abandon the active/passive distinction. He believes society will have to cope with this dilemma for some time.

Tom L. Beauchamp

A REPLY TO RACHELS ON ACTIVE AND PASSIVE EUTHANASIA *

James Rachels has recently argued that the distinction between active and passive euthanasia is neither appropriately used by the American Medical Association nor generally useful for the resolution of moral problems of euthanasia.[1] Indeed he believes this distinction—which he equates

* This paper is a heavily revised version of an article by the same title first published in T. Mappes and J. Zembaty, eds. *Social Ethics* (N.Y.: McGraw-Hill, 1976). Copyright © 1975, 1977 by Tom L. Beauchamp.

with the killing/letting die distinction—does not in itself have any moral importance. The chief object of his attack is the following statement adopted by the House of Delegates of the American Medical Association in 1973:

> The intentional termination of the life of one human being by another —mercy killing—is contrary to that for which the medical profession stands and is contrary to the policy of the American Medical Association.
> The cessation of the employment of extraordinary means to prolong the life of the body when there is irrefutable evidence that biological death is imminent is the decision of the patient and/or his immediate family. The advice and judgment of the physician should be freely available to the patient and/or his immediate family (241).

Rachels constructs a powerful and interesting set of arguments against this statement. In this paper I attempt the following: (1) to challenge his views on the grounds that he does not appreciate the moral reasons which give weight to the active/passive distinction; and (2) to provide a constructive account of the moral relevance of the active/passive distinction; and (3) to offer reasons showing that Rachels may nonetheless be correct in urging that we *ought* to abandon the active/passive distinction for purposes of moral reasoning.

I

I would concede that the active/passive distinction is *sometimes* morally irrelevant. Of this Rachels convinces me. But it does not follow that it is *always* morally irrelevant. What we need, then, is a case where the distinction is a morally relevant one and an explanation why it is so. Rachels himself uses the method of examining two cases which are exactly alike except that "one involves killing whereas the other involves letting die" (243). We may profitably begin by comparing the kinds of cases governed by the AMA's doctrine with the kinds of cases adduced by Rachels in order to assess the adequacy and fairness of his cases.

The second paragraph of the AMA statement is confined to a narrowly restricted range of passive euthanasia cases, viz., those (a) where the patients are on extraordinary means, (b) where irrefutable evidence of imminent death is available, and (c) where patient or family consent is available. Rachels' two cases involve conditions notably different from these:

> In the first, Smith stands to gain a large inheritance if anything should happen to his six-year-old cousin. One evening while the child is taking his bath, Smith sneaks into the bathroom and drowns the child, and then arranges things so that it will look like an accident.
> In the second, Jones also stands to gain if anything should happen to his six-year-old cousin. Like Smith, Jones sneaks in planning to drown the

child in his bath. However, just as he enters the bathroom Jones sees the child slip and hit his head, and fall face down in the water. Jones is delighted; he stands by, ready to push the child's head back under if it is necessary, but it is not necessary. With only a little thrashing about, the child drowns all by himself, "accidentally," as Jones watches and does nothing.

Now Smith killed the child, whereas Jones "merely" let the child die. That is the only difference between them (243).

Rachels says there is no moral difference between the cases in terms of our moral assessments of Smith and Jones' behavior. This assessment seems fair enough, but what can Rachels' cases be said to prove, as they are so markedly disanalogous to the sorts of cases envisioned by the AMA proposal? Rachels concedes important disanalogies, but thinks them irrelevant:

> The point is the same in these cases: the bare difference between killing and letting die does not, in itself, make a moral difference. If a doctor lets a patient die, for humane reasons, he is in the same moral position as if he had given the patient a lethal injection for humane reasons (244).

Three observations are immediately in order. First, Rachels seems to infer that from such cases we can conclude that the distinction between killing and letting die is *always* morally irrelevant. This conclusion is fallaciously derived. What the argument in fact shows, being an analogical argument, is only that in all *relevantly similar* cases the distinction does not in itself make a moral difference. Since Rachels concedes that other cases are disanalogous, he seems thereby to concede that his argument is as weak as the analogy itself. Second, Rachels' cases involve two *unjustified* actions, one of killing and the other of letting die. The AMA statement distinguishes one set of cases of unjustified killing and another of *justified* cases of allowing to die. Nowhere is it claimed by the AMA that what makes the difference in these cases is the active/passive distinction itself. It is only implied that one set of cases, the justified set, *involves* (passive) letting die while the unjustified set *involves* (active) killing. While it is said that justified euthanasia cases are passive ones and unjustified ones active, it is not said either that what makes some acts justified is the fact of their being passive or that what makes others unjustified is the fact of their being active. This fact will prove to be of vital importance.

The third point is that in both of Rachels' cases the respective moral agents—Smith and Jones—are morally responsible for the death of the child and are morally blameworthy—even though Jones is presumably not causally responsible. In the first case death is caused by the agent, while in the second it is not; yet the second agent is no less morally responsible. While the law might find only the first homicidal, morality condemns the motives in each case as equally wrong, and it holds that the duty to save life in such cases is as compelling as the duty not to take life. I suggest that it is largely because of this equal degree of moral responsibility that there is no morally relevant difference in Rachels' cases. In the cases envisioned by the AMA, however, an agent is held to be responsible for taking life by actively killing but is not held to be morally required to preserve life, and so not responsible for death, when removing the patient from extraordinary means (under conditions a–c above). I shall elaborate this latter point momentarily. My only conclusion thus far is the negative one that Rachels' arguments rest on weak foundations. His cases are not relevantly similar to euthanasia cases and do not support his apparent conclusion that the active/passive distinction is *always* morally irrelevant.

II

I wish first to consider an argument that I believe has powerful intuitive appeal and probably is widely accepted as stating the main reason for rejecting Rachels' views. I will maintain that this argument fails, and so leaves Rachels' contentions untouched.

I begin with an actual case, the celebrated Quinlan case.[2] Karen Quinlan was in a coma, and was on a mechanical respirator which artificially sustained her vital processes and which her parents wished to cease. At least some physicians believed there was irrefutable evidence that biological death was imminent and the coma irreversible. This case, under this description, closely conforms to the passive cases envisioned by the AMA. During an interview the father, Mr. Quinlan, asserted that he did not wish to kill his daughter, but only to remove her from the machines in order to see whether she would live or would die a natural death.[3] Suppose he had said —to envision now a second and hypothetical, but parallel case—that he wished only to see her die painlessly and therefore wished that the doctor could induce death by an overdose of morphine. Most of us would think the second act, which involves active killing, morally unjustified in these circumstances, while many of us would think the first act morally justified. (This is not the place to consider whether in fact it is justified, and if so under what conditions.) What accounts for the apparent morally relevant difference?

I have considered these two cases together in order to follow Rachels' method of entertaining parallel cases where the only difference is that the one case involves killing and the other letting die. However, there is a further difference, which crops up in the euthanasia context. The difference rests in our judgments of medical fallibility and moral responsibility. Mr. Quinlan seems to think that, after all, the doctors might be wrong. There is a remote possibility that she might live without the aid of a machine. But whether or not the medical prediction of death turns out to be accurate, if she dies then no one is morally responsible for directly bringing about or causing her death, as they would be if they caused her death by killing her. Rachels finds explanations which appeal to causal conditions unsatisfactory; but perhaps this is only because he fails to see the nature of the causal link. To bring about her death is by that act to preempt the possibility of life. To "allow her to die" by removing artificial equipment is to allow for the possibility of wrong diagnosis or incorrect prediction and hence to absolve oneself of moral responsibility for the taking of life under false assumptions. There may, of course, be utterly no empirical possibility of recovery in some cases since recovery would violate a law of nature. However, judgments of empirical impossibility in medicine are notoriously problematic—the reason for emphasizing medical fallibility. And in all the hard cases we do not *know* that recovery is empirically impossible, even if good *evidence* is available.

The above reason for invoking the active/passive distinction can now be generalized: Active termination of life removes all possibility of life for the patient, while passively ceasing extraordinary means may not. This is not trivial since patients have survived in several celebrated cases where, in knowledgeable physicians' judgments, there was "irrefutable" evidence that death was imminent.[4]

One may, of course, be entirely responsible and culpable for another's death either by killing him or by letting him die. In such cases, of which Rachels' are examples, there is no morally significant difference between killing and letting die precisely because whatever one does, omits, or refrains from doing does not absolve one of responsibility. Either active or passive involvement renders one responsible for the death of another, and both involvements are equally wrong for the same principled moral reason: it is (prima facie) morally wrong to bring about the death of an innocent person capable of living whenever the causal intervention or negligence is intentional. (I use causal terms here because causal involvement need not be active, as when by one's negligence one is nonetheless causally responsible.) But not all cases of killing and letting die fall under this same moral principle. One is sometimes culpable for killing, because morally responsible as the agent for death, as when one pulls the plug on a respirator sustaining a recovering patient (a murder). But one is sometimes not culpable for letting die because not morally responsible as agent, as when one pulls the plug on a respirator sustaining an irreversibly comatose and unrecoverable patient (a routine procedure, where one is *merely* causally responsible).[5] Different degrees and means of involvement assess different degrees of responsibility, and our assessments of culpability can become intricately complex. The only point which now concerns us, however, is that because different moral principles may govern very similar circumstances, we are sometimes morally culpable for killing but not for letting die. And to many people it will seem that in passive cases we are not morally responsible for causing death, though we are responsible in active cases.

This argument is powerfully attractive. Although I was once inclined to accept it in virtually the identical form just developed,[6] I now think that, despite its intuitive appeal, it cannot be correct. It is true that different degrees and means of involvement entail different degrees of responsibility, but it does not follow that we are *not* responsible and therefore are absolved of possible culpability in *any* case of intentionally allowing to die. We are responsible and *perhaps* culpable in either active or passive cases. Here Rachels' argument is entirely to the point: It is not primarily a question of greater or lesser responsibility by an active or a passive means that should determine culpability. Rather, the question of culpability is decided by the moral *justification* for choosing either a passive or an active means. What the argument in the previous paragraph overlooks is that one might be unjustified in using an active means or unjustified in using a passive means, and hence be culpable in the use of either; yet one might be justified in using an active means or justified in using a passive means, and hence not be culpable in using either. Fallibility might just as well be present in a judgment to use one means as in a judgment to use another. (A judgment to allow to die is just as subject to being based on *knowledge which is fallible* as a judgment to kill.) Moreover, in either case, it is a matter of what one knows and believes, and not a matter of a particular kind of causal connection or causal chain. If we kill the patient, then we are certainly causally responsible for his death. But, similarly, if we cease treatment, and the patient dies, the patient might have recovered if treatment had been continued. The patient might have been saved in either case, and hence there is no morally relevant difference between the two cases. It is, therefore, simply beside the point that "one is sometimes culpable for killing . . . but one is sometimes not culpable for letting die"—as the above argument concludes.

Accordingly, despite its great intuitive appeal and frequent mention, this argument from responsibility fails.

III

There may, however, be more compelling arguments against Rachels, and I wish now to provide what I believe is the most significant argument that can be adduced in defense of the active/passive distinction. I shall develop this argument by combining (1) so-called wedge or slippery slope arguments with (2) recent arguments in defense of rule utilitarianism. I shall explain each in turn and show how in combination they may be used to defend the active/passive distinction.

(1) *Wedge arguments* proceed as follows: if killing were allowed,

even under the guise of a merciful extinction of life, a dangerous wedge would be introduced which places all "undesirable" or "unworthy" human life in a precarious condition. Proponents of wedge arguments believe the initial wedge places us on a slippery slope for at least one of two reasons: (i) It is said that our justifying principles leave us with no principled way to avoid the slide into saying that all sorts of killings would be justified under similar conditions. Here it is thought that once killing is allowed, a firm line between justified and unjustified killings cannot be securely drawn. It is thought best not to redraw the line in the first place, for redrawing it will inevitably lead to a downhill slide. It is then often pointed out that as a matter of historical record this is precisely what has occurred in the darker regions of human history, including the Nazi era, where euthanasia began with the best intentions for horribly ill, non-Jewish Germans and gradually spread to anyone deemed an enemy of the people. (ii) Second, it is said that our basic principles against killing will be gradually eroded once some form of killing is legitimated. For example, it is said that permitting voluntary euthanasia will lead to permitting involuntary euthanasia, which will in turn lead to permitting euthanasia for those who are a nuisance to society (idiots, recidivist criminals, defective newborns, and the insane, e.g.). Gradually other principles which instill respect for human life will be eroded or abandoned in the process.

I am not inclined to accept the first reason (i).[7] If our justifying principles are themselves justified, then any action they warrant would be justified. Accordingly, I shall only be concerned with the second approach (ii).

(2) *Rule utilitarianism* is the position that a society ought to adopt a rule if its acceptance would have better consequences for the common good (greater social utility) than any comparable rule could have in that society. Any action is right if it conforms to a valid rule and wrong if it violates the rule. Sometimes it is said that alternative rules should be measured against one another, while it has also been suggested that whole moral *codes* (complete sets of rules) rather than individual rules should be compared. While I prefer the latter formulation (Brandt's), this internal dispute need not detain us here. The important point is that a particular rule or a particular code of rules is morally justified if and only if there is no other competing rule or moral code whose acceptance would have a higher utility value for society, and where a rule's acceptability is contingent upon the consequences which would result if the rule were made current.

Wedge arguments, when conjoined with rule utilitarian arguments, may be applied to euthanasia issues in the following way. We presently subscribe to a no-active-euthanasia rule (which the AMA suggests we retain). Imagine now that in our society we make current a restricted-active-euthanasia rule (as Rachels seems to urge). Which of these two moral rules would, if enacted, have the consequence of maximizing social utility? Clearly a restricted-active-euthanasia rule would have *some* utility value, as Rachels notes, since some intense and uncontrollable suffering would be eliminated. However, it may not have the highest utility value in the structure of our present code or in any imaginable code which could be made current, and therefore may not be a component in the ideal code for our society. If wedge arguments raise any serious questions at all, as I think they do, they rest in this area of whether a code would be weakened or strengthened by the addition of active euthanasia principles. For the disutility of introducing legitimate killing into one's moral code (in the form of active euthanasia rules) may, in the long run, outweigh the utility of doing so, as a result of the eroding effect such a relaxation would have on rules in the code which demand respect for human life. If, for example, rules permitting active killing were introduced, it is not implausible to suppose that destroying defective newborns (a form of involuntary euthanasia) would become an accepted and common practice, that as population increases occur the aged will be even more neglectable and neglected than they now are, that capital punishment for a wide variety of crimes would be increasingly tempting, that some doctors would have appreciably reduced fears of actively injecting fatal doses whenever it seemed to them propitious to do so, and that laws of war against killing would erode in efficacy even beyond their already abysmal level.

A hundred such possible consequences might easily be imagined. But these few are sufficient to make the larger point that such rules permitting killing could lead to a general reduction of respect for human life. Rules against killing in a moral code are not *isolated* moral principles; they are pieces of a web of rules against killing which forms the code. The more threads one removes, the weaker the fabric becomes. And if, as I believe, moral principles against active killing have the deep and continuously civilizing effect of promoting respect for life, and if principles which allow passively letting die (as envisioned in the AMA statement) do not themselves cut against this effect, then this seems an important reason for the maintenance of the active/passive distinction. (By the logic of the above argument passively letting die would also have to be prohibited if a rule permitting it had the serious adverse consequence of eroding acceptance of rules protective of respect for life. While this prospect seems to me improbable, I can hardly claim to have refuted those conservatives who would claim that even rules which sanction letting die place us on a precarious slippery slope.)

A troublesome problem, however, confronts my use of utilitarian and wedge arguments. Most all of us would agree that both killing and letting die are justified under some conditions. Killings in self-defense and in "just" wars are widely accepted as justified because the conditions excuse the killing. If society can withstand these exceptions to moral rules prohibiting killing, then why is it not plausible to suppose society can accept another excusing exception in the form of justified active euthanasia? This is an important and worthy objection, but not a decisive one. The defenseless and the dying are significantly different classes of persons from aggressors who attack individuals and/or nations. In the case of aggressors, one does not confront the question whether their lives are no longer *worth living*. Rather, we reach the judgment that the aggressors' morally blameworthy actions justify counteractions. But in the case of the dying and the otherwise ill, there is no morally blameworthy action to justify our own. Here we are required to accept the judgment that their lives are no longer *worth living* in order to believe that the termination of their lives is justified. It is the latter sort of judgment which is feared by those who take the wedge argument seriously. We do not now permit and never have permitted the taking of morally blameless lives. I think this is the key to understanding why recent cases of intentionally allowing the death of defective newborns (as in the now famous case at the Johns Hopkins Hospital) have generated such protracted controversy. Even if such newborns could not have led meaningful lives (a matter of some controversy), it is the wedged foot in the door which creates the most intense worries. For if we once take a decision to allow a restricted infanticide justification or any justification at all on grounds that a life is not meaningful or not worth living, we have qualified our moral rules against killing. That this qualification is a matter of the utmost seriousness needs no argument. I mention it here only to show why the wedge argument may have moral force even though we *already* allow some very different conditions to justify intentional killing.

There is one final utilitarian reason favoring the preservation of the active/passive distinction.[8] Suppose we distinguish the following two types of cases of wrongly diagnosed patients:

1. Patients wrongly diagnosed as hopeless, and who will survive even if a treatment *is* ceased (in order to allow a natural death).
2. Patients wrongly diagnosed as hopeless, and who will survive only if the treatment is *not ceased* (in order to allow a natural death).

If a social rule permitting only passive euthanasia were in effect, then doctors and families who "allowed death" would lose only patients in class 2, not those in class 1; whereas if active euthanasia were permitted, at least some patients in class 1 would be needlessly lost. Thus, the consequence of a no-active-euthanasia rule would be to save some lives which could not be saved if both forms of euthanasia were allowed. This reason is not a *decisive* reason for favoring a policy of passive euthanasia, since these classes (1 and 2) are likely to be very small and since there might be counterbalancing reasons (extreme pain, autonomous expression of the patient, etc.) in favor of active euthanasia. But certainly it is *a* reason favoring only passive euthanasia and one which is morally relevant and ought to be considered along with other moral reasons.

IV

It may still be insisted that my case has not touched Rachels' leading claim, for I have not shown, as Rachels puts it, that it is "the bare difference between killing and letting die that makes the difference in these cases" (244). True, I have not shown this, and in my judgment it cannot be shown. But this concession does not require capitulation to Rachels' argument. I adduced a case which is at the center of our moral intuition that killing is morally different (in at least some cases) from letting die; and I then attempted to account for at least part of the grounds for this belief. The grounds turn out to be other than the *bare* difference, but nevertheless *make* the distinction morally relevant. The identical point can be made regarding the voluntary/involuntary distinction, as it is commonly applied to euthanasia. It is not the bare difference between voluntary euthanasia (i.e., euthanasia with patient consent) and involuntary euthanasia (i.e., without patient consent) that makes one justifiable and one not. Independent moral grounds based on, for example, respect for autonomy or beneficence, or perhaps justice will alone make the moral difference.

In order to illustrate this general claim, let us presume that it is sometimes justified to kill another person and sometimes justified to allow another to die. Suppose, for example, that one may kill in self-defense and may allow to die when a promise has been made to someone that he would be allowed to die. Here conditions of self-defense and promising justify actions. But suppose now that someone *A* promises in exactly similar circumstances to kill someone *B* at *B*'s request, and also that someone *C* allows someone *D* to die in an act of self-defense. Surely *A* is obliged equally to kill or to let die if he promised; and surely *C* is permitted to let *D* die if it is a matter of defending *C*'s life. If this analysis is correct, then it follows that killing is sometimes right, sometimes wrong, depending on the circumstances, and the same is true of letting die. It is the justifying reasons which make the difference whether an action is right, not merely the kind of action it is.

Now, *if* letting die led to disastrous conclusions but killing did not, then letting die but not killing would be wrong. Consider, for example, a possible world in which dying would be indefinitely prolongable even if all extraordinary therapy were removed and the patient were allowed to die. Suppose that it costs over one million dollars to let each patient die, that nurses consistently commit suicide from caring for those being "allowed to die," that physicians are constantly being successfully sued for malpractice for allowing death by cruel and wrongful means, and that hospitals are uncontrollably overcrowded and their wards filled with communicable diseases which afflict only the dying. Now suppose further that killing in this possible world is quick, painless, and easily monitored. I submit that in this world we would believe that *killing is morally acceptable but that allowing to die is morally unacceptable*. The point of this example is again that it is the circumstances that make the difference, not the bare difference between killing and letting die.

It is, however, worth noticing that there is nothing in the AMA statement which says that the bare difference between killing and letting die itself and alone makes the difference in our differing moral assessments of rightness and wrongness. Rachels forces this interpretation on the statement. Some philosophers may have thought bare difference makes the difference, but there is scant evidence that the AMA or any thoughtful ethicist *must* believe it in order to defend the relevance and importance of the active/passive distinction. When this conclusion is coupled with my earlier argument that from Rachels' paradigm cases it follows only that the active/passive distinction is sometimes, but not always, morally irrelevant, it would seem that his case against the AMA is rendered highly questionable.

V

There remains, however, the important question as to whether we *ought* to accept the distinction between active and passive euthanasia, now that we are clear about (at least one way of drawing) the moral grounds for its invocation. That is, should we employ the distinction in order to judge some acts of euthanasia justified and others not justified? Here, as the hesitant previous paragraph indicates, I am uncertain. This problem is a substantive moral issue—not merely a conceptual one—and would require at a minimum a lengthy assessment of wedge arguments and related utilitarian considerations. In important respects empirical questions are involved in this assessment. We should like to know, and yet have hardly any evidence to indicate, what the consequences would be for our society if we were to allow the use of active means to produce death. The best hope for making such an assessment has seemed to some to rest in analogies to suicide and capital punishment statutes. Here it may reasonably be asked whether recent liberalizations of laws limiting these forms of killing have served as the thin end of a wedge leading to a breakdown of principles protecting life or to widespread violations of moral principles. Nonetheless, such analogies do not seem to me promising, since they are still fairly remote from the pertinent issue of the consequences of allowing active humanitarian killing of one person by another.

It is interesting to notice the outcome of the Kamisar-Williams debate on euthanasia—which is almost exclusively cast by both writers in a consequential, utilitarian framework.[9] At one crucial point in the debate, where possible consequences of laws permitting euthanasia are under discussion, they exchange "perhaps" judgments:

> I [Williams] will return Kamisar the compliment and say: "Perhaps." We are certainly in an area where no solution is going to make things quite easy and happy for everybody, and all sorts of embarrassments may be conjectured. But these embarrassments are not avoided by keeping to the present law: we suffer from them already.[10]

Because of the grave difficulties which stand in the way of making accurate predictions about the impact of liberalized euthanasia laws—especially those that would permit active killing—it is not surprising that those who debate the subject would reach a point of exchanging such "perhaps" judgments. And that is why, so it seems to me, we are uncertain whether to perpetuate or to abandon the active-passive distinction in our moral thinking about euthanasia. I think we *do* perpetuate it in medicine, law, and ethics because we are still somewhat uncertain about the conditions under which *passive* euthanasia should be permitted by law (which is one form of social *rule*). We are unsure about what the consequences will be of the California "Natural Death Act" and all those similar acts passed by other states which have followed in its path. If no untoward results occur, and the balance of the results seems favorable, then we will perhaps be less concerned about further liberalizations of euthanasia laws. If untoward results do occur (on a widespread scale), then we would be most reluctant to accept further liberalizations and might even abolish natural death acts.

In short, I have argued in this section that euthanasia in its active and its passive forms presents us with a dilemma which can be developed by using powerful consequentialist arguments on each side, yet there is little clarity concerning the proper resolution of the dilemma precisely because of our uncertainty regarding proclaimed consequences.

VI

I reach two conclusions at the end of these several arguments. First, I think Rachels is incorrect in arguing that the distinction between active and passive is (always) morally irrelevant. It may well be relevant, and for moral reasons—the reasons adduced in section III above. Second, I think nonetheless that Rachels may ultimately be shown correct in his contention that we ought to dispense with the active-passive distinction—for reasons adduced in sections IV–V. But if he is ultimately judged correct, it will be because we have come to see that some forms of active killing have generally acceptable social consequences, and not primarily because of the arguments he adduces in his paper—even though *something* may be said for each of these arguments. Of course, in one respect I have conceded a great deal to Rachels. The bare difference argument is vital to his position, and I have fully agreed to it. On the other hand, I do not see that the bare difference argument does play or need play a major role in our moral thinking—or in that of the AMA.

Notes

1. "Active and Passive Euthanasia," *New England Journal of Medicine* 292 (January 9, 1975), 78–80. [All page references in parentheses refer to Rachels's article as reprinted in this chapter.]
2. As recorded in the Opinion of Judge Robert Muir, Jr., Docket No. C-201-75 of the Superior Court of New Jersey, Chancery Division, Morris County (November 10, 1975). The relevant sections of this document are reprinted below.
3. See Judge Muir's Opinion, p. 18—a slightly different statement but on the subject.
4. This problem of the strength of evidence also emerged in the Quinlan trial, as physicians disagreed whether the evidence was "irrefutable." Such disagreement, when added to the problems of medical fallibility and causal responsibility just outlined, provides in the eyes of some one important argument against the *legalization* of active euthanasia, as perhaps the AMA would agree. Cf. Kamisar's arguments in this chapter.
5. Among the moral reasons why one is held to be responsible in the first sort of case and not responsible in the second sort are, I believe, the moral grounds for the active/passive distinction under discussion in this section.
6. In *Social Ethics,* as cited in the permission note to this article.
7. An argument of this form, which I find unacceptable for reasons given below, is Arthur Dyck, "Beneficent Euthanasia and Benemortasia: Alternative Views of Mercy," in M. Kohl, ed., *Beneficent Euthanasia* (Buffalo: Prometheus Books, 1975), pp. 120f.
8. I owe most of this argument to James Rachels, whose comments on an earlier draft of this paper led to several significant alterations.
9. Williams bases his pro-euthanasia argument on the prevention of two consequences: (1) loss of liberty and (2) cruelty. Kamisar bases his anti-euthanasia position on three projected consequences of euthanasia laws: (1) mistaken diagnosis, (2) pressured decisions by seriously ill patients, and (3) the wedge of the laws will lead to legalized involuntary euthanasia. Kamisar admits that individual acts of euthanasia are sometimes justified. It is the rule that he opposes. He is thus clearly a rule-utilitarian, and I believe Williams is as well (cf. his views on children and the senile). Their assessments of wedge arguments are, however, radically different.
10. Glanville Williams, "Mercy-Killing Legislation—A Reioinder," *Minnesota Law Review,* 43, no. 1 (1958), 5.

An answer to some problems about passive euthanasia involving infants is provided by John Robertson and Norman Fost in the next selection. The following is their own abstract of their argument: "The recent increase in reporting of passive euthanasia of defective newborn infants has not been accompanied by extensive analysis of the legality of the practice or the appropriateness of current law. There appears to be criminal liability on several grounds for parents, physicians, nurses, and administrators. Such liability may include charges of homicide by omission, child neglect, and failure to report child neglect. Increasing public exposure of the practice increases the probability that such prosecutions may be brought. Individuals involved in such decisions should be aware of their possible legal liability. If existing legal policy is inappropriate, it should be changed through open discussion and not subverted through private action. Two alternative policies are described [in this selection]: establishment of criteria for the class of infants who can be allowed to die or a better process of decision making. We conclude that a commitment to process would be preferable."

John A. Robertson
Norman Fost

PASSIVE EUTHANASIA OF DEFECTIVE NEWBORN INFANTS: LEGAL AND MORAL CONSIDERATIONS *

Parents and physicians now face a dilemma when infants with Down syndrome, myelomeningocele, and other birth defects require medical or surgical attention merely to stay alive. If parents withhold consent for medical care and the physician acquiesces, the infant may die. To provide the appropriate medical care, however, may maintain the existence of a being with only minimal capacity for personal development and human interaction.

Withholding treatment seems to have become a widespread, if not frequent, event. Widely publicized cases have arisen in Maine,[1] Arizona,[2] New York,[3] Denver,[4] and Los Angeles.[5] Duff and Campbell[6] reported 43 instances over a two-year period in the newborn unit of a university medical center. A number of eminent physicians recently appeared before the Senate Subcommittee on Health and at that time justified the practice.[7] Leading textbooks and journals discuss indications for withholding treatment.[8, 9]

Although the growing visibility of the practice has generated much ethical debate, discussion of the legality of the practice and the appro-

* Reproduced with permission from *J. Pediatr.*, 88 (1976), 883–89; copyrighted by The C. V. Mosby Company, St. Louis, Missouri, U. S. A.

priateness of current law has been minimal. This absence is unfortunate for several reason. The first and most important is that parents, physicians, and nurses may be risking criminal liability without awareness of the legal ramifications of their decisions. Physicians can hardly assist parents to reach an informed choice concerning treatment if they do not also disclose that their choice may have serious legal consequences. Also, analysis of the law may expose inconsistencies or inadequacies, and thus point the way to changes that will enhance the certitude and security of future decision making. Finally, the traditional legal concern with procedures for balancing conflicting interests may point the way to a reasonable solution to a perplexing dilemma of modern medicine.

This article briefly reviews the potential criminal liability of parents, physicians, and nurses involved in the decision to withhold ordinary care from defective newborn infants. Finding that any or all of them may be subject to criminal prosecution for murder, manslaughter, neglect, child abuse, or conspiracy, we then discuss some issues relevant to an evaluation of these policies. Finally, we propose a third approach to the problem which avoids the excesses of present law and present practices. *The authors do not contend that the criminal liability here enumerated should necessarily be pursued,* nor is it clear that as a practical matter that this would occur. Rather, we are concerned with elucidating the legal issues so that participants in such decisions can be fully informed, and legal policy, where desirable, altered.

LIABILITY OF PARENTS

Generally, homicide by omission occurs when a person's failure to discharge a *legal* duty to another person causes that person's death.[11] If the required action is intentionally withheld, the crime is either first- or second-degree murder, depending on the extent of premeditation and deliberation.[11] When the omission occurs through gross carelessness or disregard of the consequences of failing to act, the crime is involuntary manslaughter.[11]

In the case of a defective infant the withholding of essential care would appear to present a possible case of homicide by omission on the part of parents, physicians, and nurses, with the degree of homicide depending on the extent of premeditation. Following a live birth, the law generally presumes that personhood exists and that there is entitlement to the usual legal protections, whatever the specific physical and mental characteristics of the infant may be.[12, 13] Every state imposes on parents a legal duty to provide necessary medical assistance to a helpless minor child.[14, 15] If they withhold such care and the child dies, they may be prosecuted for manslaughter or murder, as has frequently occurred when parents have refused or neglected to obtain medical care for nondefective children.[16, 17] Although no parent has yet been prosecuted for withholding care from defective neonates, the well-recognized rule would appear equally applicable to nontreatment of defective infants. Defenses based on religious grounds, or even on poverty, if public assistance is available, have been specifically rejected, and other legal defenses, such as the defense of necessity, may not apply.[16, 18, 19] While care may be omitted as "extraordinary" if there is only a minimal chance of survival, when survival is likely, treatment cannot be withheld simply because of cost or the future social disutility of the infant.[19]

In addition to homicide, parents may also be liable under statutes that make it criminal for a parent to neglect to support or to provide necessities, to furnish medical attention, to maltreat, to be cruel to, or to endanger the child's life or health.[19]

Liability of Attending Physician

The attending physician who counsels the parents to withhold treatment, or who merely acquiesces in their decision and takes no steps to save the child's life, may also incur criminal liability. Since withholding needed medical care by the parents would in many states constitute child abuse or neglect, the physician who knows of the situation and fails to report the case to proper authorities would commit a crime in the 20 or so states where failure to report child abuse is a crime.[20, 21] While failure to report is only a misdemeanor, under the common law "misdemeanor-manslaughter rule" a person whose misdemeanor causes the death of another is guilty of manslaughter.[11] Since reporting might have led to appointment of a guardian and thus saved the child's life, the physician who fails to report could be guilty of manslaughter.

The physician may also be guilty of homicide by omission (by the same reasoning discussed under Parental Liability), because he has breached a legal duty to care for the child and thereby caused the child's death. The legal duty of the physician would be to intervene directly by carrying out the procedure, or at least to report the case to public or judicial authorities who may then intervene to save the child. The sources of this duty are several. One is the child abuse-reporting statutes, which impose a legal duty to report instances of parental neglect even in those states where failure to report is not criminal.

The duty may also derive from the physician's initial undertaking of care of the child. Although it may appear that by refusing consent the parents have terminated the physician's legal duty to care for the child, there are at least three possible grounds for arguing that the parents are not able to terminate the physician's obligations to the infant-patient, once the doctor-patient relationship has begun, if the patient will be substantially harmed by his withdrawal.

1. The first argument is based on the law of contract. The attending physician has contracted with the parents to provide care for a third party, the infant. Ordinarily the contract for services will be made with an obstetrician, a general practitioner, and/or a pediatrician before or at birth to provide all necessary medical care. When the child is born, this contractual obligation to provide services begins. Under the law of third-party beneficiary contracts, the parties contracting for services to another cannot terminate the obligation to a minor, if the minor would be thereby substantially harmed.[19, 22, 23] Since the parents are powerless to terminate the physician's obligation to care for the child, the physician would have a legal duty to take such steps as are necessary to protect the interests of the child. If emergency treatment were required, the physician would be privileged to proceed without parental consent.[24] In most cases and where feasible, the physician's duty would be better fulfilled by seeking the appointment of a guardian who could then consent to treatment.

The attending physician's contractual duty to care for the child despite parental denial of consent would not exist if the physician clearly agreed to treat the child only if normal, or, if the parents in engaging the physician made their agreement subject to modification in case of a defective birth.[22] However, neither parents nor physicians are likely in prenatal consultations to be so specific. Prosecution could, of course, change prevailing practices.

2. Even if the contract theory were rejected, physicians would still have a legal duty to care for the child on the traditional tort doctrine that one who assumes the care of another, whether gratuitously or not, cannot terminate such care if the third person would be hurt thereby.[11] This rule is based on the idea that one who undertakes care prevents others who might have come to the infant's aid from doing so.[11] Again, the physician could withdraw or not treat only if he has taken steps to notify public or hospital authorities, which would protect the child by leading to the appointment of a guardian.

3. It could be argued that the physician would have a legal duty to protect the child on the ground that he has placed the child in peril through his role as a source of information for the parents. A person who puts another in peril, even innocently and without malice, incurs a legal duty to act to protect the imperiled person.[11, 25-27] By giving the parents adverse prognostic information regarding the infant's handicaps, the economic and psychologic burdens to be faced by the parents, and so on, he may be the immediate cause of nontreatment of the infant, by leading the parents to a decision they would not otherwise have made or perhaps even considered. Under this theory even a consultant might be liable if he communicated information which led to a nontreatment decision and death, particularly if the information was incorrect or unfairly presented and then he took no action to save the child.[19]

In addition to liability for homicide by omission or under the misdemeanor-manslaughter rule, the physician may also be subject to homicide liability as an accessory; an accessory is one who ". . . counsels, encourages or aids or abets another to commit a felony."[11] This would be clearest in a case in which the physician counseled or encouraged the parents to withhold treatment. If omission of care by the parent is criminal, then the physician's liability as an accessory follows. If the physician were indifferent to the child's fate, or preferred that it would live but felt obligated to provide the parents with all the facts, it is less likely he would be culpable, since the requisite intent would be lacking.[19, 28, 29]

The attending physician may be guilty of conspiracy to commit homicide or violate the child abuse or neglect laws. Conspiracy is an agreement between two or more parties to achieve an unlawful objective, with (in most jurisdictions) an overt action toward that end.[11] If parents and physician agree that a defective newborn infant should die, and take any action toward that end, conspiracy could exist. Similarly, a staff conference on a particular case could amount to conspiracy, if the attending physician and others agreed that medical or surgical procedures should be withheld from the child.[19]

LIABILITY OF OTHER PHYSICIANS AND NURSES

Physicians other than the attending physician, such as consultants, house officers, and administrative personnel, might also incur criminal liability under the statutes and common-law principles reviewed above.

Nurses who participate or acquiesce in parental decisions to withhold treatment may also be at risk. While a nurse's care is subordinate to the orders of a physician, her legal duty is not fulfilled simply by carrying out physician orders with requisite skill and judgment. In some cases she is required to act independently or directly counter to the physician, if protection of the patient requires it.[32-34] At the very least, she might be obligated to inform her supervisor. A finding consistent with this view was reached in *Goff* v. *Doctors Hospital of San Jose*[35] where two nurses, the attending physician, and the hospital were held civilly liable when a patient died from postpartum cervical hemorrhage. The nurses were aware the mother was in peril but did not contact the attending physician, because they thought he would not come. The court found that they had a duty to report the situation to a superior.

THE POSSIBILITY OF PROSECUTION

The existence of potential criminal liability is no guarantee that parents, physicians, nurses, and hospitals will in fact be prosecuted, nor that any prosecution will be successful. Parents who have actively killed defective children have often been acquitted (though not always),[36] and no parent has been prosecuted for withholding care from, as opposed to actively killing, a defective newborn infant.[36] Similarly, the only physicians prosecuted for homicide in euthanasia situations involved terminally ill patients, and both were acquitted.[36-38] No doctor has yet been prosecuted for passive euthanasia of a defective newborn infant.

The infrequency of past criminal prosecutions, however, may not be a reliable guide for the future. As the practice becomes more openly acknowledged, pressure may build to prosecute and some prosecution is likely, if only to clarify the law. The manslaughter conviction of a Boston physician for allegedly killing a viable fetus after removal from the uterus during a lawfully performed hysterotomy illustrates the dangers of ignoring the legal issues, and the politics of the process by which a prosecution might be initiated.[13] Physicians, parents, and others may decide that they are willing to risk prosecution, or believe that the law should be broken. Such a position entails risks, and one cannot safely predict from past experience that criminal liability will never in practice be imposed.

PRACTICAL IMPLICATIONS FOR PHYSICIANS AND HOSPITALS

Parents and health-professionals with experience in the complex and heart-wrenching decisions involving defective newborn infants might justifiably react to this legal synopsis with shock and rage. Such decisions are made by people trying to do what they think is best under extremely difficult circumstances. The suggestion that such sincere and well-intended decisions might be criminal is offensive.

The authors do not intend to suggest, in this review, that such criminal charges should be made, nor do we intend to comment, pro or con, on the ethical issues involved in such decisions. Our primary purpose is to suggest that criminal charges *could* be brought, given a susceptible case and a prosecutor willing to pursue it. Some legal scholars might reasonably disagree with the validity of such charges, and we would not predict that such proceedings would necessarily end in conviction. Many would have moral objections to the initiation of such a trial, whatever the law. But few would dispute that such a case could be brought to court and, conceivably, to conviction. The experiences of Dr. Edelin[13] and the participants in the Quinlan cases[10] demonstrate dramatically how parents and physicians involved in medical decisions which have occurred countless times without judicial interference can find themselves unexpectedly at the center of a raging controversy.

What are the implications of these possibilities for physicians and hospitals caring for such infants and desirous of avoiding prosecution? First, physicians could consider informing parents that criminal liability might attach to a nontreatment decision, so that parents could be sufficiently informed of the risk to seek legal advice. In addition, such parents might be informed that even if they do not wish to keep the child, they are legally obligated, at least until parental rights are formally terminated, to provide it with needed medical care. If the parents insist on risking prosecution, the physician might then inform them that he is legally obligated to take steps toward saving the infant's life. In some jurisdictions it would be sufficient to report the matter to the child welfare or other authorities prescribed in the child abuse-reporting laws; in others the physician or the hospital might have to initiate neglect proceedings. The parents cannot terminate the physician's legal duties by withholding consent or even by discharging him. The law does not permit a physician to avoid criminal liability by submitting to the wishes of the parents and doing nothing, if this will lead to injury or death of the infant.

To avoid liability, hospitals could adopt rules prohibiting medical staff from not treating defective newborn infants, or, at least, for following certain procedures when faced with those decisions. The procedure could include reporting such cases to hospital authorities who would then seek a judicial ruling authorizing treatment. Resort to judicial approval, however burdensome and painful in this situation, could perform several useful functions. It would shield parents, physicians, nurses, and hospitals from criminal liability, pass the burden of a difficult decision to a more impartial process, and provide an opportunity to test or challenge the law before rather than after criminal prosecution. If a court ruled for or against treatment, the decision could be appealed to state appellate courts, which could define more precisely the duties involved and, conceivably, permit nontreatment in specific cases. While time would not permit appellate review of most cases, such issues of broad public policy which are sure to recur can be reviewed even though the specific controversy has been resolved by death or treatment.[39]

EVALUATION OF LEGAL POLICY

Many persons who have experienced the dilemma of caring for defective newborn infants would disagree with current law. Duff and Campbell,[6] for instance, argue that "if working out these dilemmas in ways we suggest is in violation of the law . . . the law should be changed." They would grant parents and their physicians the final discretion to decide whether a defective infant should be treated, and hence live or die[6]:

> We believe the burdens of decision making must be borne by families and their professional advisors because they are most familiar with the respective situations. Since families primarily must live with and are most affected by the decision, it therefore appears that society and the health

professions should provide only general guidelines for decision making. Moreover, since variations between situations are so great, and the situations themselves so complex, it follows that much latitude in decision-making should be expected and tolerated.

What law, if any, should govern this situation? Ideally, the law should provide clear rules and predictable enforcement while resolving conflicting interests in a way consistent with prevailing moral, personal, professional, and economic values. Satisfactory law in respect to the defective-infant dilemma depends on the answers to two questions. First, is there a definable class of human offspring from whom, under prevailing moral standards, ordinary medical care may be withheld without their consent? If withholding care can never be justified, the sole policy question is whether the existing legal structures best implement that goal or whether a new offense and penalty structure should be created. The second question arises after one concludes that withholding care in some instances may be morally justified or socially desirable, and asks who among parents, physicians, and other decision makers is best equipped to decide when care is to be withheld? Here policy will focus on criteria, procedures, and decision-making processes for implementing a social policy of involuntary passive euthanasia.

It is the first question over which moral and policy issue is most keenly joined and which is therefore most crucial. Supporters of present law argue that there is no reasonable basis for allocating the right to life among human offspring on the basis of physical and mental characteristics, or social contribution—that all are persons and all deserve the legal protections and rights accorded persons.[19, 40] Many defective newborn infants in fact are capable of achieving some meaningful existence; even if they are not, the social and other costs of maintaining them is but a minute portion of health expenditures.[19] State assistance may be available to parents of modest means, and, in any event, parents who do not wish to keep a defective child are free to terminate their legal obligations. Furthermore, a policy of allocating rights according to personal characteristics, capacity, or social utility requires an arbitrary choice among personal and social characteristics reflective of social, cultural, or racial bias which is easly abused and inconsistent with a democratic society.[42] Determining the right to life by the net social utility of a person's future pitches one onto a slippery slope, the bottom of which holds no person or value sacred as against social utility.

Opponents of the law argue that not only may we reasonably and carefully distinguish between human offspring by their capacities, but we can draw narrow boundaries which do not set us onto the slippery slope where all values are subject to social worth assessments. Given high social and personal costs in keeping alive human beings with only marginal ability for personal development or interaction, the delineation of such a class is justified. Proponents of this view need not hold that every child with Down syndrome or myelomeningocele should not be treated. Only that in some cases, such as anencephaly or myelomeningocele with an extremely unfavorable prognosis,[9] the defects are so extensive that nontreatment is morally and socially justified.

DUE PROCESS AND DECISION MAKING

A choice between these two positions depends ultimately on deeply held philosophical and religious views and is only partially susceptible to rational argument and marshalling of evidence. Rather than attempt to persuade the reader to any one personal view or analyze the ethical issues of specific cases, we suggest that even if after reflection one decides that there is a class of defective newborn infants from whom treatment can be justifiably withheld, it does not follow that parents and physicians should be the sole judge in each case of who shall survive.

The question of specifying the class of defectives and circumstances in which treatment may be justifiably withheld remains. The claim is not that treatment may be withheld from any infant, or even from all infants with some defect, but rather that in some circumstances infants with certain kinds of anomalies should or need not be treated.[43] How then is that class and those circumstances to be identified? What checks or safeguards should exist to be sure that an infant meets those criteria?

The position offered by Duff and Campbell[6]—that parents and physicians should have absolute discretion to decide whether an infant should live or die—appears to go too far. Simply because nontreatment decisions are acceptable in some circumstances of extreme defect, it does not follow that parents and physicians should *always* be free to decide whether all defective infants should live or die. Otherwise they may decide not to treat infants with less extensive defects, whom few persons would agree should die. Indeed, there is no reason to think that parents and physicians would always consider all the factors relevant to a nontreatment decision and reach a socially justified choice. (1) The emotional trauma and conflict of giving birth to a defective newborn infant may make the parents incapable of careful consideration of the issues.[44, 45] (2) Given their own, often conflicting interests, parents and physicians might not scrutinize all factors or balance them out in a fair way.[19] Thus, many parents might decide against treating a baby with Down syndrome, and the physician might agree, even though neither social, financial, nor psychic cost in a particular instance would justify nontreatment. (3) Neither parents nor physicians can claim the special expertise in making complex ethical-social judgments which warrant giving them such broad authority.[46]

What is needed, then, is either a set of authoritative criteria describing the limited circumstances in which ordinary care may be withheld from defective newborn infants, or a process of decision making which minimizes the risk of abuses or mistakes. We do not here attempt to articulate those criteria, other than to point out that if nontreatment is ever justified, it is because the nature of the defect, developmental potential, cost to parent and society, etc. seems overwhelmingly to argue against treatment. Such criteria could be set forth for assessment by the medical and lay community and would have to be revised frequently to incorporate changing medical and social facts. Only in scrutinizing our reasons can we be sure that these decisions are in fact morally defensible. This would reduce the risk of arbitrary decision making and assure that infants are not being allowed to die for specious reasons. One problem concerns the process by which criteria would be formulated. Would a national commission, a legislature, or professional bodies be convened for this purpose? A second major difficulty with specific criteria is the almost limitless and unpredictable complexity of individual cases. Also, defining or articulating criteria in an open public way does lend legitimacy to the practice of taking life on grounds of social utility.

An alternative to the articulation of specific criteria would be a requirement for a better *process* of decision making. A concern with process demonstrates the solemnity of the commitment to life, and the exceptional nature of any deviation from that commitment. In addition, process can assure that criteria are being accurately applied, that limits exist, and that the possibilities of conflicts of interest are minimized.

The essence of due process is to maximize the probability that decisions will be made impartially after full consideration of all relevant facts and interests, rather than on the uncontested perceptions and self-interest of one party.[19, 48] Such a process can be helpful, even if only advisory to parents and physicians, by exposing or sensitizing them to considerations which they might have ignored on their own. A legal conception of due process would entail turning over decision making to someone more likely to be disinterested than the parents or their private physician and assuring that the interests of the child are fully represented in that forum.[19] Alternative decision makers might include one or a group of physicians, a judge, or a mixed lay and medical committee: they could consider the need for decisions and reasons to be stated in writing, and in some cases, judicial review.[19] Although the notion of a "God committee" has been much maligned,[47] experience with institutional "human subjects" committees in recent years suggests that groups can be formed which will improve the ethical acceptability of controversial and complex medical decisions. One last alternative would be a strictly post hoc institutional review process of specific decisions, within the limits of confidentiality, similar to review of other hospital practices as occurs with tissue committees, clinicopathologic conferences, and the like. One objection to this approach is that whatever change it produces is slow, and unjustified deaths might result in the interim.

A crucial theoretical problem in requiring due process would be the setting of limits within which the process must be invoked. If no defective infant can be allowed to die without due process, why should any non-consenting patient be allowed to die? A requirement for inclusion of all such cases would involve a *reductio ad absurdum,* namely, review of every pediatric patient who dies under the care of a physician, since life can almost always be extended to some degree. The public concern over the defective newborn infant, however, does not seem to extend to patients who are terminally ill and allowed to die.

Judicialization of medical decision making is often inappropriate, but where long life is at stake, the forms and procedure of due process may serve to focus the precise issues and increase impartiality. Such process would limit the cases of passive euthanasia to the clearest ones, and thereby limit the precedent-expanding significance of nontreatment.

Unless those who favor nontreatment are willing to subject their selection criteria to critical scrutiny, the practice could be presumed unjustified, and present legal policy continued. If, as Duff and Campbell [6] say, the law needs to be changed, this should not be done unofficially in newborn nurseries but in the traditional open forums, such as legislatures or courtrooms. By claiming the right to act in ignorance or defiance of existing legal principles and statutes, the physician, parent, nurse, or hospital administrator claims a right which he would not ascribe to others.

We believe that resolution of this controversy by a criminal proceeding would not be desirable. We also believe that public opinion would be supportive of such decisions being made outside of the courts, providing the public could be assured that the possibility of abuse is minimal. Such reassurance would at the least depend on a process of institutional or professional review. Alternatively, test cases could be brought anonymously through the legal system. Whatever the mechanism, public scrutiny and involvement is unlikely to disappear and the medical community can probably help patients best by actively participating in the structuring of a resolution, rather than responding to thrusts initiated by others.

Notes

1. Boston Globe, Feb. 25, 1974, p. 1, col. 1.
2. New York Times, Jan. 18, 1974, p. 32, col. 8.
3. Newark Star Ledger, Oct. 3, 1973, p. 32, col. 8.
4. Time, March 25, 1974, p. 84.
5. Trubo R: An act of mercy: Euthanasia today, Los Angeles: Nash, 1973.
6. Duff RS, and Campbell AGM: Moral and ethical dilemmas in the special-care nursery, N Engl J. Med 289:890, 1973.

7. New York Times, June 12, 1974, p. 18, col. 4.

8. Ingraham FD, and Matson DD: Neurosurgery of infancy and childhood, Springfield, Ill., 1954, Charles C Thomas, Publisher, pp. 35–39.

9. Lorber J: Results of treatment of myelomenigocele, Dev Med Child Neurol 13:279, 1971.

10. In Re Karen Quinlan, An Alleged Incompetent. Sup. Ct. N.J. Chancery Division, Morris Cty., Docket No. C-201-75, Nov 10, 1975.

11. LaFave W. and Scott A: Handbook of Criminal law, St. Paul, 1972, West Publishing Company, pp. 182–191.

12. People v. Chavez, 77 Cal. App. 2d 621, 176 P.2d 92, 1947.

13. Robertson JA: Medical ethics in the courtroom, Hastings Center Report 4:1, 1974.

14. Cal. Penal Code 270: 14 (West, 1970).

15. N.J. Stat. Ann tit. 9, 6–1 (West, 1960).

16. State v. Stehr, 92 Neb. 755, 139 N.W. 676 (1913).

17. Craig v. State, 220 Md. 590, 155 A.2d 684 (1959).

18. People v. Pierson, 176 N.Y. 201, 68 N.E. 243 (1903).

19. Robertson JA: Involuntary euthanasia of defective newborns: A legal analysis, Stanford Law Review, 27:213, 1975.

20. Vt. Stat. Ann. tit. 13, 1304, 1974.

21. Cal. Penal Code 273a(1) (West 1970).

22. Rhodes v. Rhodes, 266 S.E. 2d 790 (Ky Ct. App., 1954).

23. Plunkett v. Atkins, 371, P.2d 727 (Okla. Sup. Ct., 1962).

24. Jackovach v. Yokum, 237 N.W. 444 (S. Ct., Iowa 1931).

25. Jones v. State, 220 Ind. 384, 43 N.E. 2d 1017, 1942.

26. King v. Commonwealth, 285 Ky. 654, 148 S.W. 2d 1044, 1941.

27. Depue v. Flateau, 100 Minn. 299, 111 N.W. 2d 1, 1907.

28. Nye and Nissen v. United States, 336 U.S. 613, 1949.

29. Hicks v. United States, 395 F. 2d 468 (8th Cir. 1968).

30. Paulsen M: Child abuse reporting laws: The shape of the legislation, Colum L Rev 67:1, 1967.

31. Purcell v. Zimbelman, 18 Ariz. App. 75, 500 P.2d 535 (Ct. App. 1972).

32. Hubuda v. Trustees of Rex Hospital Inc., 3 N.D. App. 11, 164 S.E. 2d 17 (Ct. App. 1968).

33. Byrd v. Marion Gen. Hosp. 202 N.C. 337, 162, S.E. 738 (1932).

34. Monogue v. Rutland Hospital, 119 Vt. 336, 125 A. 2d 796 (1956).

35. 166 Cal. App. 2d 314, 333 P. 2d 29, 1958.

36. Sanders J: Euthanasia: None dare call it murder, J Crim Law Crim Pol Sci 60:351, 1969.

37. New York Times, Jan. 13, 1974, p. 44, col 4.

38. New York Times, Feb. 10, 1974, p. 98, col 3.

39. Roe v. Wade: 93 S. Ct. 705, 1973.

40. Grunberg F· Who lives and dies? New York Times, April 22, 1974, p 35, col 2.

41. Ames MD, and Schut L: Results of treatment of 171 consecutive myelo-meningoceles, 1963–1968, Pediatrics, 50:466, 1972.

42. Bok S: Ethical problems of abortion, Hastings Center Studies 2:33, 1974.

43. McCormick RA: To save or let die—the dilemma of modern medicine, JAMA 229:172, 1974.
44. Fletcher J: Attitudes toward defective newborns, Hastings Center Studies, 2:21, 1974.
45. Mandelbaum A, and Wheeler ME: The meaning of a defective child to parents. Social Casework 41:360, 1960.
46. Potter R: The paradoxical preservation of principle, Vill L Rev 13:784, 1968.
47. Freeman E: The "God Committee," N Y Times Mag, May 21, 1972.
48. Fost N: How decisions are made: A physician's view, Proceedings of the Skytop Conference on Ethical Issues in Spinal Bifida (in press).

Robertson and Fost have mentioned some of the moral, medical, and legal pitfalls in the practice of passive euthanasia for defective newborns. H. Tristram Engelhardt, Jr., raises some very general questions about the sanctity of life and the rights of persons. He argues that there is a spectrum of increasing value to life, from plant life to higher animal forms. He then distinguishes human *personal* life from human *biological* life, so that some humans are not persons. He argues that neither fetuses nor infants are persons in the strict sense, for they are not rational, self-conscious beings. Still, children are highly valued because of their social roles. He advances several different arguments to show that in the case of deformed infants, "Parents become the obvious ones to decide concerning the treatment of their very young children, as long as that choice does not erode the care of children generally. . . . And parents can properly refuse life-prolonging treatment for their deformed infants if such treatment would entail a substantial investment of their economic and psychological resources." These decisions must always be balancing ones, and Engelhardt does not grant a moral right to refuse such treatment simply because the parent so chooses. (The reader may wish to note that the implications of this paper reach far beyond the problem of euthanasia.)

H. T. Engelhardt, Jr.

MEDICINE AND THE CONCEPT OF PERSON *

Recent advances in medicine and the biomedical sciences have raised a number of ethical issues that medical ethics or, more broadly, bioethics

* An earlier version of this paper was read as a part of the Matchette Foundation Series, "The Expanding Universe of Modern Medicine," The Kennedy Institute and the Department of Philosophy, Georgetown University, Washington, D.C., November 19, 1974. I wish to express my debt to George Agich, Thomas J. Bole, III, Edmund L. Erde, Laurence B. McCullough, and John Moskop for their discussion and criticism of the ancestral drafts of this paper.

have treated. Ingredient in such considerations, however, are fundamentally conceptual and ontological issues. To talk of the sanctity of life, for example, presupposes that one knows (1) what life is, and (2) what makes for its sanctity. More importantly, to talk of the rights of persons presupposes that one knows what counts as a person. In this paper I will provide an examination of the concept of person and will argue that the terms "human life" and even "human person" are complex and heterogeneous terms. I will hold that human life has more than one meaning and that there is more than one sense of human person. I will then indicate how the recognition of these multiple meanings has important implications for medicine.

I. Kinds of Life and Sanctity of Life

Whatever is meant by life's being sacred, it is rarely held that all life is equally sacred. Most people would find the life of bacteria, for example, to be less valuable or sacred than the life of fellow humans. In fact, there appears to be a spectrum of increasing value to life (I will presume that the term sanctity of life signifies that life has either special values or rights). All else being equal, plants seem to be valued less than lower animals, lower animals less than higher animals (such as primates other than humans), and humans are usually held to have the highest value. Moreover, distinctions are made with respect to humans. Not all human life has the same sanctity. The issue of brain-death, for example, turns on such a distinction. Brain-dead, but otherwise alive, human beings do not have the sanctity of normal adult human beings. That is, the indices of brain-death have been selected in order to measure the death of a person. As a legal issue, it is a question of when a human being ceases to be a person before the law. In a sense, the older definition of death measured the point at which organismic death occurred, when there was a complete cessation of vital functions.[1] The life of the human organism was taken as a necessary condition for being a person, and, therefore, such a definition allowed one to identify cases in which humans ceased to be persons.

The brain-oriented concept of death is more directly concerned with human *personal* life.[2] It makes three presuppositions: (1) that being a person involves more than mere vegetative life, (2) that merely vegetative life may have value but it has no rights, (3) that a sensory-motor organ such as the brain is a necessary condition for the possibility of experience and action in the world, that is, for being a person living in the world. Thus in the absence of the possibility of brain-function, one has the absence of the possibility of personal life—that is, the person is dead. Of course, the presence of some brain activity (or more than vegetative function) does not imply the presence of a person—a necessary condition for the life of a person is not a sufficient condition for the life of a person. The brain-oriented concept of death is of philosophical significance, for, among other things, it implies a distinction between human biological life and human personal life, between the life of a human organism and the life of a human person. That human biological life continues after brain death is fairly clear: the body continues to circulate blood, the kidneys function; in fact, there is no reason why the organism would not continue to be cross-fertile (e.g., produce viable sperm) and, thus, satisfy yet one more criterion for biological life. Such a body can be a biologically integrated reproductive unit even if the level of integration is very low. And, if such a body is an instance of human biological but not human personal life, then it is open to use merely as a subject of experimentation without the constraints of a second status as a person. Thus Dr. Willard Gaylin has argued that living but brain-dead bodies could provide an excellent source of subjects for medical experimentation and education [3] and recommends "sustaining life in the brain-dead." [4] To avoid what would otherwise be an oxymoronic position, he is legitimately pressed to distinguish, as he does in fact, between "aliveness" and "personhood," [5] or, to use more precise terminology, between human biological and human personal life. In short, a distinction between the status of human biological and personal life is presupposed.

We are brought then to a set of distinctions: first, human life must be distinguished as human personal and human biological life. Not all instances of human biological life are instances of human personal life. Brain-dead (but otherwise alive) human beings, human gametes, cells in human cell cultures, all count as instances of human biological life. Further, not only are some humans not persons, there is no reason to hold that all persons are humans, as the possibility of extraterrestrial self-conscious life suggests.

Second, the concept of the sanctity of life comes to refer in different ways to the value of biological life and the dignity of persons. Probably much that is associated with arguments concerning the sanctity of life really refers to the dignity of the life of persons. In any event, there is no unambiguous sense of being simply "pro-life" or a defender of the sanctity of life—one must decide what sort of life one wishes to defend and on what grounds. To begin with, the morally significant difference between biological and personal life lies in the fact, to use Kant's idiom, that persons are ends in themselves. Rational, self-conscious agents can make claims to treatment as ends in themselves because they can experience themselves, can know that they experience themselves, and can determine and control the circumstances of such experience. Self-conscious agents are self-determining and can claim respect as such. That is, they can claim the right to be respected as free agents. Such a claim is to the effect that self-respect and mutual respect turn on self-determination, on the fact that self-conscious beings are necessary for the existence of a moral order—a kingdom of ends, a community based on mutual self-respect, not force. Only self-conscious agents can be held accountable for their actions and thus be bound together solely in terms of mutual respect of each other's autonomy.

What I intend here is no more than an exegesis of what we could mean by "respecting persons." Kant, for example, argued that rational beings are "persons, because their very nature [as rational beings] points them out as ends in themselves." [6] In this fashion, Kant developed a distinction between things that have only "a worth *for us*" and persons "whose existence is an end in itself." [7] As a result, Kant drew a stark and clear distinction between persons and non-persons. "A person is [a] subject whose actions are capable of being imputed [that is, one who can act responsibly]. Accordingly, moral personality is nothing but the freedom of a rational being under moral laws (whereas psychological personality is merely the capacity to be conscious of the identity of one's self in the various conditions of one's existence). . . . [In contrast], a thing is that which is not capable of any imputation [that is, of acting responsibly]." [8] To be respected as a moral agent is precisely to be respected as a free self-conscious being capable of being blamed and praised, of being held responsible for its actions. The language of respect in the sense of recognizing others as free to determine themselves (i.e., as ends in themselves) rather than as beings to be determined by others (i.e., to be used as means, instruments to goods and values) turns upon acknowledging others as free, as moral agents.

This somewhat obvious exegesis (or tautological point) is an account of the nature of the language of obligation. Talk of obligation functions (1) to remind us that certain actions cannot be reconciled with the notion of a moral community, and (2) to enjoin others to pursue particular values or goods. The only actions that strictly contradict the notion of a moral community are those that are incompatible with the notion of such a community—actions that treat moral agents as if they were objects. Morality as mutual respect of autonomy (i.e., more than conjoint pursuit of particular goods or goals) can be consistently pursued only if persons in the strict sense (i.e., self-conscious agents, entities able to be self-legislative) are treated with respect for their autonomy. Though we may treat other entities with a form of respect, that respect is never central to the notion of a community of moral agents. Insofar as we identify persons with moral agents, we exclude from the range of the concept person those entities which are not self-conscious. Which is to say, only those beings are unqualified bearers of rights and duties who can both claim to be acknowledged as having a dignity beyond a value (i.e., as being ends in themselves) and can be responsible for their actions. Of course, this strict sense of person is not unlike that often used in the law.[9] And, as Kant suggests in the passage above, it requires as well an experience of self-identity through time.

It is only respect for persons in this strict sense that cannot be violated without contradicting the idea of a moral order in the sense of the living with others on the basis of a mutual respect of autonomy. The point to be emphasized is a distinction between value and dignity, between biological life and personal life. These distinctions provide a basis for the differentiation between biological or merely animal life, and personal life, and turn on the rather commonsense criterion of respect being given that which can be respected—that is, blamed or praised. Moral treatment comes to depend, not implausibly, on moral agency. The importance of such distinctions for medicine is that they can be employed in treating medical ethical issues. As arguments, they are attempts to sort out everyday distinctions between moral agents, other animals, and just plain things. They provide a conceptual apparatus based on the meaning of obligations as respect due that which can have obligations.

The distinctions between human biological life and human personal life, and between the value of human biological life and the dignity of human personal life, involve a basic conceptual distinction that modern medical science presses as an issue of practical importance. Medicine after all is not merely the enterprise of preserving human life—if that were the case, medicine would confuse human cell cultures with patients who are persons. In fact, a maxim "to treat patients as persons" presupposes that we do or can indeed know who the persons are. These distinctions focus not only on the newly problematic issue of the definition of death, but on the question of abortion as well: issues that turn on when persons end and when they begin. In the case of the definition of death, one is saying that even though genetic continuity, organic function, and reproductive capability may extend beyond brain death, personal life does not. Sentience in an appropriate embodiment is a necessary condition for being a person.[10] One, thus, finds that persons die when this embodiment is undermined.

With regard to abortion, many have argued similarly that the fetus is not a person, though it is surely an instance of human biological life. Even if the fetus is a human organism that will probably be genetically and organically continuous with a human person, it is not yet such a person.[11] Simply put, fetuses are not rational, self-conscious beings—that is, given a strict definition of persons, fetuses do not qualify as persons. One sees this when comparing talk about dead men with talk about fetuses. When speaking of a dead man, one knows of whom one speaks, the one who died, the person whom one knew before his death. But in speaking of the fetus, one has no such person to whom one can refer. There is not yet a person, a "who," to whom one can refer in the case of the fetus (compare: one can keep promises to dead men but not to men yet unborn). In short, the fetus in no way singles itself out as, or shows itself to be, a person. This conclusion has theoretical advantages, since many zygotes never implant and some divide into two.[12] It offers as well a moral clarification of the practice of using intrauterine contraceptive devices and abortion. Whatever these practices involve, they do not involve the taking of the life of a person.[13] This position in short involves recurring to a distinction forged by both Aristotle and St. Thomas—between biological life and personal life,[14] between life that has value and life that has dignity.

But this distinction does too much, as the arguments by Michael Tooley on behalf of infanticide show.[15] By the terms of the argument, infants, as well as fetuses, are not persons—thus, one finds infants as much open to infanticide as fetuses are left open to abortion. The question then is whether one can recoup something for infants or perhaps even for fetuses. One might think that a counterargument, or at least a mitigating argument, could be made on the basis of potentiality—the potentiality of infants or the potentiality of fetuses. That argument, though, fails because one must distinguish the potentialities of a person from the potentiality to become a person. If, for example, one holds that a fetus has the potentiality of a person, one begs the very question at issue—whether fetuses are persons. But, on the other hand, if one succeeds in arguing that a fetus or infant has the potentiality to become a person, one has conceded the point that the fetus or infant is not a person. One may value a dozen eggs or a handful of acorns because they can become chickens or oak trees. But a dozen eggs is not a flock of chickens, a handful of acorns is not a stand of oaks. In short, the potentiality of X's to become Y's may cause us to value X's very highly because Y's are valued very highly, but until X's are Y's they do not have the value of Y's.[16]

Which is to say, given our judgments concerning brain-dead humans and concerning zygotes, embryos, and fetuses, we are left in a quandary with regard to infants. How, if at all, are we to understand them to be persons, beings to whom we might have obligations? One should remember that these questions arise against the backdrop of issues concerning the disposition of deformed neonates—whether they should all be given maximal treatment, or whether some should be allowed to die, or even have their deaths expedited.[17]

In short, though we have sorted out a distinction between the value of human biological life and the dignity of human personal life, this distinction does not do all we want, or rather it may do too much. That is, it goes against an intuitive appreciation of children, even neonates, as not being open to destruction on request. We may not in the end be able to support that intuition, for it may simply be a cultural prejudice; but I will now try to give a reasonable exegesis of its significance.

II. Two Concepts of Person

I shall argue in this section that a confusion arises out of a false presupposition that we have only one concept of person: we have at least two concepts (probably many more) of person. I will restrict myself to examining the two that are most relevant here. First, there is the sense of person that we use in identifying moral agents: individual, living bearers of rights and duties. That sense singles out entities who can participate in the language of morals, who can make claims and have those claims respected: the strict sense we have examined above. We would, for example, understand "person" in this sense to be used properly if we found another group of self-conscious agents in the universe and called them persons even if they were not human, though it is a term that usually applies to normal adult humans. This sense of person I shall term the strict sense, one which is used in reference to self-conscious, rational agents. But what of the respect accorded to infants and other examples of non-self-conscious or not-yet-self-conscious human life? How are such entities to be understood?

A plausible analysis can, I believe, be given in terms of a second concept or use of person—a social concept or social role of person that is invoked when certain instances of human biological life are treated as if they were persons strictly, even though they are not. A good example is the mother-child or parent-child relationship in which the infant is treated as a person even though it is not one strictly. That is, the infant is treated as if it had the wants and desires of a person—its cries are treated as a call for food, attention, care, etc., and the infant is socialized, placed within a social structure, the family, and becomes a child. The shift is from merely biological to social significance. The shift is made on the basis that the infant is a human and is able to engage in a minimum of social interaction. With regard to the latter point, severely anencephalic infants may not qualify for the role *person* just as brain-dead adults would fail to qualify; both lack the ability to engage in minimal social interaction.[18] This use of person is, after all, one employed with instances of human biological life that are enmeshed in social roles as if they were persons. Further, one finds a difference between the biological mother-fetus relation and the social mother-child relation. The first relation can continue whether or not there is social recognition of the fetus, the second cannot. The mother-child relation is essentially a social practice.[19]

This practice can be justified as a means of preserving trust in families, of nurturing important virtues of care and solicitude towards the weak, and of assuring the healthy development of children. Further, it has a special value because it is difficult to determine specifically when in human ontogeny persons strictly emerge. Socializing infants into the role *person* draws the line conservatively. Humans do not become persons strictly until sometime after birth. Moreover, there is a considerable value in protecting anything that looks and acts in a reasonably human fashion, especially when it falls within an established human social role as infants do within the role *child*. This ascription of the role *person* constitutes a social practice that allows the rights of a person to be imputed to forms of human life that can engage in at least a minimum of social interaction. The interest is in guarding anything that could reasonably play the role *person* and thus to strengthen the social position of persons generally.

The social sense of person appears as well to structure the treatment of the senile, the mentally retarded, and the otherwise severely mentally infirm. Though they are not moral agents, persons strictly, they are treated as if they were persons. The social sense of person identifies their place in a social relationship with persons strictly. It is, in short, a practice that gives to instances of human biological life the status of persons. Unlike persons strictly, who are bearers of both rights and duties, persons in the social sense have rights but no duties. That is, they are not morally responsible agents, but are treated with respect (i.e., rights are imputed to them) in order to establish a practice of considerable utility to moral agents: a society where kind treatment of the infirm and weak is an established practice. The central element of the utility of this practice lies in the fact that it is often difficult to tell when an individual is a person strictly (i.e., how senile need one be in order no longer to be able to be a person strictly), and persons strictly might need to fear concerning their treatment (as well as the inadvertent mistreatment of other persons strictly) were such a practice not established. The social sense of person is a way of treating certain instances of human life in order to secure the life of persons strictly.

To recapitulate, we value children and our feelings of care for them, and we seek ways to make these commitments perdure. That is, social roles are ways in which we give an enduring fabric to our often inconstant passions. This is not to say that the social role person is merely a convention. To the contrary, it represents a fabric of ways of nurturing the high value we place on human life, especially the life that will come to be persons such as we. That fabric constitutes a practice of giving great value to instances of human biological life that can in some measure act as if they were persons, so that (1) the dignity of persons strictly is guarded against erosion during the various vicissitudes of health and disease, (2) virtues of care and attention to the dependent are nurtured, and (3) important social goals such as the successful rearing of children (and care of the aged) succeed. In the case of infants, one can add in passing a special consideration (4) that with luck they will become persons strictly, and that actions taken against infants could injure the persons they will eventually become.[20]

It should be stressed that the social sense of person is primarily a utilitarian construct. A person in this sense is not a person strictly, and hence not an unqualified object of respect. Rather, one treats certain instances of human life as person for the good of those individuals who are persons strictly. As a consequence, exactly where one draws the line between persons in the social sense and merely human biological life is not crucial as long as the integrity of persons strictly is preserved. Thus there is a somewhat arbitrary quality about the distinction between fetuses and infants. One draws a line where the practice of treating human life as human personal life is practical and useful. Birth, including the production of a viable fetus through an abortion procedure, provides a somewhat natural line at which to begin to treat human biological life as human personal life. One might retort, Why not include fetuses as persons in a social sense? The answer is, Only if there are good reasons to do so in terms of utility. One would have to measure the utility of abortions for the convenience of women and families, for the prevention of the birth of infants with serious genetic diseases, and for the control of population growth against whatever increased goods would come from treating fetuses as persons. In addition, there would have to be consideration of the woman's right to choose freely concerning her body, and this would weigh heavily against any purely utilitarian considerations for restricting abortions. Early abortions would probably have to be allowed in any case in order to give respect due to the woman as a moral agent. But if these considerations are met, the exact point at which the line is drawn between a fetus and an infant is arbitrary in that utility considerations rarely produce absolute lines of demarcation. The best that one can say is that treating infants as persons in a social sense supports many central human values that abortion does not undermine, and that allowing at least early abortions acknowledges a woman's freedom to determine whether or not she wishes to be a mother.

One is thus left with at least two concepts of person. On the one hand, persons strictly can and usually do identify themselves as such—they are self-conscious, rational agents, respect for whom is part of valuing freedom, assigning blame and praise, and understanding obligation. That is, one's duty to respect persons strictly is the core of morality itself. The social concept of person is, on the other hand, more mediate, it turns on central values but is not the same as respect for the dignity of persons strictly. It allows us to value highly certain but not all instances of human biological life, without confusing that value with the dignity of persons strictly. That is, we can maintain the distinction between human biological and human personal life. We must recognize, though, that some human biological life is treated as human personal life even though it does not involve the existence of a person in the strict sense.

III. CONCLUSIONS

I wish to conclude now with a number of reflections reviewing the implications of distinguishing between human biological and human personal life, and between social and strict senses of person. First, it would seem that one can appreciate the general value of human biological life as just that. Human sperm, human ova, human cell cultures, human zygotes, embryos, and fetuses can have value, but they lack the dignity of persons. They are thus, all else being equal, open to socially justifiable experimentation in a way persons in either the strict or social sense should never be. That is, they can be used as means merely.

With infants, one finds human biological life already playing the social role of person. An element of this is the propriety of parents' controlling the destiny of their very young children insofar as this does not undermine the role *child*. That is, parents are given broad powers of control over their children as long as they do not abuse them, because very young children do in fact live in and through their families. Very young children are more in the possession of their families than in their own possession— they are not self-possessed, they are not yet moral agents. They do not yet belong to themselves. In fact, though persons strictly have both rights and duties, persons in the social sense are given moral rights but have no duties. Moreover, others must act in their behalf, since they are not self-determining entities. And when they act in their behalf, they need not do so in a manner that respects them as moral agents (i.e., there is no moral autonomy to respect), but in terms of what in general would be their best interests. Further, the duty to pursue those best interests can be defeated.

At least some puzzles about parental choice with regard to the treatment of their deformed infants or experimentation on their very young children can be resolved in these terms. Parents become the obvious ones to decide concerning the treatment of their very young children as long as that choice does not erode the care of children generally, or injure the persons strictly those children will become. And parents can properly refuse life-prolonging treatment for their deformed infants if such treatment would entail a substantial investment of their economic and psychological resources. They can be morally justified if they calculate expenses against the expected life-style of the child if treated, and the probability of success. Such a utility calculus is justified (i.e., it is in accord with general social interests in preserving the role child) insofar as it involves a sufficiently serious acknowledgment of the value of the role child (i.e., as long as such choices are not capricious and there is a substantial hardship involved so that such investment is "not worth it")[21] in order to maintain the practice of the social sense of person. Further, one can justify social intervention in the form of legal injunctions to treat where such calculations by the parents are not convincing.

As to using very young children in experiments, they can be used in a fashion that adults may not, since they are not persons strictly. By that I mean someone can consent on their behalf when the risk is minimal, the value pursued substantial, when such experiments cannot in fact be performed on adults, and when such treatment does not erode the use of the social sense of person. One might picture here the trial of rubella vaccine on children that was not intended to be of direct benefit to those children, especially those who would grow to be misanthropic bachelors and thus never want to protect fetuses from damage. Nor need one presume anything except that most small children who are vaccinated have in some fashion been coerced or coopted into being vaccinated.

Consequently, with very young children one need not respect caprice in order to maintain the social sense of person. With free agents that is a different matter. Part of the freedom of self-determination is the latitude to act with caprice. For example, adults should be able, all else being equal, to refuse life-prolonging treatment; very young children should not. Surely difficult issues arise with older children and adolescents.[22] But the problems of dealing with free choice on the part of older children and adolescents attest to the validity of the rule rather than defeating it. With adults one is primarily concerned with the dignity of free agents, and what is problematic with respect to adolescents is that they are very much free agents.[23] In contrast, with small children one is concerned with their value (and the value of the social sense of person) and with not damaging the persons the children will become. In intermediate cases (i.e., older children) one must respect what freedom and self-possession does exist.

In summary, fetuses appear in no sense to be persons, children appear in some sense to be persons, normal adult humans show themselves to be persons. Is anything lost by these distinctions? I would argue not and that only clarity is gained. For those who hold some variety of homunculus theory of potentiality, it may appear that something is lost, for example, by saying that infants are not persons strictly. But how they could be such is, on the view I have advanced, at best a mystery. In this respect I would like to add a caveat lest in some fashion my distinction between persons strictly and persons socially be taken to imply that those humans who are only (!) persons socially are somehow set in jeopardy. It is one thing to say that an entity lacks the dignity of being a person strictly, and another thing to say that it does not have great value. For example, the argument with regard to the social role *child* has been that a child is a person socially because it does indeed have great value and because the social sense of person has general value. Children receive the social sense of person because we value children, and moreover because the social sense of person has a general utility in protecting persons strictly. In short, there is no universal way of speaking of the sanctity of life; some life (personal life) has dignity, all life can have value, and human biological life that plays the social role person has a special value and is treated as human personal life.

What I have offered is, in short, an examination of the ways in which the biomedical sciences have caused the concept of person to be reexamined, and some of the conclusions of these examinations. These analyses lead us to speak not only of human biological versus human personal life, of strict versus social concepts of person, but to distinguish, with regard to the sanctity of life, the value of biological life, the dignity of strictly personal life, and the care due to human biological life that can assume the social role of a person.

Notes

1. *Black's Law Dictionary*, 4th ed., rev., s.v. "death."
2. For the first such statutory definition of death see: "Definition of Death," Kan. Stat. Ann., secs. 77–202 (1970).
3. Willard Gaylin, "Harvesting the Dead," *Harper's Magazine*, 249 (September 1974), 23–30.
4. *Ibid.*, p. 28.
5. *Ibid.*
6. Immanuel Kant, *Fundamental Principles of the Metaphysic of Morals*, in *Kant's Critique of Practical Reason and Other Works on the Theory of Ethics*, trans. Thomas K. Abbott, 6th ed. (1873; rpt. London: Longmans, Green and Co., 1909), p. 46; *Kants gesammelte Schriften*, 23 vols., Preussische Akademie der Wissenschaften, eds. (Berlin: Walter de Gruyter, 1902–1956), IV, 428.
7. *Ibid.*
8. Immanuel Kant, *The Metaphysical Principals of Virtue: Part II of The Metaphysics of Morals*, trans. James Ellington (New York: Bobbs-Merrill, 1964), p. 23; Akademie Textausgabe, VI, 223.
9. *Black's Law Dictionary*, 4th ed., rev., s.v. "person."
10. Strictly, the present brain-oriented definition of death distinguishes between a vegetative level of biological life and all higher levels. Report of the Ad Hoc Committee of the Harvard Medical School to Examine the Definition of Brain Death, "An Definition of Irreversible Coma," *Journal of the American Medical Association*, 205 (August 5, 1968), 85–88; Report of the Ad Hoc Committee of the American Electroencephalographic Society on EEG Criteria for Determination of Cerebral Death, "Cerebral Death and the Electroencephalogram," *Journal of the American Medical Association*, 209 (September 8, 1969), 1505–10. The point of this definition (at least in part) is to be conservative, not to make the mistake of prematurely pronouncing someone dead. On that ground, it is better to draw the line between vegetative life and sentient life, rather than between sentient life and self-conscious life. Moreover, non-self-conscious human life can, as will be argued, be treated as a person in other than a strict sense of that concept.
11. I have treated these issues more fully elsewhere. H. Tristram Engelhardt, Jr., "The Ontology of Abortion," *Ethics*, 84 (April 1974), 217–34.
12. If one held that zygotes were persons (i.e., that persons begin at conception), one would have to account for how persons can split into two (i.e., monozygous twins), and for the fact that perhaps half of all persons die

in utero. That is, there is evidence to indicate that perhaps up to 50 percent of all zygotes never implant. Arthur T. Hertig, "Human Trophoblast: Normal and Abnormal," *American Journal of Clinical Pathology,* 47 (March 1967), 249–68.

13. That is, even if such practices might involve some disvalue, it would surely not be that of taking the life of a person. Also, one must recognize that if intrauterine contraceptive devices act by preventing the implantation of the zygote, they would count as a form of abortion.

14. Both Aristotle and St. Thomas held that human persons developed at some point after conception. See Aristotle, *Historia Animalium,* Book II, Chapter 3, 583 b, and St. Thomas Aquinas, *Summa Theologica,* Part 1, Q 118, art. 2, reply to obj. 2. See also St. Thomas Aquinas, *Opera Omnia,* XXVI (Paris: Vives, 1875), in *Aristoteles Stagiritae: Politicorum seu de Rebus Civilibus,* Book II, Lectio XII, p. 484, and *Opera Omnia,* XI, *Commentum in Quartum Librum Sententiarium Magistri Petri Lombardi,* Distinctio XXXI, Expositio Textus, p. 127.

15. Michael Tooley, "A Defense of Abortion and Infanticide," in *The Problem of Abortion,* ed. Joel Feinberg (Belmont, Calif.: Wadsworth Publishing Company, 1973), pp. 51–91.

16. One might think that a counterexample exists in the case of sleeping persons. That is, a person while asleep is not self-conscious and rational, and would seem in the absence of a doctrine of potentiality not to be a person and to be therefore open to being used by others. A sleeping person is, though, a person in three senses in which a fetus or infant is not. First, in speaking of the sleeping person, one can know of whom one speaks in the sense of having previously known him before sleep. One therefore can know whose rights would be violated should that "person" be killed while asleep. His right to his life would *in part* be analogous to a dead man's right to have a promise kept that had been made to him when he was a self-conscious living person. In contrast, the fetus is not yet a person, an entity to whom, for example, promises can be made in anything but a metaphorical sense. Second, the sleeping man has a concrete presence in the world that is uniquely his, a fully intact functioning brain. Though asleep, the fully developed physical presence of the person continues. Third, the gap of sleep will be woven together by the life of the person involved: he goes to sleep expecting to awake and awakes to bring those past expectations into his present life. In short, one is not dealing with the potentiality of something to become a person, but with the potentiality of a person to resume his life after sleep.

17. See, for example, John M. Freeman, "To Treat or Not to Treat," *Practical Management of Meningomyelocele,* ed. John Freeman (Baltimore: University Park Press, 1974), pp. 13–22, and John Lorber, "Selective Treatment of Myelomeningocele: To Treat or Not to Treat," *Pediatrics,* 53 (March 1974), 307–8. Arguments such as Professor Tooley's imply that one may fairly freely employ positive or negative euthanasia in such cases, in that infants are not yet persons. Tooley, "A Defense of Abortion and Infanticide," p. 91.

18. It is important to note that severely anencephalic infants and braindead adults fail to be persons in a social sense because they lack the ability for social interaction, not because they lack the potentiality to become persons.

Markedly senile individuals can thus be persons socially long after they are no longer persons strictly.

19. H. Tristram Engelhardt, Jr., "The Ontology of Abortion," pp. 230–32.

20. That is, once one is committed to refraining from killing infants because of a general interest in the value of the role *child,* one is committed to caring for infants so as not to injure the persons (strict) who will develop out of those infants. If one were to treat infants poorly, one would set into motion a chain of events that would injure the persons who would come to exist in the future (i.e., the persons such injured infants would become). But this presupposes that one has already decided on other grounds that infants should not be subject to infanticide. S. I. Benn fails to make this point; see "Abortion, Infanticide, and Respect for Persons," in *The Problem of Abortion,* p. 102.

21. It is not merely that it is difficult to impose a positive duty upon parents when that positive duty would involve great hardship, but that the actual object of that duty is not a person strictly.

22. See, for example, John E. Schowalter et al., "The Adolescent Patient's Decision to Die," *Pediatrics,* 51 (January 1973), 97–103; and Robert M. Veatch, ed., "Case Studies in Bioethics, Case No. 315," *Hastings Center Report,* 4 (September 1974), 8–10.

23. The issue with adolescents is not that they are not persons, but that special claims to act paternalistically can be made in their regard by parents.

Several of the selections thus far have made reference to the nationally famous case of Karen Ann Quinlan. Legal opinions by the presiding judges in the Superior and Supreme Courts in New Jersey are reprinted as the next selections. While formally these opinions are legal ones, many of the *moral* arguments found in previous selections recur here supporting a judicial decision. Judge Muir argues against allowing Karen Quinlan's parents to order that the respirator that was maintaining her life be turned off. Joseph Quinlan, the father of comatose, 21-year-old Karen Quinlan, asked to be appointed legal guardian of the person and property of his daughter (for reasons of mental incompetency). Her life processes were sustained by a mechanical respirator, and her father asked the court to authorize discontinuance of all "extraordinary" therapeutic procedures affecting her life processes. Justice Muir refuses to grant the father's requests. He argues that Karen Quinlan is alive, by legal and medical definitions, and that since prevailing medical opinion holds that the use of life-sustaining equipment should continue, there is a *duty* (probably moral, medical, and legal) to continue using it. Judge Muir also appeals to the idea that the state has an interest in preserving life and that there is no constitutional right to die that a parent can assert in a proxy manner in the child's behalf. Judge Muir, for these reasons, reaches the conclusion that removal of the respirator would be an act of homicide.*

Justice Robert Muir, Jr.

OPINION IN THE MATTER OF KAREN QUINLAN *

Dr. Morse, . . . a neurologist, asserted with medical certainty that Karen Quinlan is not brain-dead. He identified the Ad Hoc Committee of Harvard Medical School Criteria as the ordinary medical standard for determining brain death and that Karen satisfied none of the criteria. These criteria are set forth in a 1968 report entitled "Report of the Ad Hoc Committee of Harvard Medical School to Examine the Definition of Brain Death": A Definition of "Irreversible Coma," 205 J.A.M.A. 85 (1968).

The report reflects that it is concerned "only with those comatose individuals who have discernible central nervous system activity" and the problem of determining the characteristics of a permanently non-functioning brain. The criteria as established are:

1. Unreceptivity and Unresponsitivity—There is a total unawareness to externally applied stimuli and inner need and complete unresponsiveness. . . . Even the most intensely painful stimuli evoke no vocal or other response, not even a groan, withdrawal of a limb, or quickening of respiration.

2. No Movements or Breathing—Observations covering a period of at least one hour by physicians is adequate to satisfy the criteria of no spontaneous muscular movement or spontaneous respiration or response to stimuli such as a pain, touch, sound or light. After the patient is on a mechanical respirator, the total absence of spontaneous breathing may be established by turning off the respirator for three minutes and observing whether there is any effort on the part of the subject to breathe spontaneously. . . .

3. No Reflexes—Irreversible coma with abolition of central nervous system activity is evidenced in part by the absence of elicitable reflexes. The pupil will be fixed and dilated and will not respond to a direct source of bright light. Since the establishment of a fixed, dilated pupil is clear-cut in clinical practice, there would be no uncertainty as to its presence. Ocular movement (to head turning and to irrigation of ears with ice water) and blinking are absent. There is no evidence of postural activity (deliberate or other). Swallowing, yawning, vocalization are in abeyance. Corneal and pharyngeal reflexes are absent.

As a rule the stretch of tendon reflexes cannot be elicited; i.e., tapping the tendons of the biceps, triceps, and pronator muscles, quadriceps and gastrocnemius muscles with reflex hammer elicits no contraction of the respective muscles. Plantar or noxious stimulation gives no response.

4. Flat Electroencephalogram—Of great confirmatory value is the flat or isoelectric EEG. . . .

* *In re Quinlan,* 137 N.J. super 227 (1975).

All tests must be repeated at least 24 hours later with no change.

The validity of such data as indications of irreversible cerebral damage depends on the exclusion of two conditions: hypothermia (temperature below 90°F.) or central nervous system depressants, such as barbiturates.

Dr. Morse reflected carefully in his testimony on Karen's prognosis. He described her condition as a chronic or "persistent vegetative state." Dr. Fred Plum, a creator of the phrase, describes its significance by indicating the brain as working in two ways. "We have an internal vegetative regulation which controls body temperature, which controls breathing, which controls to a considerable degree blood pressure, which controls to some degree heart rate, which controls chewing, swallowing and which controls sleeping and waking. We have a more highly developed brain, which is uniquely human, which controls our relation to the outside world, our capacity to talk, to see, to feel, to sing, to think. . . . Brain death necessarily must mean the death of both of these functions of the brain, vegetative and the sapient. Therefore, the presence of any function which is regulated or governed or controlled by the deeper parts of the brain which in layman's terms might be considered purely vegetative would mean that the brain is not biologically dead.". . .

Dr. Morse states Karen Quinlan will not return to a level of cognitive function (i.e., that she will be able to say "Mr. Coburn I'm glad you are my guardian."). What level or plateau she will reach is unknown. He does not know of any course of treatment that can be given and cannot see how her condition can be reversed but is unwilling to say she is in an irreversible state or condition. He indicated there is a possibility of recovery but that level is unknown particularly due to the absence of pre-hospital history. . . .

Mrs. Quinlan and the children were the first to conclude Karen should be removed from the respirator. Mrs. Quinlan, working at the local parish church, had ongoing talks with Father Trapasso, who supported her conclusion and indicated that it was a permissible practice within the tenets of Roman Catholic teachings.

Mr. Quinlan was slower in making his decision. His hope for recovery continued despite the disheartening medical reports. Neither his wife nor Father Trapasso made any attempt to influence him. A conflict existed between letting her natural body functioning control her life and the hope for recovery. . . .

Once having made the determination, the Quinlans approached hospital officials to effectuate their decision. . . .

The Quinlans on July 31, 1975, signed the following:

> We authorize and direct Doctor Morse to discontinue all extraordinary measures, including the use of a respirator for our daughter Karen Quinlan.

We acknowledge that the above named physician has thoroughly discussed the above with us and that the consequences have been fully explained to us. Therefore, we hereby RELEASE from any and all liability the above named physician, associates and assistants of his choice, Saint Clare's Hospital and its agents and employees.

The Quinlans, upon signing the release, considered the matter decided. Dr. Morse, however, felt he could not and would not agree to the cessation of the respirator assistance. . . . After checking on other medical case histories, he concluded to terminate the respirator would be a substantial deviation from medical tradition, that it involved ascertaining "quality of life," and that he would not do so.

Karen Quinlan is quoted as saying she never wanted to be kept alive by extraordinary means. The statements attributed to her by her mother, sister and a friend are indicated to have been made essentially in relation to instances where close friends or relatives were terminally ill. In one instance, an aunt, in great pain, was terminally ill from cancer. In another instance, the father of a girl friend was dying under like circumstances. In a third circumstance, a close family friend was dying of a brain tumor. Mrs. Quinlan testified her daughter was very full of life, that she loved life and did not want to be kept alive in any way she would not enjoy life to the fullest. . . .

All defendants rely on *John F. Kennedy Memorial Hospital* v. *Heston,* 58 N.J. 576 (1971) to challenge the constitutional claims asserting no constitutional right to die exists and arguing a compelling State interest in favor of preserving human life.

They all, essentially, contend, since Karen Quinlan is medically and legally alive, the Court should not authorize termination of the respirator, that to do so would be homicide and an act of euthanasia.

The doctors suggest the decision is one more appropriately made by doctors than by a court of law and that under the circumstances of this case a decision in favor of the plaintiff would require ascertainment of quality of life standards to serve as future guide lines.

The Prosecutor, if plaintiff is granted the relief sought, requests a declaratory judgment "with regard to the effect of the homicide statutes and his duty of enforcement."

The hospital also seeks a declaratory judgment that the criteria outlined by the Ad Hoc Committee of the Harvard Medical School to Examine the Definition of Brain Death be sanctioned as the ordinary medical standards for determination of brain death. . . .

Karen Quinlan is by legal and medical definition alive. She is not dead by the Ad Hoc Committee of Harvard Medical School standards nor by the traditional definition, the stoppage of blood circulation and related vital functions. The quality of her living is described as a persistent vegetative state, a description that engenders total sorrow and despair in an emotional sense. She does not exhibit cognitive behavior (i.e., the process of knowing or perceiving). Those qualities unique to man, the higher mental functions, are absent. Her condition is categorized as irreversible and the chance of returning to discriminate functioning remote. Nevertheless, while her condition is neurologically activated, due to the absence of a pre-hospital history, and in light of medical histories showing other comatose patients surviving longer coma periods, there is some medical qualification on the issue of her returning to discriminative functioning and on whether she should be removed from the respirator. There is a serious question whether she can live off the respirator and survive (at least two physicians indicated she could not). It is also apparent that extensive efforts to wean her from the respirator created a danger of more extensive brain injury. There is no treatment suggested. . . .

None of the doctors testified there was *no* hope. The hope for recovery is remote but no doctor talks in the absolute. Certainly he cannot and be credible in light of the advancements medical science has known and the inexactitudes of medical science.

There *is* a duty to continue the life assisting apparatus, if within the treating physician's opinion, it should be done. Here Dr. Morse has refused to concur in the removal of Karen from the respirator. It is his considered position that medical tradition does not justify that act. There is no mention in the doctor's refusal of concern over criminal liability and the Court concludes that such is not the basis for his determination. It is significant that Dr. Morse, a man who demonstrated strong empathy and compassion, a man who has directed care that impressed all the experts, is unwilling to direct Karen's removal from the respirator.

The assertion that Karen would elect, if competent, to terminate the respirator requires careful examination.

She made these statements at the age of twenty. In the words of her mother, she was full of life. She made them under circumstances where another person was suffering, suffering in at least one instance from severe pain. While perhaps it is not too significant, there is no evidence she is now in pain. . . .

The conversations with her mother and friends were theoretical ones. She was not personally involved. It was not under the solemn and sobering fact that death is a distinct choice, see *In re Estate of Brooks*, 32 Ill. 2d 361, 205 N.E.2d 435 (1965). Karen Quinlan while she was in complete control of her mental faculties to reason out the staggering magnitude of the decision not to be "kept alive" did not make a decision. This is not the situation of a Living Will which is based upon a concept of informed consent.

While the repetition of the conversations indicates an awareness of the problems of terminal illness, the elements involved—the vigor of youth that espouses the theoretical good and righteousness, the absence of being presented the question as it applied to her—are not persuasive to establish a probative weight sufficient to persuade this Court that Karen Quinlan would elect her own removal from the respirator. . . .

It is also noted the concept of the Court's power over a person suffering under a disability is to *protect* and aid the best interests. . . . Here the authorization sought, if granted, would result in Karen's death. The natural processes of her body are not shown to be sufficiently strong to sustain her by themselves. The authorization, therefore, would be to permit Karen Quinlan to die. This is not protection. It is not something in her best interests, in a temporal sense, and it is in a temporal sense that I must operate whether I believe in life after death or not. The single most important temporal quality Karen Ann Quinlan has is life. This Court will not authorize that life to be taken from her. . . .

The Common Law concept of homicide, the unlawful killing of one person by another, is reflected in our codified law. N.J.S.A. 2A:113-1, 2 and 5. The intentional taking of another's life, regardless of motive, is sufficient grounds for conviction. *State* v. *Ehlers,* 98 N.J.L. 236, 240–241 (E. & A. 1922); See *People* v. *Conley,* 64 Cal. 2d 310, 411 P.2d 911, 49 Cal. Rptr. 815 (Sup. Ct. 1966). Humanitarian motives cannot justify the taking of a human life. See *State* v. *Ehlers, supra,* at 240–241. The fact that the victim is on the threshold of death or in terminal condition is no defense to a homicide charge. *State* v. *Mally,* 139 Mont. 599, 366 P.2d 868, 873 (Sup. Ct. 1961).

New Jersey has adopted the principles of the Common Law against homicide. While some of the aforecited decisions are from other jurisdictions, they are reflections of the Common Law and therefore dispositive of the manner this State would treat like circumstances. It is a reasonable construction that the law of this State would preclude the removal of Karen Quinlan from the respirator. As such, a Court of Equity must follow the positive statutory law; it cannot supersede it.

A significant amount of the legal presentation to the court has involved whether the act of removing Karen from the respirator constitutes an affirmative act, or could be considered an act of omission. An intricate discussion on semantics and form is not required since the substance of the sought for authorization would result in the taking of the life of Karen Quinlan when the law of the State indicates that such an authorization would be a homicide. . . .

There is no constitutional right to die that can be asserted by a parent for his incompetent adult child. . . .

In *John F. Kennedy Memorial Hospital* v. *Heston,* 58 N.J. 576 (1971), Justice Weintraub indicated "it seems correct to say there is no constitutional right to die." [at 580] In doing so, the Court recognized the

State's interest in preserving life. Equally, this Court recognizes the State's interest in preserving life, particularly in this instance where the Court sits in the capacity of *parens patriae*. There is a presumption that one chooses to go on living. The presumption is not overcome by the prior statements of Karen Quinlan. As previously noted, she did not make the statements as a personal confrontation. Additionally, it is not Karen who asserts her religious belief but her parents. In those instances where the parental standing to assert the religious belief has been upheld, it dealt with future life conduct of their children, not the ending of life. *Wisconsin* v. *Yoder* (1972); *Pierce* v. *Society of Sisters* (1925).

The right to life and the preservation of it are "interests of the highest order" and this Court deems it constitutionally correct to deny Plaintiff's request.

Judges often find themselves in as much disagreement as do ethicists. In the next selection Justice C. J. Hughes of the Supreme Court of New Jersey overturns the lower-court decision by Judge Muir. Judge Hughes' legal and moral reasoning often contrasts with that of Judge Muir. For example, in perhaps the single most important position advanced in his opinion, Judge Hughes states that "the focal point of decision should be the prognosis as to the reasonable possibility of return to cognitive and sapient life, as distinguished from the forced continuance of that biological existence to which Karen seems to be doomed." Whereas Judge Muir seemed to find little if any difference between an act of ceasing life-saving therapy and homicide, Judge Hughes finds them quite distinct acts. For this reason, and also because he is willing to appoint Joseph Quinlan the guardian capable of making the critical decisions, Judge Hughes' position seems more like the American Medical Association position, previously criticized by Rachels. It might be worthy of notice, however, that Judge Hughes does not dispute Judge Muir's contentions that Karen Quinlan is alive and that she does not have a constitutional right to die that is exercisable by her parents.

Justice C. J. Hughes

IN THE MATTER OF KAREN QUINLAN *

The matter [of Karen Quinlan] is of transcendent importance, involving questions related to the definition and existence of death, the prolongation of life through artificial means developed by medical technology

* *In re Quinlan,* 70 N.J. 10, 335 A.2d 647 (1976).

undreamed of in past generations of the practice of the healing arts; the impact of such durationally indeterminate and artificial life prolongation on the rights of the incompetent, her family and society in general; the bearing of constitutional right and the scope of judicial responsibility, as to the appropriate response of an equity court of justice to the extraordinary prayer for relief of the plaintiff. Involved as well is the right of the plaintiff, Joseph Quinlan, to guardianship of the person of his daughter.

Among his "factual and legal contentions" under such Pretrial Order was the following:

    I. Legal and Medical Death
        (a) Under the existing legal and medical definitions of death recognized by the State of New Jersey, Karen Ann Quinlan is dead.

This contention, made in the context of Karen's profound and allegedly irreversible coma and physical debility, was discarded during trial by the following stipulated amendment to the Pretrial Order:

    Under any legal standard recognized by the State of New Jersey and also under standard medical practice, Karen Ann Quinlan is presently alive.

Other amendments to the Pretrial Order made at the time of trial expanded the issues before the court. The Prosecutor of Morris County sought a declaratory judgment as to the effect any affirmation by the court of a right in a guardian to terminate life-sustaining procedures would have with regard to enforcement of the criminal laws of New Jersey with reference to homicide. . . .

Essentially then, appealing to the power of equity, and relying on claimed constitutional rights of free exercise of religion, of privacy and of protection against cruel and unusual punishment, Karen Quinlan's father sought judicial authority to withdraw the life-sustaining mechanisms temporarily preserving his daughter's life, and his appointment as guardian of her person to that end. His request was opposed by her doctors, the hospital, the Morris County Prosecutor, the State of New Jersey, and her guardian *ad litem*. . . .

THE FACTUAL BASE

The experts believe that Karen cannot now survive without the assistance of the respirator; that exactly how long she would live without it is unknown; that the strong likelihood is that death would follow soon after its removal, and that removal would also risk further brain damage and would curtail the assistance the respirator presently provides in warding off infection.

It seemed to be the consensus not only of the treating physicians but also of the several qualified experts who testified in the case, that removal from the respirator would not conform to medical practices, standards and traditions.

The further medical consensus was that Karen in addition to being comatose is in a chronic and persistent "vegetative" state, having no awareness of anything or anyone around her and existing at a primitive reflex level. Although she does have some brain stem function (ineffective for respiration) and has other reactions one normally associates with being alive, such a moving, reacting to light, sound and noxious stimuli, blinking her eyes, and the like, the quality of her feeling impulses is unknown. She grimaces, makes stereotyped cries and sounds and has chewing motions. Her blood pressure is normal. . . .

Karen is described as emaciated, having suffered a weight loss of at least 40 pounds, and undergoing a continuing deteriorative process. Her posture is described as fetal-like and grotesque; there is extreme flexion-rigidity of the arms, legs and related muscles and her joints are severely rigid and deformed. . . .

Several basic findings in the physical area are mandated. Severe brain and associated damage, albeit of uncertain etiology, has left Karen in a chronic and persistent vegetative state. No form of treatment which can cure or improve that condition is known or available. As nearly as may be determined, considering the guarded area of remote uncertainties characteristic of most medical science predictions, she can *never* be restored to cognitive or sapient life. Even with regard to the vegetative level and improvement therein (if such it may be called) the prognosis is extremely poor and the extent unknown if it should in fact occur.

She is debilitated and moribund and although fairly stable at the time of argument before us (no new information having been filed in the meanwhile in expansion of the record), no physician risked the opinion that she could live more than a year and indeed she may die much earlier. . . .

Developments in medical technology have obfuscated the use of the traditional definition of death. Efforts have been made to define irreversible coma as a new criterion for death, such as by the 1968 report of the Ad Hoc Committee of the Harvard Medical School. . . .

But, as indicated, it was the consensus of medical testimony in the instant case that Karen, for all her disability, met none of these criteria, nor indeed any comparable criteria extant in the medical world and representing, as does the Ad Hoc Committee report, according to the testimony in this case, prevailing and accepted medical standards.

We have adverted to the "brain death" concept and Karen's disassociation with any of its criteria, to emphasize the basis of the medical decision made by Dr. Morse. When plaintiff and his family, finally reconciled to the certainty of Karen's impending death, requested the withdrawal of life support mechanisms, he demurred. His refusal was based upon his conception of medical standards, practice and ethics described in the medical testimony. . . .

CONSTITUTIONAL AND LEGAL ISSUES

At the outset we note the dual role in which plaintiff comes before the Court. He not only raises, derivatively, what he perceives to be the constitutional and legal rights of his daughter Karen, but he also claims certain rights independently as parent.

Although generally a litigant may assert only his own constitutional rights, we have no doubt that plaintiff has sufficient standing to advance both positions. . . .

The Right of Privacy

It is the issue of the constitutional right of privacy that has given us most concern. . . .

Although the Constitution does not explicitly mention a right of privacy, Supreme Court decisions have recognized that a right of personal privacy exists and that certain areas of privacy are guaranteed under the Constitution. . . .

The Court in *Griswold* found the unwritten constitutional right of privacy to exist in the penumbra of specific guarantees of the Bill of Rights "formed by emanations from those guarantees that help give them life and substance." 381 U.S. at 484, 85 S.Ct. at 1681, 14 L.Ed. 2d at 514. Presumably this right is broad enough to encompass a patient's decision to decline medical treatment under certain circumstances, in much the same way as it is broad enough to encompass a woman's decision to terminate pregnancy under certain conditions. . . .

The claimed interests of the State in this case are essentially the preservation and sanctity of human life and defense of the right of the physician to administer medical treatment according to his best judgment. In this case the doctors say that removing Karen from the respirator will conflict with their professional judgment. The plaintiff answers that Karen's present treatment serves only a maintenance function. . . . We think that the State's interest *contra* weakens and the individual's right to privacy grows as the degree of bodily invasion increases and the prognosis dims. Ultimately there comes a point at which the individual's rights overcome the State interest. It is for that reason that we believe Karen's choice, if she were competent to make it, would be vindicated by the law. Her prognosis is extremely poor—she will never resume cognitive life. And the bodily invasion is very great—she requires 24 hour intensive nursing care, antibiotics, the assistance of a respirator, a catheter and feeding tube.

Our affirmation of Karen's independent right of choice, however, would ordinarily be based upon her competency to assert it. The sad truth, however, is that she is grossly incompetent and we cannot discern her supposed choice based on the testimony of her previous conversations with friends, where such testimony is without sufficient probative weight. 137 N.J. Super. at 260. Nevertheless we have concluded that Karen's right of privacy may be asserted on her behalf by her guardian under the peculiar circumstances here present.

If a putative decision by Karen to permit this non-cognitive, vegetative existence to terminate by natural forces is regarded as a valuable incident of her right of privacy, as we believe it to be, then it should not be discarded solely on the basis that her condition prevents her conscious exercise of the choice. The only practical way to prevent destruction of the right is to permit the guardian and family of Karen to render their best judgment, subject to the qualifications hereinafter stated, as to whether she would exercise it in these circumstances. If their conclusion is in the affirmative this decision should be accepted by a society the overwhelming majority of whose members would, we think, in similar circumstances, exercise such a choice in the same way for themselves or for those closest to them. It is for this reason that we determine that Karen's right of privacy may be asserted in her behalf, in this respect, by her guardian and family under the particular circumstances presented by this record.

Regarding Mr. Quinlan's right of privacy, we agree with Judge Muir's conclusion that there is no parental constitutional right that would entitle him to a grant of relief *in propria persona.* . . .

The Medical Factor

Having declared the substantive legal basis upon which plaintiff's rights as representative of Karen must be deemed predicated, we face and respond to the assertion on behalf of defendants that our premise unwarrantably offends prevailing medical standards. We thus turn to consideration of the medical decision supporting the determination made below, conscious of the paucity of pre-existing legislative and judicial guidance as to the rights and liabilities therein involved.

> A significant problem in any discussion of sensitive medical-legal issues is the marked, perhaps unconscious, tendency of many to distort what the law is, in pursuit of an exposition of what they would like the law to be. Nowhere is this barrier to the intelligent resolution of legal controversies more obstructive than in the debate over patient rights at the end of life. Judicial refusals to order lifesaving treatment in the face of contrary claims of bodily self-determination or free religious exercise are too often cited in support of a preconceived "right to die," even though the patients, wanting to live, have claimed no such right. Conversely, the assertion of

a religious or other objection to lifesaving treatment is at times condemned as attempted suicide, even though suicide means something quite different in the law. [Byrn, "Compulsory Lifesaving Treatment for the Competent Adult," 44 FORDHAM L. REV., 1 (1975)].

Perhaps the confusion there adverted to stems from mention by some courts of statutory or common law condemnation of suicide as demonstrating the state's interest in the preservation of life. We would see, however, a real distinction between the self-infliction of deadly harm and a self-determination against artificial life support or radical surgery, for instance, in the face of irreversible, painful and certain imminent death. . . .

The medical obligation is related to standards and practice prevailing in the profession. The physicians in charge of the case, as noted above, declined to withdraw the respirator. That decision was consistent with the proofs below as to the then existing medical standards and practices. Under the law as it then stood, Judge Muir was correct in declining to authorize withdrawal of the respirator.

However, in relation to the matter of the declaratory relief sought by plaintiff as representative of Karen's interests, we are required to reevaluate the applicability of the medical standards projected in the court below. The question is whether there is such internal consistency and rationality in the application of such standards as should warrant their constituting an ineluctable bar to the effectuation of substantive relief for plaintiff at the hands of the court. We have concluded not.

In regard to the foregoing it is pertinent that we consider the impact on the standards both of the civil and criminal law as to medical liability and the new technological means of sustaining life irreversibly damaged.

The modern proliferation of substantial malpractice litigation and the less frequent but even more unnerving possibility of criminal sanctions would seem, for it is beyond human nature to suppose otherwise, to have bearing on the practice and standards as they exist. The brooding presence of such possible liability, it was testified here, had no part in the decision of the treating physicians. As did Judge Muir, we afford this testimony full credence. But we cannot believe that the stated factor has not had a strong influence on the standards, as the literature on the subject plainly reveals. . . .

We glean from the record here that physicians distinguish between curing the ill and comforting and easing the dying; that they refuse to treat the curable as if they were dying or ought to die, and that they have sometimes refused to treat the hopeless and dying as if they were curable. In this sense, as we were reminded by the testimony of Drs. Korein and Diamond, many of them have refused to inflict an undesired prolongation of the process of dying on a patient in irreversible condition when it is clear that such "therapy" offers neither human nor humane benefit. We think these attitudes represent a balanced implementation of a profoundly realistic perspective on the meaning of life and death and that they respect the whole Judeo-Christian tradition of regard for human life. . . .

The evidence in this case convinces us that the focal point of decision should be the prognosis as to the reasonable possibility of return to cognitive and sapient life, as distinguished from the forced continuance of that biological vegetative existence to which Karen seems to be doomed.

In summary of the present Point of this opinion, we conclude that the state of the pertinent medical standards and practices which guided the attending physicians in this matter is not such as would justify this Court in deeming itself bound or controlled thereby in responding to the case for declaratory relief established by the parties on the record before us.

Alleged Criminal Liability

. . . We conclude that there would be no criminal homicide in the circumstances of this case. We believe, first, that the ensuing death would not be homicide but rather expiration from existing natural causes. Secondly, even if it were to be regarded as homicide, it would not be unlawful.

These conclusions rest upon definitional and constitutional bases. The termination of treatment pursuant to the right of privacy is, within the limitations of this case, *ipso facto* lawful. Thus, a death resulting from such an act would not come within the scope of the homicide statutes proscribing only the unlawful killing of another. There is a real and in this case determinative distinction between the unlawful taking of the life of another and the ending of artificial life-support systems as a matter of self-determination.

Furthermore, the exercise of a constitutional right such as we have here found is protected from criminal prosecution. See *Stanley* v. *Georgia, supra,* 394 U.S. at 559, 89 S.Ct. at 1245, 22 L.Ed. 2d at 546. We do not question the State's undoubted power to punish the taking of human life, but that power does not encompass individuals terminating medical treatment pursuant to their right of privacy. See *id.* at 568, 89 S.Ct. at 1250, 22 L.Ed. 2d at 551. The constitutional protection extends to third parties whose action is necessary to effectuate the exercise of that right where the individuals themselves would not be subject to prosecution or the third parties are charged as accessories to an act which could not be a crime. . . .

The Guardianship of the Person

The trial court was apparently convinced of the high character of Joseph Quinlan and his general suitability as guardian under other circumstances, describing him as "very sincere, moral, ethical and religious." The court felt, however, that the obligation to concur in the medical care and treatment of his daughter would be a source of anguish to him and would distort his "decision-making processes." We disagree, for we sense from the whole record before us that while Mr. Quinlan feels a natural grief, and understandably sorrows because of the tragedy which has befallen his daughter, his strength of purpose and character far outweighs these sentiments and qualifies him eminently for guardianship of the person as well as the property of his daughter. Hence we discern no valid reason to overrule the statutory intendment of preference to the next of kin.

CONCLUSION

We therefore remand this record to the trial court to implement (without further testimonial hearing) the following decisions:

1. To discharge, with the thanks of the Court for his service, the present guardian of the person of Karen Quinlan, Thomas R. Curtin, Esquire, a member of the Bar and an officer of the court.
2. To appoint Joseph Quinlan as guardian of the person of Karen Quinlan with full power to make decisions with regard to the identity of her treating physicians.

We repeat for the sake of emphasis and clarity that upon the concurrence of the guardian and family of Karen, should the responsible attending physicians conclude that there is no reasonable possibility of Karen's ever emerging from her present comatose condition to a cognitive, sapient state and that the life-support apparatus now being administered to Karen should be discontinued, they shall consult with the hospital "Ethics Committee" or like body of the institution in which Karen is then hospitalized. If that consultative body agrees that there is no reasonable possibility of Karen's ever emerging from her present comatose condition to a cognitive, sapient state, the present life-support system may be withdrawn and said action shall be without any civil or criminal liability therefor, on the part of any participant, whether guardian, physician, hospital or others.

By the above ruling we do not intend to be understood as implying that a proceeding for judicial declaratory relief is necessarily required for the implementation of comparable decisions in the field of medical practice.

Modified and remanded.

Judge Muir and Judge Hughes have given us important court decisions about euthanasia. Judicial decisions, however, are only one sort of legal remedy. Another occurs through the legislative process. The following law was passed in California in 1976 as a "natural death act." The bill allows terminal patients to cease medical care for themselves by means of a "Directive to Physicians" signed in advance. The bill asserts that adult patients have a "fundamental right to control" such decisions affecting them. The bill, however, covers only terminal cases where death is imminent, the process of dying is natural, and there is no deliberate act that directly causes death.

State of California

NATURAL DEATH ACT

LEGISLATIVE COUNSEL'S DIGEST

AB 3060, Keene.   Cessation of medical care for terminal patients.

No existing statute prescribes a procedure whereby a person may provide in advance for the withholding or withdrawal of medical care in the event the person should suffer a terminal illness or mortal injury.

This bill would expressly authorize the withholding or withdrawal of life-sustaining procedures, as defined, from adult patients afflicted with a terminal condition, as defined, where the patient has executed a directive in the form and manner prescribed by the bill. Such a directive would generally be effective for 5 years from the date of execution unless sooner revoked in a specified manner. This bill would relieve physicians, licensed health professionals acting under the direction of a physician, and health facilities from civil liability, and would relieve physicians and licensed health professionals acting under the direction of a physician from criminal prosecution or charges of unprofessional conduct, for withholding or withdrawing life-sustaining procedures in accordance with the provisions of the bill.

The bill would provide that such a withholding or withdrawal of life-sustaining procedures shall not constitute a suicide nor impair or invalidate life insurance, and the bill would specify that the making of such a directive shall not restrict, inhibit, or impair the sale, procurement, or issuance of life insurance or modify existing life insurance. The bill would provide that health insurance carriers, as prescribed, could not require execution of a directive as a condition for being insured for, or receiving, health care services.

The bill would make it a misdemeanor to willfully conceal, cancel, deface, obliterate, or damage the directive of another without the declarant's consent. Any person, not justified or excused by law, who falsifies or forges the directive of another or willfully conceals or withholds personal knowledge of a prescribed revocation with the intent to cause a withholding or withdrawal of life-sustaining procedures contrary to the wishes of the declarant and thereby causes life-sustaining procedures to be withheld or withdrawn, and death to thereby be hastened, would be subject to prosecution for unlawful homicide.

This bill would also provide that, notwithstanding Section 2231 of the Revenue and Taxation Code, there shall be no reimbursement nor appropriation made by this bill for a specified reason.

The people of the State of California do enact as follows:

SECTION 1.   Chapter 3.9 (commencing with Section 7185) is added to Part 1 of Division 7 of the Health and Safety Code, to read:

CHAPTER 3.9.   NATURAL DEATH ACT

7185.   This act shall be known and may be cited as the Natural Death Act.

7186.   The Legislature finds that adult persons have the fundamental right to control the decisions relating to the rendering of their own medical care, including the decision to have life-sustaining procedures withheld or withdrawn in instances of a terminal condition.

The Legislature further finds that modern medical technology has made possible the artificial prolongation of human life beyond natural limits.

The Legislature further finds that, in the interest of protecting individual autonomy, such prolongation of life for persons with a terminal condition may cause loss of patient dignity and unnecessary pain and suffering, while providing nothing medically necessary or beneficial to the patient.

The Legislature further finds that there exists considerable uncertainty in the medical and legal professions as to the legality of terminating the use or application of life-sustaining procedures where the patient has voluntarily and in sound mind evidenced a desire that such procedures be withheld or withdrawn.

In recognition of the dignity and privacy which patients have a right to expect, the Legislature hereby declares that the laws of the State of California shall recognize the right of an adult person to make a written directive instructing his physician to withhold or withdraw life-sustaining procedures in the event of a terminal condition.

7187.   The followng definitions shall govern the construction of this chapter:

(a) "Attending physician" means the physician selected by, or assigned to, the patient who has primary responsibility for the treatment and care of the patient.

(b) "Directive" means a written document voluntarily executed by the declarant in accordance with the requirements of Section 7188. The directive, or a copy of the directive, shall be made part of the patient's medical records.

(c) "Life-sustaining procedure" means any medical procedure or intervention which utilizes mechanical or other artificial means to sustain, restore, or supplant a vital function, which, when applied to a qualified patient, would serve only to artificially prolong the moment of death and where, in the judgment of the attending physician, death is imminent whether or not such procedures are utilized. "Life-sustaining procedure" shall not include the administration of medication or the performance of any medical procedure deemed necessary to alleviate pain.

(d) "Physician" means a physician and surgeon licensed by the Board of Medical Quality Assurance or the Board of Osteopathic Examiners.

(e) "Qualified patient" means a patient diagnosed and certified in writing to be afflicted with a terminal condition by two physicians, one of whom shall be the attending physician, who have personally examined the patient.

(f) "Terminal condition" means an incurable condition caused by injury, disease, or illness, which, regardless of the application of life-sustaining procedures, would, within reasonable medical judgment, produce death, and where the application of life-sustaining procedures serve only to postpone the moment of death of the patient.

7188.   Any adult person may execute a directive directing the withholding or withdrawal of life-sustaining procedures in a terminal condition. The directive shall be signed by the declarant in the presence of two witnesses not related to the declarant by blood or marriage and who would not be entitled to any portion of the estate of the declarant upon his decease under any will of the declarant or codicil thereto then existing or, at the time of the directive, by operation of law then existing. In addition, a witness to a directive shall not be the attending physician, an employee of the attending physician or a health facility in which the declarant is a patient, or any person who has a claim against any portion of the estate of the declarant upon his decease at the time of the execution of the directive. The directive shall be in the following form:

DIRECTIVE TO PHYSICIANS

Directive made this _____ day of _____ (month, year).

I _____, being of sound mind, willfully, and voluntarily make known my desire that my life shall not be artificially prolonged under the circumstances set forth below, do hereby declare:

1. If at any time I should have an incurable injury, disease, or illness certified to be a terminal condition by two physicians, and where the application of life-sustaining procedures would serve only to artificially prolong the moment of my death and where my physician determines that my death is imminent whether or not life-sustaining procedures are utilized,

I direct that such procedures be withheld or withdrawn, and that I be permitted to die naturally.

2. In the absence of my ability to give directions regarding the use of such life-sustaining procedures, it is my intention that this directive shall be honored by my family and physician(s) as the final expression of my legal right to refuse medical or surgical treatment and accept the consequences from such refusal.

3. If I have been diagnosed as pregnant and that diagnosis is known to my physician, this directive shall have no force or effect during the course of my pregnancy.

4. I have been diagnosed and notified at least 14 days ago as having a terminal condition by _____ M.D., whose address is _____, and whose telephone number is _____. I understand that if I have not filled in the physician's name and address, it shall be presumed that I did not have a terminal condition when I made out this directive.

5. This directive shall have no force or effect five years from the date filled in above.

6. I understand the full import of this directive and I am emotionally and mentally competent to make this directive.

Signed _____

City, County and State of Residence _____

The declarant has been personally known to me and I believe him or her to be of sound mind.

Witness _____

Witness _____

7188.5.   A directive shall have no force or effect if the declarant is a patient in a skilled nursing facility as defined in subdivision (c) of Section 1250 at the time the directive is executed unless one of the two witnesses to the directive is a patient advocate or ombudsman as may be designated by the State Department of Aging for this purpose pursuant to any other applicable provision of law. The patient advocate or ombudsman shall have the same qualifications as a witness under Section 7188.

The intent of this section is to recognize that some patients in skilled nursing facilities may be so insulated from a voluntary decisionmaking role, by virtue of the custodial nature of their care, as to require special assurance that they are capable of willfully and voluntarily executing a directive.

7189.   (a) A directive may be revoked at any time by the declarant, without regard to his mental state or competency, by any of the following methods:

(1) By being canceled, defaced, obliterated, or burnt, torn, or otherwise destroyed by the declarant or by some person in his presence and by his direction.

(2) By a written revocation of the declarant expressing his intent to revoke, signed and dated by the declarant. Such revocation shall become effective only upon communication to the attending physician by the declarant or by a person acting on behalf of the declarant. The attending physician shall record in the patient's medical record the time and date when he received notification of the written revocation.

(3) By a verbal expression by the declarant of his intent to revoke the directive. Such revocation shall become effective only upon communication to the attending physician by the declarant or by a person acting on behalf of the declarant. The attending physician shall record in the patient's medical record the time, date, and place of the revocation and the time, date, and place, if different, of when he received notification of the revocation.

(b) There shall be no criminal or civil liability on the part of any person for failure to act upon a revocation made pursuant to this section unless that person has actual knowledge of the revocation.

7189.5.   A directive shall be effective for five years from the date of execution thereof unless sooner revoked in a manner prescribed in Section 7189. Nothing in this chapter shall be construed to prevent a declarant from reexecuting a directive at any time in accordance with the formalities of Section 7188, including reexecution subsequent to a diagnosis of a terminal condition. If the declarant has executed more than one directive, such time shall be determined from the date of execution of the last directive known to the attending physician. If the declarant becomes comatose or is rendered incapable of communicating with the attending physician, the directive shall remain in effect for the duration of the comatose condition or until such time as the declarant's condition renders him or her able to communicate with the attending physician.

7190.   No physician or health facility which, acting in accordance with the requirements of this chapter, causes the withholding or withdrawal of life-sustaining procedures from a qualified patient, shall be subject to civil liability therefrom. No licensed health professional, acting under the direction of a physician, who participates in the withholding or withdrawal of life-sustaining procedures in accordance with the provisions of this chapter shall be subject to any civil liability. No physician, or licensed health professional acting under the direction of a physician, who participates in the withholding or withdrawal of life-sustaining procedures in accordance with the provisions of this chapter shall be guilty of any criminal act or of unprofessional conduct.

7191.   (a) Prior to effecting a withholding or withdrawal of life-sustaining procedures from a qualified patient pursuant to the directive, the attending physician shall determine that the directive complies with Section

7188, and, if the patient is mentally competent, that the directive and all steps proposed by the attending physician to be undertaken are in accord with the desires of the qualified patient.

(b) If the declarant was a qualified patient at least 14 days prior to executing or reexecuting the directive, the directive shall be conclusively presumed, unless revoked, to be the directions of the patient regarding the withholding or withdrawal of life-sustaining procedures. No physician, and no licensed health professional acting under the direction of a physician, shall be criminally or civilly liable for failing to effectuate the directive of the qualified patient pursuant to this subdivision. A failure by a physician to effectuate the directive of a qualified patient pursuant to this division shall constitute unprofessional conduct if the physician refuses to make the necessary arrangements, or fails to take the necessary steps, to effect the transfer of the qualified patient to another physician who will effectuate the directive of the qualified patient.

(c) If the declarant becomes a qualified patient subsequent to executing the directive, and has not subsequently reexecuted the directive, the attending physician may give weight to the directive as evidence of the patient's directions regarding the withholding or withdrawal of life-sustaining procedures and may consider other factors, such as information from the affected family or the nature of the patient's illness, injury, or disease, in determining whether the totality of circumstances known to the attending physician justify effectuating the directive. No physician, and no licensed health professional acting under the direction of a physician, shall be criminally or civilly liable for failing to effectuate the directive of the qualified patient pursuant to this subdivision.

7192. (a) The withholding or withdrawal of life-sustaining procedures from a qualified patient in accordance with the provisions of this chapter shall not, for any purpose, constitute a suicide.

(b) The making of a directive pursuant to Section 7188 shall not restrict, inhibit, or impair in any manner the sale, procurement, or issuance of any policy of life insurance, nor shall it be deemed to modify the terms of an existing policy of life insurance. No policy of life insurance shall be legally impaired or invalidated in any manner by the withholding or withdrawal of life-sustaining procedures from an insured qualified patient, notwithstanding any term of the policy to the contrary.

(c) No physician, health facility, or other health provider, and no health care service plan, insurer issuing disability insurance, self-insured employee welfare benefit plan, or nonprofit hospital service plan, shall require any person to execute a directive as a condition for being insured for, or receiving, health care services.

7193. Nothing in this chapter shall impair or supersede any legal right or legal responsibility which any person may have to effect the withholding or withdrawal of life-sustaining procedures in any lawful manner. In such respect the provisions of this chapter are cumulative.

7194. Any person who willfully conceals, cancels, defaces, obliterates, or damages the directive of another without such declarant's consent shall be guilty of a misdemeanor. Any person who, except where justified or excused by law, falsifies or forges the directive of another, or willfully conceals or withholds personal knowledge of a revocation as provided in Section 7189, with the intent to cause a withholding or withdrawal of life-sustaining procedures contrary to the wishes of the declarant, and thereby, because of any such act, directly causes life-sustaining procedures to be withheld or withdrawn and death to thereby be hastened, shall be subject to prosecution for unlawful homicide as provided in Chapter 1 (commencing with Section 187) of Title 8 of Part 1 of the Penal Code.

7195. Nothing in this chapter shall be construed to condone, authorize, or approve mercy killing, or to permit any affirmative or deliberate act or omission to end life other than to permit the natural process of dying as provided in this chapter.

SEC. 2. If any provision of this act or the application thereof to any person or circumstances is held invalid, such invalidity shall not affect other provisions or applications of the act which can be given effect without the invalid provision or application, and to this end the provisions of this act are severable.

SEC. 3. Notwithstanding Section 2231 of the Revenue and Taxation Code, there shall be no reimbursement pursuant to this section nor shall there be any appropriation made by this act because the Legislature recognizes that during any legislative session a variety of changes to laws relating to crimes and infractions may cause both increased and decreased costs to local government entities and school districts which, in the aggregate, do not result in significant identifiable cost changes.

The California Natural Death Act was subjected to intense legislative criticism before its final passage. Some of the reasons why many persons are opposed not only to this particular bill but to living wills in general are surveyed in the following selection by Richard McCormick and André Hellegers. While they agree with the objectives of the California Bill, they believe the bill will actually be counterproductive by "lessening patients' rights." They especially object to the notion that the law is used as an instrument to assure patients' rights rather than allowing the decision making to be made within the confines of the physician-patient relationship. They propose alternative legislation that is free of the "philosophical and practical problems" they find in the California Bill.

Richard A. McCormick

André E. Hellegers

LEGISLATION AND THE LIVING WILL *

Last fall, Gov. Edmund G. Brown Jr. of California signed A. B. 3060, known as the Natural Death Act, a bill that had been introduced by the State Assemblyman, Barry Keene. This historic act provides for the possibility of a written directive by an adult patient authorizing the "withholding or withdrawal of extraordinary life-sustaining procedures" in the situation of "terminal illness." The California Legislature explicitly stated the reasoning behind the motivation of the bill. It emphasized the right of adult patients to control decisions relating to their own medical care; the advance in powerful, modern life-sustaining devices; the hardships associated with some prolongation of life (loss of patient dignity, unnecessary suffering, unreasonable emotional and financial hardship on the patient's family); and, above all, the existing uncertainty in the medical and legal professions about the legality of terminating the use of life-sustaining procedures "where the patient has voluntarily and in sound mind evidenced a desire that such procedures be withheld or withdrawn." There can be little doubt that New Jersey's Karen Ann Quinlan case intensified this latter concern.

The effect of the bill is to relieve physicians, paramedical personnel and health facilities from civil liability or criminal prosecution when they act according to the provisions of the bill. Furthermore, A. B. 3060 provides that action according to such provisions shall not constitute a suicide. . . . We concentrate on three considerations: the presuppositions of such legislation, the possible consequences and an alternative solution.

PRESUPPOSITIONS

The medical profession is the servant of patients, not their master. In one sense, the living-will legislation seeks to maintain this self-determination of the patient. But in another, it dangerously abdicates this patient control. The need to write a living will to prevent the use of so-called extraordinary means implies that in some way physicians are masters of

* From *America,* 136, no. 10 (March 12, 1977), 210–13 (slightly edited). Reprinted by permission.

their patients, unless patients take legal action in advance. Thus, it raises the entire question of the locus of power in those cases where no living will has been written, either because the potential patient was too young to write a will (the child) or because the potential patient was not aware of the implications of writing, or not writing, such a will.

Our opposition, then, to living-will legislation does not stem from what such legislation seeks to achieve, namely the self-determination of the patient over his or her own fate in the face of a potentially abusive use of technology. Rather, we question whether such legislation may not result in precisely the opposite effect. We have no objection to the living will as a signal sent in advance by knowledgeable persons to their potential physicians. Indeed, such informal documents can be immensely helpful and reassuring. Our profound misgivings stem from the notion of living wills as law. The very fact that a law is deemed necessary to assure patients' rights implies, and therefore tends to reinforce, an erroneous presupposition about the locus of decision making in the physician-patient relationship.

The Karen Ann Quinlan case is a dramatic example. In that case, the Quinlan family sought to subtract their daughter from the jurisdiction of her physicians. We believe the Quinlan parents were justified in asking that the use of the respirator be stopped. Dr. Jack E. Zimmerman, director of the intensive care unit at Washington, D. C.'s George Washington University Medical Center reflected what is widely regarded as the attitude of most physicians. If Joseph Quinlan had asked physicians at the intensive care unit to turn off his daughter's respirator, Mr. Quinlan's request "would have been met." Contrarily, if her actual physicians believe the request of the Quinlan family to be frivolous, we believe the moral onus was upon those physicians to have resort to the courts to subtract Karen Ann from the guardianship of her parents. The way events developed in that case, the presumptions were that physicians have a right to treat a patient unasked, indeed, opposed. We reject that premise. We believe that, both philosophically and practically, proposed laws on death with dignity or living wills tend to enshrine the notion that physicians are masters of their patients and not their servants.

What is objectionable about such enshrinement? We believe it is both wrong in itself and threatening in its implications. It is wrong in itself because the individual, having the prime obligation for his own health care, has also thereby the right to the necessary means for such basic health care—specifically, the right of self-determination in the acceptance or rejection of treatment. When an individual puts himself into a doctor's hands, he engages the doctor's services; he does not abdicate his right to decide his own fate. Patients retain the right to refuse a physician's advice, however ill-advised they might be in doing so.

No one has made that point more clearly than Pius XII. In an address to the International Congress of Anesthesiologists on Nov. 24, 1957, the Holy Father stated: "The rights and duties of the doctor are correlative to those of the patient. The doctor, in fact, has no separate or independent right where the patient is concerned. In general, he can take action only if the patient explicitly or implicitly, directly or indirectly, gives him permission." Furthermore, Pius XII stated that when the patient, of age and *sui juris,* is unconscious, it is the right and duty of the family to make decisions based on the presumed will of the unconscious patient. Thus, he explicitly concluded that when attempts at resuscitation become too onerous, "they [the family] can lawfully insist that the doctor should discontinue these attempts, and the doctor can lawfully comply.". . .

CONSEQUENCES

The Intestate

The first consequence of the proposed legislation is the abandonment to codification of a right that human beings inherently have, i.e., to refuse to be treated by any or all physicians. The very proposal to write such legislation easily suggests the practical conclusion that that right must be acquired. That immediately raises the issue: What does the law do to or for those who have written no will? . . . Until now, no legislature has proposed the introduction of laws whereby potential patients can demand extraordinary therapy treatment, as most often legally depicted, that maintains circulation and respiration without being able to cure the disease. Must or may the physician assume, without a will, that his patient wants extraordinary means used, since the patient had an opportunity to write a will? At stake, then, is whether the onus is on the individual to write a will if he wishes to avoid excessive resuscitation.

Since the intestate—and they are likely to be the vast majority—are left unprotected in a medico-moral limbo, we fear the growth of the popular misconception that living-will legislation confers rights rather than recognizes them. This is particularly dangerous in our time because once the right to refuse treatment is construed as conferral, the traditional distinction between omission and commission (officially adopted by the American Medical Association in 1973) is threatened. In other words, if the right is not viewed as basically a natural right—with inherent moral limitations—but a conferred right, then on such a view the law could also confer the right to be killed. It is a well known fact that advocates of mercy killing strongly support so-called death-with-dignity bills.

Family

The second effect of living wills is that they tend to exclude the family from any responsibility. Advocates of living wills see this as a desirable aim, for they argue that families tend to insist on excessive treatment. On the other hand, families are theoretically more likely to know the wishes of their relatives than physicians who may never have met them in health. Moreover, many physicians hold that it is very important for a family to participate in decision making. They are, in a sense, both copatient and cophysician, copatient because they are afraid, cophysician because they would be the physician if they could. The living will essentially excludes the family from any decision making for those who have written one. As yet undetermined, even undiscussed, is the role of the family in the case of the intestate patient. If absence of a will is taken to be an indicator of the patient's desire for extraordinary means (or else he would have written a will), the family is again excluded.

Penalties and Practice

In most living-will legislation, there is no penalty attached for violation. In this case, it is not clear why the legislation is written in the first place; for a medal, an arm band or even a written document without legal force would suffice to inform a physician of the patient's general philosophy of living or dying.

In some proposals, however, violation of the declarant's wishes is a misdemeanor. The effects of this on practice are rarely discussed. To under-resuscitate a patient with a living will may lead to his death, but is unlikely to lead to a penalty since it is against overtreatment that the will is directed. Conversely, to overresuscitate a patient with a will and leave him in a state repugnant to him may save his life, but makes the physician liable for the penalty. In sum, then, where penalties are attached to the law, it is not inconceivable that those with wills will be needlessly underresuscitated and those without wills overresuscitated. Paradoxically, since it is likely that large numbers, through neglect or ignorance, will never write a will, it is not unlikely that the legislation will lead to an increase in excessive treatment rather than a decrease.

Emergencies

There is likely to be a practical problem in emergencies. It is a fact that fewer and fewer patients today have private physicians—about 25 percent by most estimates. Moreover, family physicians, with close ties to their patients, are not likely to be the ones at whom the legislation is aimed. Excessive treatment is a problem of patients outside primary care, in impersonal hospials with modern technologies. Emergency rooms in hospitals are unlikely places in which to search for wills, while having to decide, almost instantaneously, whether to resuscitate or not. It is highly unlikely that a law on living wills can work in such an emergency setting in the way it is intended, unless physicians refrain from resuscitating to be on the safe side of being penalized.

Conscience Clauses

In some states, it is proposed to add a "conscience clause" to death-with-dignity bills so that the physician need not comply. He then must transfer the patient to another doctor willing to comply. Paradoxically, unwise as we think living-will legislation is, the effect of conscience clauses only accentuates our first misgivings about such legislation. The conscience clause gives to a physician precisely those rights of possession of patients that we deny in the first place, yet that this legislation seems tacitly to assume. Physicians have always had the right to withdraw from a case if they are asked to perform acts that are incompatible with their conscience as physicians or individuals. To codify this freedom changes by implication the onus and assumes that, without taking a legal provision, the physician has lost an inherent right. So the proposed legislation assumes, philosophically, that the traditional rights of physicians to withdraw from their patients, or vice versa, do not exist and must be asserted.

ALTERNATIVE

There are two main reasons why living-will legislation might, in theory, be written: (1) because without it, patients cannot subtract themselves from physicians who will overtreat them; (2) because without it, doctors are not free to render such treatment as they wish to give and patients desire to receive. We believe that legislation is not designed above all to protect patients against the excessive zeal of physicians, but to protect physicians against existing laws that hamper their freedom to omit extraordinary means of treatment when patients and their families do not wish to undergo such treatment. In a recent poll conducted by the American Medical Association (*A.M.A. News,* January 24), 94.5 percent of the physicians polled stated that they normally try to adhere to a terminally ill patient's expressed wishes about the nature and extent of care to be provided as death approaches. More concretely, most surveyed stated that when a patient had made a no-intervention decision, a doctor should respect it. The same poll indicated that legal constraints are most often mentioned by 67.5 percent of doctors when they are asked what factors might keep them from acceding to a patient's wishes. Thus, fear may exist among physicians that to omit or cease a therapy could be construed under existing laws to constitute malpractice or even homicide.

If this be the case, we suggest that it is, both in discussion and legislation, better to face directly the issue of physician protection from existing laws rather than to imply that the problem is one of protecting patients from excessive zeal in physicians. We suggest such legislation can be written without the creation of the philosophical and practical problems alluded to above.

Without going into detail, we suggest that legislation could be written which simply states that, when a patient suffers from a fatal disease, a physician can register that fact with an appropriate hospital body that would have the right, but not the duty, to verify the fact. A mentally competent patient could then request in writing that no extraordinary treatment be applied to him. Where a patient was incompetent to act, by age or condition, the family could make a similar written request. Once the written request had been made, the legislation could stipulate that the treating physician was not subject to civil or criminal prosecution for omitting or ceasing treatment.

In those cases where it was the opinion of the physician that the patients, or their families, were needlessly or frivolously jeopardizing the patients' lives, the physician could notify the same committee, which could then have recourse to the courts to place the patient under guardianship. It should be noted that our proposal diametrically opposes the procedures followed in the Karen Ann Quinlan case, where the moral onus fell upon the parents to subtract their daughter from the jurisdiction of her physicians.

If the key problem is one of malpractice and homicide law, we suggest it be addressed directly. But we deplore the trend to do so by writing laws that too easily suggest that there is an inherent right of physicians over patients, unless those patients can assert their independence from unasked-for and uncalled-for ministrations by physicians through the mechanisms of writing a will in advance. Will not the freedom of physicians and patients be threatened by such an approach? We fear so.

SUGGESTED READINGS FOR CHAPTER 4

Books and Articles

BEAUCHAMP, TOM L. "The Moral Justification for Cessation of Extraordinary Therapeutic Procedures," in *Emerging Medical, Moral, and Legal Concerns,* ed. A. W. Siemsen, et al. New York, 1978.

BEAUCHAMP, TOM L., and WALTERS, LEROY, eds. *Contemporary Issues in Bioethics.* Encino, Calif.: Dickenson Publishing Co., 1978. Chap. 7.

BEHNKE, JOHN A., and BOK, SISSELA. *The Dilemma of Euthanasia.* Garden City, N.Y.: Doubleday Anchor Books, 1975.

BOK, SISSELA. "Personal Directions for Care at the End of Life." *New England Journal of Medicine,* 295 (August 12, 1976), 367–69.

DOWNING, A. B. *Euthanasia and the Right to Die.* New York: Humanities Press, 1970.

DYCK, ARTHUR. "An Alternative to the Ethic of Euthanasia." In Williams, Robert H., ed. *To Live and To Die: When, Why, and How.* New York: Springer-Verlag, 1973. Pp. 98–112.

ENGELHARDT, H. TRISTAM. "Euthanasia and Children: The Injury of Continued Existence." *Journal of Pediatrics,* 83 (July 1973), 170–71.

FLETCHER, GEORGE. "Prolonging Life." 42 WASHINGTON LAW REVIEW 999–1016 (1967).

FLETCHER, JOSEPH. "Ethics and Euthanasia." In Williams, Robert H., ed. *To Live and To Die: When, Why, and How.* New York: Springer-Verlag, 1973. Pp. 113–22.

FOOT, PHILIPPA. "Euthanasia." *Philosophy and Public Affairs,* 6 (Winter 1977), 85–112.

GUSTAFSON, JAMES M. "Mongolism, Parental Desires, and the Right to Life." *Perspectives in Biology and Medicine,* 16 (Summer 1973), 529–57.

HARE, R. M. "Euthanasia: A Christian View." *Philosophic Exchange,* 2 (Summer 1975), 43–52.

KOHL, MARVIN, ed. *Beneficent Euthanasia.* Buffalo: Prometheus Books, 1975.

MAGUIRE, DANIEL C. *Death By Choice.* Garden City, N.Y.: Doubleday & Company, 1974.

McCORMICK, RICHARD A. "To Save or Let Die." *Journal of the American Medical Association,* 229 (July 8, 1974), 172–76.

Massachusetts General Hospital, Clinical Care Committee. "Optimum Care for Hopelessly Ill Patients." *New England Journal of Medicine,* 295 (August 12, 1976), 362–64.

SHAW, ANTHONY. "Dilemmas of 'Informed Consent' in Children." *New England Journal of Medicine,* 289 October 25, 1973), 885–90.

VEATCH, ROBERT M. *Death, Dying and the Biological Revolution.* New Haven: Yale University Press, 1976.

WILLIAMS, GLANVILLE. "Euthanasia and Abortion." *University of Colorado Law Review,* 38 (1966).

WOOZLEY, A. D. "Euthanasia and the Principle of Harm." *Philosophy and Public Policy.* Norfolk, Va.: Teagle and Little, 1977. Pp. 93–100.

Bibliographies

CLOUSER, K. DANNER, and ZUCKER, ARTHUR, eds. *Abortion and Euthanasia: An Annotated Bibliography.* Philadelphia: Society for Health and Human Values, 1974.

Euthanasia Educational Fund. "Euthanasia—An Annotated Bibliography" (May 1970). [250 W. 57th St., New York, N.Y. 10019]

SOLLITTO, SHARMON, and VEATCH, ROBERT M., comps. *Bibliography of Society, Ethics, and the Life Sciences.* Hastings-on-Hudson, N.Y.: Institute of Society, Ethics, and the Life Sciences, 1976. Issued annually since 1973.

WALTERS, LEROY, ed. *Bibliography of Bioethics.* Detroit: Gale Research Co. Issued annually since 1975. See under "Active Euthanasia," "Allowing to Die," "Euthanasia," "Living Wills," "Prolongation of Life," "Treatment Refusal," "Voluntary Euthanasia," and "Withholding Treatment."

Encyclopedia of Bioethics Articles

ACTING AND REFRAINING—HAROLD MOORE

AGING AND THE AGED: Ethical Implications in Aging—DREW CHRISTIANSEN

DOUBLE EFFECT—WILLIAM E. MAY

INFANTICIDE—MICHAEL TOOLEY

LIFE: Value of Life—PETER SINGER

LIFE: Quality of Life—WARREN T. REICH

LIFE SUPPORT DEVICES: Philosophical Perspective—A. G. M. VAN MELSEN

PAIN AND SUFFERING: Philosophical Perspective — JEROME SHAFFER

PATERNALISM—TOM L. BEAUCHAMP

PERSON—A. G. M. VAN MELSEN

5

THE SIGNIFICANCE OF LIFE AND DEATH

INTRODUCTION

A recurrent theme in much philosophical, literary, and religious litera-ture has to do with the meaning or meaninglessness of life and death. Most of us have felt, at least occasionally, that death is an inherent evil whose ultimate victory renders life meaningless. Indeed, many persons have felt intensely and for prolonged periods that absolutely nothing about hu-man existence is really worthwhile or significant. This conviction sometimes leads to the belief that death too is a meaningless event, and even to the view that suicide is appropriate in the face of a meaningless existence. Leo Tolstoy, in his autobiographical confessions, reports that in his youth he thought such questions aimless and irrelevant, but in his older years he thought them the only important questions. Recently many philosophers have been inclined to regard these questions as Tolstoy did in his youth: as aimless, irrelevant, unanswerable, and to be covered over. But other philosophers acknowledge their importance, and in this chapter some of the most significant reflections about the meaning, purpose, and value (if any) of life and death are presented.

Death and the Meaning of Life

There are several layers of problems about the meaning of life. The first is conceptual: What does this question about meaning actually mean? If we can get clear about this conceptual matter, we can proceed to the second level: What answer, if any, can be provided to the question whether life is meaningful in the face of inevitable death?

313

There is a fairly common pattern in the way such questions emerge. Doubts that life is significant arise first. The beliefs that prompt such doubts are usually quite basic and comprehensive beliefs about the universe and human nature. To use an example of Kurt Baier's, many modern Christians no longer are able to share the belief of medieval Christianity that our "stretch on earth is only a short interlude, a temporary incarceration of the soul in the prison of the body, a brief trial and test, fated to end in death, the release from pain and suffering." When modern Christians came to doubt this factual claim about immortality, they similarly came to doubt both that "What really matters, is the life after the death of the body" and that the meaning of existence is found in the salvation of one's immortal soul.[1] In this example the loss of belief in an alleged religious truth about human life and death carries with it loss of belief that a related Christian conviction can supply the meaning of life. This example shows that many important questions about the meaning of life and death have to do with those factual beliefs which control in fundamental ways our outlook on human existence. It is perhaps not overly dramatic to say that one's fundamental convictions about human existence control one's views about the meaning of life and death.

Pessimism and the Role of Death

Much of the literature on the meaning of life and death communicates the pessimistic view that the search for meaning is doomed to failure. Nietzsche and Schopenhauer are notorious exponents of this position, and in the present chapter Tolstoy provides a graphic account of feelings that give rise to it. The theme of inevitable death plays a prominent role in his philosophy. Perhaps its most constant theme is that no matter what the joys and successes of life may be, the time always comes when death conquers. This reflection on death's ultimate victory is sometimes turned inwardly on an author's own life. But inescapably it is generalized to the entire human population, and indeed to the cosmic nature of things. It is then asked what could possibly be the point of life itself, since death inevitably conquers.

Religious Responses to Pessimism.   Two basic forms of response have been offered to such pessimistic reflections. The best known are those religious responses where it is held that God retains the values of human life and overcomes death's deprivations by the award of human immortality. Yet even among religious thinkers there is no single religious answer. They also tend more to *affirm* that there is meaning in life than to *explain* in what that meaning consists. Perhaps the single most common theme in religious literature is that by human contact with God one is assured of community with an eternal being who guides the whole of creation, of which each life is a part and to which each makes a lasting contribution. Nevertheless, as several critics have pointed out, it is not clear how such contact with God insures meaning in life, or even what the sense of "meaning" is. Even more fundamental questions have to do with the truth of the claims asserted in religious beliefs—e.g. that God exists, that his goals for creation are discoverable, and that God alone gives meaning to human life.

Nonreligious Responses to Pessimism. A second type of response focuses on the theme that the meaning of life is found in individuals' autonomously selected goals. Meaningfulness is created whenever someone selects a goal and finds fulfillment in its achievement. Whereas the religious view typically finds the meaning *of* one's life in the position it occupies in God's creation, the nonreligious response typically finds a meaning *in* one's life through one's own elected purposes (a distinction nicely developed by Kurt Baier). Whereas the religious believer tends to regard life as worth living only for its instrumental value in furthering God's purposes and not for its own sake, the nonreligious response tends to regard life as worth living for its own sake and not because of any purely instrumental value it might have. It is human inventiveness and effort, then, that give a meaning to life on the nonreligious view. In this secular, humanistic view of the universe and of human life, meaning is found in one's contribution to others, one's work, the rearing of children, etc.—and not in anything more grandiose.

Nonreligious views have been felt by many to be deficient because they fail to show that the sum of human endeavors culminates in some form of a lasting contribution. Accordingly, death still seems to many pessimists to conquer in the end. Here the typical humanist response is some form of the theme that lastingness is not the crucial matter. The crucial matter is to make of life whatever it offers and to realize that death is only its end, not something that magically erases all the values present in life. Whether or not either this humanist response or its religious alternative provides an adequate reply to the pessimist is one central issue in this chapter.

Death as an Evil

The notion that death deprives life of its meaning seems to presuppose that death is an evil. But is it? The following argument, by Epicurus, is a famous attempt to prove that death is not an evil:

> Become accustomed to the belief that death is nothing to us. For all good and evil consists in sensation, but death is deprivation of sensation. And therefore a right understanding that death is nothing to us makes the mortality of life enjoyable, not because it adds to it an infinite span of time, but because it takes away the craving for immortality. For there is nothing terrible in not living, so that the man speaks idly who says that he fears death not because it will be painful when it comes, but because it is painful in anticipation. So death, the most terrifying of all ills, is nothing to us, since so long as we exist death is not with us, but when

death comes, then we do not exist. It does not then concern either the living, or the dead, since the former it is not, and the latter are no more.

Some philosophers have contended, largely in agreement with Epicurus, that death is simply the end of life, its limit, and not something that is either good or bad. There are here again both conceptual and substantive questions of value. The conceptual question concerns what could be meant by saying that death is an evil; the substantive question asks whether death truly is an evil.

Some have argued that death is an inherent evil and even an indignity —one that must be faced for what it is, without evasion. Such views are not without practical implications for the way in which we are to treat the dying. For one thing, if the evil of death cannot be overcome or even minimized no matter what the circumstances, then it seems we ought to do all that we can under all circumstances to prolong the lives of those who are dying. Such a view could also lead to serious reservations about supporting death-with-dignity movements, such as those euthanasia societies examined in previous chapters. This view also would almost certainly lead to condemnation of acts of suicide, as well as to a special revulsion toward literature that romanticizes death or glorifies suicide.

The alternative to the view that death is an evil and an indignity is not that death is some kind of good. Rather, it is argued that death is good or evil only *relative to* the circumstances under which it occurs. It makes a difference in assessing the value of a death whether the dying person is young, whether numerous personal goals remain, what the person's physical condition is, etc. This relativistic view, like its nonrelativistic counterpart, also has practical implications, which for the most part are quite the opposite of those of the inherent-evil view. From the relativity thesis it seems to follow that there will be times when lives are not worth preserving, a view which, in turn, is likely to lead to some form of support for the euthanasia movements discussed in the previous chapters. It would also support the notion that there can be death with dignity, and it might have implications for one's views on the morality and rationality of suicide.

Some parts of this chapter are dominated by discussions of the meaning of life and death, while others focus equally on the questions whether there can be dignity in death and whether death is an inherent evil. But, as a whole, the chapter invites consideration whether there is any real significance either in life or death—an ancient and unresolved question of metaphysics, ethics, and religion.

Note

1. K. Baier, *The Meaning of Life* (Canberra: Inaugural Lecture, 1957), pp. 3–4.

We have already had reason to mention Tolstoy's interest in questions of the meaning of life and death. Tolstoy often dwelled in his novels on how to recover meaning in life when loved ones were constantly dying or when one's own death appeared to be inevitable. Tolstoy's search for meaning in the face of suffering and death are here recorded in the form of an autobiographical "confession." Tolstoy ponders two major questions: (1) Is it irrational to form intentions and purposes if in the end nothing is of significance? (This question, as derived from Tolstoy, is considered in a later selection in this chapter by R. M. Hare.) (2) Is suicide morally justified in the face of a meaningless existence? (This question, also as derived from Tolstoy, is considered by Albert Camus in the next selection.) Tolstoy finds reason for rejecting both "scientific" and "philosophical" sources of meaning in life. He finds meaning only in the life of the religious faith. Indeed, he condemns the philosophical quest for meaning as grounded on reason, whereas he believes meaning can only be found in faith. Tolstoy, then, raises sceptical or pessimistic questions about the meaning of life in the face of inevitable death but also gives a religious response to this sort of pessimism.

Leo Tolstoy

DEATH AND THE MEANING OF LIFE *

In my writings I advocated, what to me was the only truth, that it was necessary to live in such a way as to derive the greatest comfort for oneself and one's family.

Thus I proceeded to live, but five years ago something very strange began to happen with me: I was overcome by minutes at first of perplexity and then of an arrest of life, as though I did not know how to live or what to do, and I lost myself and was dejected. But that passed, and I continued to live as before. Then those minutes of perplexity were repeated oftener and oftener, and always in one and the same form. These arrests of life found their expression in ever the same questions: "Why? Well, and then?"

At first I thought that those were simply aimless, inappropriate questions. It seemed to me that that was all well known and that if I ever wanted to busy myself with their solution, it would not cost me much labour,— that now I had no time to attend to them, but that if I wanted to I should find the proper answers. But the questions began to repeat themselves oftener and oftener, answers were demanded more and more persistently, and, like dots that fall on the same spot, these questions, without any answers, thickened into one black blotch.

There happened what happens with any person who falls ill with a

* From *A Confession*, trans. Leo Wiener. New York: Thomas Y. Crowell & Co., 1899.

mortal internal disease. At first there appear insignificant symptoms of indisposition, to which the patient pays no attention; then these symptoms are repeated more and more frequently and blend into one temporally indivisible suffering. The suffering keeps growing, and before the patient has had time to look around, he becomes conscious that what he took for an indisposition is the most significant thing in the world to him,—is death.

The same happened with me. I understood that it was not a passing indisposition, but something very important, and that, if the questions were going to repeat themselves, it would be necessary to find an answer for them. And I tried to answer them. The questions seemed to be so foolish, simple, and childish. But the moment I touched them and tried to solve them, I became convinced, in the first place, that they were not childish and foolish, but very important and profound questions in life, and, in the second, that, no matter how much I might try, I should not be able to answer them. Before attending to my Samára estate, to my son's education, or to the writing of a book, I ought to know why I should do that. So long as I did not know why, I could not do anything, I could not live. Amidst my thoughts of farming, which interested me very much during that time, there would suddenly pass through my head a question like this: "All right, you are going to have six thousand desyatínas of land in the Government of Samára, and three hundred horses,—and then?" And I completely lost my senses and did not know what to think farther. Or, when I thought of the education of my children, I said to myself: "Why?" Or, reflecting on the manner in which the masses might obtain their welfare, I suddenly said to myself: "What is that to me?" Or, thinking of the fame which my works would get me, I said to myself: "All right, you will be more famous than Gógol, Púshkin, Shakespeare, Molière, and all the writers in the world,— what of it?" And I was absolutely unable to make any reply. The questions were not waiting, and I had to answer them at once; if I did not answer them, I could not live.

I felt that what I was standing on had given way, that I had no foundation to stand on, that that which I lived by no longer existed, and that I had nothing to live by.

My life came to a standstill. I could breathe, eat, drink, and sleep, and could not help breathing, eating, drinking, and sleeping; but there was no life, because there were no desires the gratification of which I might find reasonable. If I wished for anything, I knew in advance that, whether I gratified my desire or not, nothing would come of it. If a fairy had come and had offered to carry out my wish, I should not have known what to say. If in moments of intoxication I had, not wishes, but habits of former desires, I knew in sober moments that that was a deception, that there was nothing to wish for. I could not even wish to find out the truth, because I guessed what it consisted in. The truth was that life was meaningless. It was as though I had just been living and walking along, and had come to an abyss, where I saw clearly that there was nothing ahead but perdition. And it was impossible to stop and go back, and impossible to shut my eyes, in order that I might not see that there was nothing ahead but suffering and imminent death,—complete annihilation.

What happened to me was that I, a healthy, happy man, felt that I could not go on living,—an insurmountable force drew me on to find release from life. I cannot say that I *wanted* to kill myself.

The force which drew me away from life was stronger, fuller, more general than wishing. It was a force like the former striving after life, only in an inverse sense. I tended with all my strength away from life. The thought of suicide came as naturally to me as had come before the ideas of improving life. That thought was so seductive that I had to use cunning against myself, lest I should rashly execute it. I did not want to be in a hurry, because I wanted to use every effort to disentangle myself: if I should not succeed in disentangling myself, there would always be time for that. And at such times I, a happy man, hid a rope from myself so that I should not hang myself on a cross-beam between two safes in my room, where I was by myself in the evening, while taking off my clothes, and did not go out hunting with a gun, in order not to be tempted by any easy way of doing away with myself. I did not know myself what it was I wanted: I was afraid of life, strove to get away from it, and, at the same time, expected something from it.

All that happened with me when I was on every side surrounded by what is considered to be complete happiness. I had a good, loving, and beloved wife, good children, and a large estate, which grew and increased without any labour on my part. I was respected by my neighbours and friends, more than ever before, was praised by strangers, and, without any self-deception, could consider my name famous. With all that, I was not deranged or mentally unsound,—on the contrary, I was in full command of my mental and physical powers, such as I had rarely met with in people of my age: physically I could work in a field, mowing, without falling behind a peasant; mentally I could work from eight to ten hours in succession, without experiencing any consequences from the strain. And while in such condition I arrived at the conclusion that I could not live, and, fearing death, I had to use cunning against myself, in order that I might not take my life.

This mental condition expressed itself to me in this form: my life is a stupid, mean trick played on me by somebody. Although I did not recognize that "somebody" as having created me, the form of the conception that some one had played a mean, stupid trick on me by bringing me into the world was the most natural one that presented itself to me.

Involuntarily I imagined that there, somewhere, there was somebody who was now having fun as he looked down upon me and saw me, who had lived for thirty or forty years, learning, developing, growing in body and mind, now that I had become strengthened in mind and had reached that summit of life from which it lay all before me, standing as a complete fool on that summit and seeing clearly that there was nothing in life and never would be. And that was fun to him—

But whether there was or was not that somebody who made fun of me, did not make it easier for me. I could not ascribe any sensible meaning to a single act, or to my whole life. I was only surprised that I had not understood that from the start. All that had long ago been known to everybody. Sooner or later there would come diseases and death (they had come already) to my dear ones and to me, and there would be nothing left but stench and worms. All my affairs, no matter what they might be, would sooner or later be forgotten, and I myself should not exist. So why should I worry about all these things? How could a man fail to see that and live,— that was surprising! A person could live only so long as he was drunk; but the moment he sobered up, he could not help seeing that all that was only a deception, and a stupid deception at that! Really, there was nothing funny and ingenious about it, but only something cruel and stupid.

Long ago has been told the Eastern story about the traveller who in the steppe is overtaken by an infuriated beast. Trying to save himself from the animal, the traveller jumps into a waterless well, but at its bottom he sees a dragon who opens his jaws in order to swallow him. And the unfortunate man does not dare climb out, lest he perish from the infuriated beast, and does not dare jump down to the bottom of the well, lest he be devoured by the dragon, and so clutches the twig of a wild bush growing in a cleft of the well and holds on to it. His hands grow weak and he feels that soon he shall have to surrender to the peril which awaits him at either side; but he still holds on and sees two mice, one white, the other black, in even measure making a circle around the main trunk of the bush to which he is clinging, and nibbling at it on all sides. Now, at any moment, the bush will break and tear off, and he will fall into the dragon's jaws. The traveller sees that and knows that he will inevitably perish; but while he is still clinging, he sees some drops of honey hanging on the leaves of the bush, and so reaches out for them with his tongue and licks the leaves. Just so I hold on to the branch of life, knowing that the dragon of death is waiting inevitably for me, ready to tear me to pieces, and I cannot understand why I have fallen on such suffering. And I try to lick that honey which used to give me pleasure; but now it no longer gives me joy, and the white and the black mouse day and night nibble at the branch to which I am holding on. I clearly see the dragon, and the honey is no longer sweet to me. I see only the inevitable dragon and the mice, and am unable to turn my glance away from them. That is not a fable, but a veritable, indisputable, comprehensible truth.

The former deception of the pleasures of life, which stifled the terror of the dragon, no longer deceives me. No matter how much one should say to me, "You cannot understand the meaning of life, do not think, live!" I am unable to do so, because I have been doing it too long before. Now I cannot help seeing day and night, which run and lead me up to death. I see that alone, because that alone is the truth. Everything else is a lie.

The two drops of honey that have longest turned my eyes away from the cruel truth, the love of family and of authorship, which I have called an art, are no longer sweet to me.

"My family—" I said to myself, "but my family, my wife and children, they are also human beings. They are in precisely the same condition that I am in: they must either live in the lie or see the terrible truth. Why should they live? Why should I love them, why guard, raise, and watch them? Is it for the same despair which is in me, or for dullness of perception? Since I love them, I cannot conceal the truth from them,—every step in cognition leads them up to this truth. And the truth is death."

"Art, poetry?" For a long time, under the influence of the success of human praise, I tried to persuade myself that that was a thing which could be done, even though death should come and destroy everything, my deeds, as well as my memory of them; but soon I came to see that that, too, was a deception. It was clear to me that art was an adornment of life, a decoy of life. But life lost all its attractiveness for me. How, then, could I entrap others? So long as I did not live my own life, and a strange life bore me on its waves; so long as I believed that life had some sense, although I was not able to express it,—the reflections of life of every description in poetry and in the arts afforded me pleasure, and I was delighted to look at life through this little mirror of art; but when I began to look for the meaning of life, when I experienced the necessity of living myself, that little mirror became either useless, superfluous, and ridiculous, or painful to me. I could no longer console myself with what I saw in the mirror, namely, that my situation was stupid and desperate. It was all right for me to rejoice so long as I believed in the depth of my soul that life had some sense. At that time the play of lights—of the comical, the tragical, the touching, the beautiful, the terrible in life—afforded me amusement. But when I knew that life was meaningless and terrible, the play in the little mirror could no longer amuse me. No sweetness of honey could be sweet to me, when I saw the dragon and the mice that were nibbling down my support.

That was not all. If I had simply comprehended that life had no meaning, I might have known that calmly,—I might have known that that was my fate. But I could not be soothed by that. If I had been like a man living in a forest from which he knew there was no way out, I might have lived; but I was like a man who had lost his way in the forest, who was overcome by terror because he had lost his way, who kept tossing about in his desire to come out on the road, knowing that every step got him only more entangled, and who could not help tossing.

That was terrible. And, in order to free myself from that terror, I wanted to kill myself. I experienced terror before what was awaiting me,— I knew that that terror was more terrible than the situation itself, but I could not patiently wait for the end. No matter how convincing the reflection was that it was the same whether a vessel in the heart should break or something should burst, and all should be ended, I could not wait patiently for the end. The terror of the darkness was too great, and I wanted as quickly as possible to free myself from it by means of a noose or a bullet. It was this feeling that more than anything else drew me on toward suicide. . . .

"Well, I know," I said to myself, "all which science wants so persistently to know, but there is no answer to the question about the meaning of my life." But in the speculative sphere I saw that, in spite of the fact that the aim of the knowledge was directed straight to the answer of my question, or because of that fact, there could be no other answer than what I was giving to myself: "What is the meaning of my life?"—"None." Or, "What will come of my life?"—"Nothing." Or, "Why does everything which exists exist, and why do I exist?"—"Because it exists."

Putting the question to the one side of human knowledge, I received an endless quantity of exact answers about what I did not ask: about the chemical composition of the stars, about the movement of the sun toward the constellation of Hercules, about the origin of species and of man, about the forms of infinitely small, imponderable particles of ether; but the answer in this sphere of knowledge to my question what the meaning of my life was, was always: "You are what you call your life; you are a temporal, accidental conglomeration of particles. The interrelation, the change of these particles, produces in you that which you call life. This congeries will last for some time; then the interaction of these particles will cease, and that which you call life and all your questions will come to an end. You are an accidentally cohering globule of something. The globule is fermenting. This fermentation the globule calls its life. The globule falls to pieces, and all fermentation and all questions will come to an end." Thus the clear side of knowledge answers, and it cannot say anything else, if only it strictly follows its principles.

With such an answer it appears that the answer is not a reply to the question. I want to know the meaning of my life, but the fact that it is a particle of the infinite not only gives it no meaning, but even destroys every possible meaning.

Those obscure transactions, which this side of the experimental, exact science has with speculation, when it says that the meaning of life consists in evolution and the coöperation with this evolution, because of their obscurity and inexactness cannot be regarded as answers.

The other side of knowledge, the speculative, so long as it sticks strictly to its fundamental principles in giving a direct answer to the question, everywhere and at all times has answered one and the same: "The world is something infinite and incomprehensible. Human life is an incomprehensible part of this incomprehensible *all*." Again I exclude all those transactions between the speculative and the experimental sciences, which form the whole ballast of the half-sciences, the so-called science of jurisprudence and the political and historical sciences. Into these sciences are just as irregularly introduced the concepts of evolution and perfection, but with this difference, that there it is the evolution of everything, while here it is the evolution of the life of man. The irregularity is one and the same: evolution, perfection in the infinite, can have neither aim nor direction, and answers nothing in respect to my question.

I lived for a long time in this madness, which, not in words, but in deeds, is particularly characteristic of us, the most liberal and learned of men. But, thanks either to my strange, physical love for the real working class, which made me understand it and see that it is not so stupid as we suppose, or to the sincerity of my conviction, which was that I could know nothing and that the best that I could do was to hang myself,—I felt that if I wanted to live and understand the meaning of life, I ought naturally to look for it, not among those who had lost the meaning of life and wanted to kill themselves, but among those billions departed and living men who had been carrying their own lives and ours upon their shoulders. And I looked around at the enormous masses of deceased and living men,—not learned and wealthy, but simple men,—and I saw something quite different. I saw that all these billions of men that lived or had lived, all, with rare exceptions, did not fit into my subdivisions, and that I could not recognize them as not understanding the question, because they themselves put it and answered it with surprising clearness. Nor could I recognize them as Epicureans, because their lives were composed rather of privations and suffering than of enjoyment. Still less could I recognize them as senselessly living out their meaningless lives, because every act of theirs and death itself was explained by them. They regarded it as the greatest evil to kill themselves. It appeared, then, that all humanity was in possession of a knowledge of the meaning of life, which I did not recognize and which I contemned. It turned out that rational knowledge did not give any meaning to life, excluded life, while the meaning which by billions of people, by all humanity, was ascribed to life was based on some despised, false knowledge.

The rational knowledge in the person of the learned and the wise denied the meaning of life, but the enormous masses of men, all humanity, recognized this meaning in an irrational knowledge. This irrational knowledge was faith, the same that I could not help but reject. That was God as one and three, the creation in six days, devils and angels, and all that which I could not accept so long as I had not lost my senses.

My situation was a terrible one. I knew that I should not find anything on the path of rational knowledge but the negation of life, and there, in faith, nothing but the negation of reason, which was still more impossible than the negation of life. From the rational knowledge it followed that life was an evil and men knew it,—it depended on men whether they should cease living, and yet they lived and continued to live, and I myself lived, though I had known long ago that life was meaningless and an evil. From faith it followed that, in order to understand life, I must renounce reason, for which alone a meaning was needed.

Albert Camus raises many of the same questions as Tolstoy, and manifests many of the same attitudes. But in the end he is fundamentally opposed to Tolstoy's resorting to religion. Camus begins this selection (and indeed his whole book, *The Myth of Sisyphus*) with the following startling comment: "There is but one truly serious philosophical problem, and that is suicide. Judging whether life is or is not worth living amounts to answering the fundamental question of philosophy." Camus sees a clear connection between the justification of suicide, if life is meaningless, and the justification of continuing in life, if it is meaningful. In order, then, to decide whether or not one ought to commit suicide, one must first ascertain whether life is meaningful. Camus spends a great deal of time trying to get his readers to feel the sense of absurdity that plagues both him and Tolstoy. He explores several possible answers to his questions. He rejects the pessimistic view that life is totally absurd and hence not worth living, and also rejects the religious and philosophical responses that find meaning in some feature of the non-human universe. He takes the middle way of declaring the universe itself absurd but our existence capable of being given meaning by pursuit of our own projects. Camus believes that his answer "resolves" the problem of suicide.

Albert Camus

AN ABSURD REASONING *

There is but one truly serious philosophical problem, and that is suicide. Judging whether life is or is not worth living amounts to answering the fundamental question of philosophy. All the rest—whether or not the world has three dimensions, whether the mind has nine or twelve categories —comes afterwards. These are games; one must first answer. And if it is true, as Nietzsche claims, that a philosopher, to deserve our respect, must

---

* From *The Myth of Sisyphus and Other Essays*, trans. Justin O'Brien. Copyright © 1955. New York: Alfred A. Knopf, Inc. Reprinted by permission of Alfred A. Knopf, Inc. and Hamish Hamilton Ltd.

preach by example, you can appreciate the importance of that reply, for it will precede the definitive act. These are facts the heart can feel; yet they call for careful study before they become clear to the intellect.

If I ask myself how to judge that this question is more urgent than that, I reply that one judges by the actions it entails. I have never seen anyone die for the ontological argument. Galileo, who held a scientific truth of great importance, abjured it with the greatest ease as soon as it endangered his life. In a certain sense, he did right. That truth was not worth the stake. Whether the earth or the sun revolves around the other is a matter of profound indifference. To tell the truth, it is a futile question. On the other hand, I see many people die because they judge that life is not worth living. I see others paradoxically getting killed for the ideas or illusions that give them a reason for living (what is called a reason for living is also an excellent reason for dying). I therefore conclude that the meaning of life is the most urgent of questions. How to answer it? On all essential problems (I mean thereby those that run the risk of leading to death or those that intensify the passion of living) there are probably but two methods of thought: the method of La Palisse and the method of Don Quixote. Solely the balance between evidence and lyricism can allow us to achieve simultaneously emotion and lucidity. In a subject at once so humble and so heavy with emotion, the learned and classical dialectic must yield, one can see, to a more modest attitude of mind deriving at once and the same time from common sense and understanding.

Suicide has never been dealt with except as a social phenomenon. On the contrary, we are concerned here, at the outset, with the relationship between individual thought and suicide. An act like this is prepared within the silence of the heart, as is a great work of art. The man himself is ignorant of it. One evening he pulls the trigger or jumps. Of an apartment-building manager who had killed himself I was told that he had lost his daughter five years before, that he had changed greatly since, and that that experience had "undermined" him. A more exact word cannot be imagined. Beginning to think is beginning to be undermined. Society has but little connection with such beginnings. The worm is in man's heart. That is where it must be sought. One must follow and understand this fatal game that leads from lucidity in the face of existence to flight from light.

There are many causes for a suicide, and generally the most obvious ones were not the most powerful. Rarely is suicide committed (yet the hypothesis is not excluded) through reflection. What sets off the crisis is almost always unverifiable. Newspapers often speak of "personal sorrows" or of "incurable illness." These explanations are plausible. But one would have to know whether a friend of the desperate man had not that very day addressed him indifferently. He is the guilty one. For that is enough to precipitate all the rancors and all the boredom still in suspension.

But if it is hard to fix the precise instant, the subtle step when the mind opted for death, it is easier to deduce from the act itself the consequences it implies. In a sense, and as in melodrama, killing yourself amounts to confessing. It is confessing that life is too much for you or that you do not understand it. Let's not go too far in such analogies, however, but rather return to everyday words. It is merely confessing that that "is not worth the trouble." Living, naturally, is never easy. You continue making the gestures commanded by existence for many reasons, the first of which is habit. Dying voluntarily implies that you have recognized, even instinctively, the ridiculous character of that habit, the absence of any profound reason for living, the insane character of that daily agitation, and the uselessness of suffering.

What, then, is that incalculable feeling that deprives the mind of the sleep necessary to life? A world that can be explained even with bad reasons is a familiar world. But, on the other hand, in a universe suddenly divested of illusions and lights, man feels an alien, a stranger. His exile is without remedy since he is deprived of the memory of a lost home or the hope of a promised land. This divorce between man and his life, the actor and his setting, is properly the feeling of absurdity. All healthy men having thought of their own suicide, it can be seen, without further explanation, that there is a direct connection between this feeling and the longing for death. . . .

The subject of this essay is precisely this relationship between the absurd and suicide, the exact degree to which suicide is a solution to the absurd. The principle can be established that for a man who does not cheat, what he believes to be true must determine his action. Belief in the absurdity of existence must then dictate his conduct. It is legitimate to wonder, clearly and without false pathos, whether a conclusion of this importance requires forsaking as rapidly as possible an incomprehensible condition. I am speaking, of course, of men inclined to be in harmony with themselves.

Like great works, deep feelings always mean more than they are conscious of saying. The regularity of an impulse or a repulsion in a soul is encountered again in habits of doing or thinking, is reproduced in consequences of which the soul itself knows nothing. Great feelings take with them their own universe, splendid or abject. They light up with their passion an exclusive world in which they recognize their climate. There is a universe of jealousy, of ambition, of selfishness, or of generosity. A universe—in other words, a metaphysic and an attitude of mind. What is true of already specialized feelings will be even more so of emotions basically as indeterminate, simultaneously as vague and as "definite," as remote and as "present" as those furnished us by beauty or aroused by absurdity.

At any streetcorner the feeling of absurdity can strike any man in the face. As it is, in its distressing nudity, in its light without effulgence, it is elusive. But that very difficulty deserves reflection. It is probably true that a man remains forever unknown to us and that there is in him something irreducible that escapes us. But *practically* I know men and recognize them by their behavior, by the totality of their deeds, by the consequences caused in life by their presence. Likewise, all those irrational feelings which offer no purchase to analysis. I can define them *practically,* appreciate them *practically,* by gathering together the sum of their consequences in the domain of the intelligence, by seizing and noting all their aspects, by outlining their universe. It is certain that apparently, though I have seen the same actor a hundred times, I shall not for that reason know him any better personally. Yet if I add up the heroes he has personified and if I say that I know him a little better at the hundredth character counted off, this will be felt to contain an element of truth. For this apparent paradox is also an apologue. There is a moral to it. It teaches that a man defines himself by his make-believe as well as by his sincere impulses. There is thus a lower key of feelings, inaccessible in the heart but partially disclosed by the acts they imply and the attitudes of mind they assume. It is clear that in this way I am defining a method. But it is also evident that that method is one of analysis and not of knowledge. For methods imply metaphysics; unconsciously they disclose conclusions that they often claim not to know yet. Similarly, the last pages of a book are already contained in the first pages. Such a link is inevitable. The method defined here acknowledges the feeling that all true knowledge is impossible. Solely appearances can be enumerated and the climate make itself felt.

Perhaps we shall be able to overtake that elusive feeling of absurdity in the different but closely related worlds of intelligence, of the art of living, or of art itself. The climate of absurdity is in the beginning. The end is the absurd universe and that attitude of mind which lights the world with its true colors to bring out the privileged and implacable visage which that attitude has discerned in it.

All great deeds and all great thoughts have a ridiculous beginning. Great works are often born on a streetcorner or in a restaurant's revolving door. So it is with absurdity. The absurd world more than others derives its nobility from that abject birth. In certain situations, replying "nothing" when asked what one is thinking about may be pretense in a man. Those who are loved are well aware of this. But if that reply is sincere, if it symbolizes that odd state of soul in which the void becomes eloquent, in which the chain of daily gestures is broken, in which the heart vainly seeks the link that will connect it again, then it is as it were the first sign of absurdity.

It happens that the stage sets collapse. Rising, streetcar, four hours in the office or the factory, meal, streetcar, four hours of work, meal, sleep, and Monday Tuesday Wednesday Thursday Friday and Saturday according to the same rhythm—this path is easily followed most of the time. But one day the "why" arises and everything begins in that weariness tinged with amazement. "Begins"—this is important. Weariness comes at the end of the acts of a mechanical life, but at the same time it inaugurates the impulse of consciousness. It awakens consciousness and provokes what follows. What follows is the gradual return into the chain or it is the definitive awakening. At the end of the awakening comes, in time, the consequence: suicide or recovery. In itself weariness has something sickening about it. Here, I must conclude that it is good. For everything begins with consciousness and nothing is worth anything except through it. There is nothing original about these remarks. But they are obvious; that is enough for a while, during a sketchy reconnaissance in the origins of the absurd. Mere "anxiety," as Heidegger says, is at the source of everything.

Likewise and during every day of an unillustrious life, time carries us. But a moment always comes when we have to carry it. We live on the future: "tomorrow," "later on," "when you have made your way," "you will understand when you are old enough." Such irrelevancies are wonderful, for, after all, it's a matter of dying. Yet a day comes when a man notices or says that he is thirty. Thus he asserts his youth. But simultaneously he situates himself in relation to time. He takes his place in it. He admits that he stands at a certain point on a curve that he acknowledges having to travel to its end. He belongs to time, and by the horror that seizes him, he recognizes his worst enemy. Tomorrow, he was longing for tomorrow, whereas everything in him ought to reject it. That revolt of the flesh is the absurd.

A step lower and strangeness creeps in: perceiving that the world is "dense," sensing to what a degree a stone is foreign and irreducible to us, with what intensity nature or a landscape can negate us. At the heart of all beauty lies something inhuman, and these hills, the softness of the sky, the outline of these trees at this very minute lose the illusory meaning with which we had clothed them, henceforth more remote than a lost paradise. The primitive hostility of the world rises up to face us across millennia. For a second we cease to understand it because for centuries we have understood in it solely the images and designs that we had attributed to it beforehand, because henceforth we lack the power to make use of that artifice. The world evades us because it becomes itself again. That stage scenery masked by habit becomes again what it is. It withdraws at a distance from us. Just as there are days when under the familiar face of a woman, we see as a stranger her we had loved months or years ago, perhaps we shall come even to desire what suddenly leaves us so alone. But the time has not yet come. Just one thing: that denseness and that strangeness of the world is the absurd.

Men, too, secrete the inhuman. At certain moments of lucidity, the mechanical aspect of their gestures, their meaningless pantomime makes silly everything that surrounds them. A man is talking on the telephone behind a glass partition; you cannot hear him, but you see his incomprehensible dumb show: you wonder why he is alive. This discomfort in the face of man's own inhumanity, this incalculable tumble before the image of what we are, this "nausea," as a writer of today calls it, is also the absurd. Likewise the stranger who at certain seconds comes to meet us in a mirror, the familiar and yet alarming brother we encounter in our own photographs is also the absurd. . . .

Now I can broach the notion of suicide. It has already been felt what solution might be given. At this point the problem is reversed. It was previously a question of finding out whether or not life had to have a meaning to be lived. It now becomes clear, on the contrary, that it will be lived all the better if it has no meaning. Living an experience, a particular fate, is accepting it fully. Now, no one will live this fate, knowing it to be absurd, unless he does everything to keep before him that absurd brought to light by consciousness. Negating one of the terms of the opposition on which he lives amounts to escaping it. To abolish conscious revolt is to elude the problem. The theme of permanent revolution is thus carried into individual experience. Living is keeping the absurd alive. Keeping it alive is, above all, contemplating it. Unlike Eurydice, the absurd dies only when we turn away from it. One of the only coherent philosophical positions is thus revolt. It is a constant confrontation between man and his own obscurity. It is an insistence upon an impossible transparency. It challenges the world anew every second. Just as danger provided man the unique opportunity of seizing awareness, so metaphysical revolt extends awareness to the whole of experience. It is that constant presence of man in his own eyes. It is not aspiration, for it is devoid of hope. That revolt is the certainty of a crushing fate, without the resignation that ought to accompany it.

This is where it is seen to what a degree absurd experience is remote from suicide. It may be thought that suicide follows revolt—but wrongly. For it does not represent the logical outcome of revolt. It is just the contrary by the consent it presupposes. Suicide, like the leap, is acceptance at its extreme. Everything is over and man returns to his essential history. His future, his unique and dreadful future—he sees and rushes toward it. In its way, suicide settles the absurd. It engulfs the absurd in the same death. But I know that in order to keep alive, the absurd cannot be settled. It escapes suicide to the extent that it is simultaneously awareness and rejection of death. It is, at the extreme limit of the condemned man's last thought, that shoelace that despite everything he sees a few yards away, on the very brink of his dizzying fall. The contrary of suicide, in fact, is the man condemned to death.

That revolt gives life its value. Spread out over the whole length of a life, it restores its majesty to that life. To a man devoid of blinders, there is no finer sight than that of the intelligence at grips with a reality that transcends it. The sight of human pride is unequaled. No disparagement is of any use. That discipline that the mind imposes on itself, that will conjured up out of nothing, that face-to-face struggle have something exceptional about them. To impoverish that reality whose inhumanity constitutes man's majesty is tantamount to impoverishing him himself. I understand then why the doctrines that explain everything to me also debilitate me at the same time. They relieve me of the weight of my own life, and yet I must carry it alone. At this juncture, I cannot conceive that a skeptical metaphysics can be joined to an ethics of renunciation.

Consciousness and revolt, these rejections are the contrary of renunciation. Everything that is indomitable and passionate in a human heart quickens them, on the contrary, with its own life. It is essential to die unreconciled and not of one's own free will. Suicide is a repudiation. The absurd man can only drain everything to the bitter end, and deplete himself. The absurd is his extreme tension, which he maintains constantly by solitary effort, for he knows that in that consciousness and in that day-to-day revolt he gives proof of his only truth, which is defiance. This is a first consequence. . . .

But what does life mean in such a universe? Nothing else for the moment but indifference to the future and a desire to use up everything that is given. Belief in the meaning of life always implies a scale of values, a choice, our preferences. Belief in the absurd, according to our definitions, teaches the contrary. But this is worth examining.

Knowing whether or not one can live *without appeal* is all that interests me. I do not want to get out of my depth. This aspect of life being given me, can I adapt myself to it? Now, faced with this particular concern, belief in the absurd is tantamount to substituting the quantity of experiences for the quality. If I convince myself that this life has no other aspect than that of the absurd, if I feel that its whole equilibrium depends on that perpetual opposition between my conscious revolt and the darkness in which it struggles, if I admit that my freedom has no meaning except in relation to its limited fate, then I must say that what counts is not the best living but the most living. It is not up to me to wonder if this is vulgar or revolting, elegant or deplorable. Once and for all, value judgments are discarded here in favor of factual judgments. I have merely to draw the conclusions from what I can see and to risk nothing that is hypothetical. Supposing that living in this way were not honorable, then true propriety would command me to be dishonorable.

The most living; in the broadest sense, that rule means nothing. It calls for definition. It seems to begin with the fact that the notion of quantity has not been sufficiently explored. For it can account for a large share of human experience. A man's rule of conduct and his scale of values have no meaning except through the quantity and variety of experiences he has been in a position to accumulate. Now, the conditions of modern life impose on the majority of men the same quantity of experiences and consequently the same profound experience. To be sure, there must also be taken into consideration the individual's spontaneous contribution, the "given" element in him. But I cannot judge of that, and let me repeat that my rule here is to get along with the immediate evidence. I see, then, that the individual character of a common code of ethics lies not so much in the ideal importance of its basic principles as in the norm of an experience that it is possible to measure. To stretch a point somewhat, the Greeks had the code of their leisure just as we have the code of our eight-hour day. But already many men among the most tragic cause us to foresee that a longer experience changes this table of values. They make us imagine that adventurer of the everyday who through mere quantity of experiences would break all records (I am purposely using this sports expression) and would thus win his own code of ethics. Yet let's avoid romanticism and just ask ourselves what such an attitude may mean to a man with his mind made up to take up his bet and to observe strictly what he takes to be the rules of the game.

Breaking all the records is first and foremost being faced with the world as often as possible. How can that be done without contradictions and without playing on words? For on the one hand the absurd teaches that all experiences are unimportant, and on the other it urges toward the greatest quantity of experiences. How, then, can one fail to do as so many of those men I was speaking of earlier—choose the form of life that brings us the most possible of that human matter, thereby introducing a scale of values that on the other hand one claims to reject?

But again it is the absurd and its contradictory life that teaches us. For the mistake is thinking that that quantity of experiences depends on the circumstances of our life when it depends solely on us. Here we have to be over-simple. To two men living the same number of years, the world always provides the same sum of experiences. It is up to us to be conscious of them Being aware of one's life, one's revolt, one's freedom, and to the maximum, is living, and to the maximum. Where lucidity dominates, the scale of values becomes useless. Let's be even more simple. Let us say that the sole obstacle, the sole deficiency to be made good, is constituted by premature death. Thus it is that no depth, no emotion, no passion, and no sacrifice could render equal in the eyes of the absurd man (even if he wished it so) a conscious life of forty years and a lucidity spread over sixty years. Madness and death are his irreparables. Man does not choose. The absurd and the extra life it involves *therefore do not depend on man's will,* but on its contrary, which is death. Weighing words carefully, it is altogether a question of luck. One just has to be able to consent to this. There will never be any substitute for twenty years of life and experience.

By what is an odd inconsistency in such an alert race, the Greeks claimed that those who died young were beloved of the gods. And that is true only if you are willing to believe that entering the ridiculous world of the gods is forever losing the purest of joys, which is feeling, and feeling on this earth. The present and the succession of presents before a constantly conscious soul is the ideal of the absurd man. But the word "ideal" rings false in this connection. It is not even his vocation, but merely the third consequence of his reasoning. Having started from an anguished awareness of the inhuman, the meditation on the absurd returns at the end of its itinerary to the very heart of the passionate flames of human revolt.

Thus I draw from the absurd three consequences, which are my revolt, my freedom, and my passion. By the mere activity of consciousness I transform into a rule of life what was an invitation to death—and I refuse suicide. I know, to be sure, the dull resonance that vibrates throughout these days. Yet I have but a word to say: that it is necessary. . . .

The preceding merely defines a way of thinking. But the point is to live.

THE MYTH OF SISYPHUS

The gods had condemned Sisyphus to ceaselessly rolling a rock to the top of a mountain, whence the stone would fall back of its own weight. They had thought with some reason that there is no more dreadful punishment than futile and hopeless labor. . . .

You have already grasped that Sisyphus is the absurd hero. He *is*, as much through his passions as through his torture. His scorn of the gods, his hatred of death, and his passion for life won him that unspeakable penalty in which the whole being is exerted toward accomplishing nothing. This is the price that must be paid for the passions of this earth. . . .

If this myth is tragic, that is because its hero is conscious. Where would his torture be, indeed, if at every step the hope of succeeding upheld him? The workman of today works every day in his life at the same tasks, and this fate is no less absurd. But it is tragic only at the rare moments when it becomes conscious. Sisyphus, proletarian of the gods, powerless and rebellious, knows the whole extent of his wretched condition: it is what he thinks of during his descent. The lucidity that was to constitute his torture at the same time crowns his victory. There is no fate that cannot be surmounted by scorn. . . .

All Sisyphus' silent joy is contained therein. His fate belongs to him. His rock is his thing. Likewise, the absurd man, when he contemplates his torment, silences all the idols. In the universe suddenly restored to its silence, the myriad wondering little voices of the earth rise up. Unconscious, secret calls, invitations from all the faces, they are the necessary reverse and price of victory. There is no sun without shadow, and it is essential to know the night. The absurd man says yes and his effort will henceforth be unceasing. If there is a personal fate, there is no higher destiny, or at least there is but one which he concludes is inevitable and despicable. For the rest, he knows himself to be the master of his days. At that subtle moment when man glances backward over his life, Sisyphus returning toward his rock, in that slight pivoting he contemplates that series of unrelated actions which becomes his fate, created by him, combined under his memory's eye and soon sealed by his death. Thus, convinced of the wholly human origin of all that is human, a blind man eager to see who knows that the night has no end, he is still on the go. The rock is still rolling.

I leave Sisyphus at the foot of the mountain! One always finds one's burden again. But Sisyphus teaches the higher fidelity that negates the gods and raises rocks. He too concludes that all is well. This universe henceforth without a master seems to him neither sterile nor futile. Each atom of that stone, each mineral flake of that night-filled mountain, in itself forms a world. The struggle itself toward the heights is enough to fill a man's heart. One must imagine Sisyphus happy.

Richard Taylor begins the following selection with a consideration of the Sisyphus myth with which Camus concluded. Taylor analyzes this myth in order to reach a conclusion about the nature of meaning: "Meaninglessness is essentially endless pointlessness, and meaningfulness is therefore the opposite." The creation of objectives and finding achievement in them is thus the key for Taylor to the introduction of meaning into one's life. To the argument that there is no ultimate meaning if our objectives do not eventuate in something lasting, Taylor responds that the search for ultimate preservation of values is misguided: The point of living, he says, is simply to be living according to the desires intrinsic to one's own nature—not according to some other, extrinsic, goal. Taylor's humanist response is thus very much like Camus', yet it is largely devoid of the pessimistic and disquieting feelings of despair and absurdity which prompt both Camus and Tolstoy to their reflections.

Richard Taylor

THE MEANING OF LIFE *

The question whether life has any meaning is difficult to interpret, and the more one concentrates his critical faculty on it the more it seems to elude him, or to evaporate as any intelligible question. One wants to turn

---

* From *Good and Evil* by Richard Taylor, copyright © 1970 by Richard Taylor. Reprinted with permission of Macmillan Publishing Co., Inc.

it aside, as a source of embarrassment, as something that, if it cannot be abolished, should at least be decently covered. And yet I think any reflective person recognizes that the question it raises is important, and that it ought to have a significant answer.

If the idea of meaningfulness is difficult to grasp in this context, so that we are unsure what sort of thing would amount to answering the question, the idea of meaninglessness is perhaps less so. If, then, we can bring before our minds a clear image of meaningless existence, then perhaps we can take a step toward coping with our original question by seeing to what extent our lives, as we actually find them, resemble that image, and draw such lessons as we are able to from the comparison.

Meaningless Existence

A perfect image of meaninglessness, of the kind we are seeking, is found in the ancient myth of Sisyphus. Sisyphus, it will be remembered, betrayed divine secrets to mortals, and for this he was condemned by the gods to roll a stone to the top of a hill, the stone then immediately to roll back down, again to be pushed to the top by Sisyphus, to roll down once more, and so on again and again, *forever*. Now in this we have the picture of meaningless, pointless toil, of a meaningless existence that is absolutely *never* redeemed. It is not even redeemed by a death that, if it were to accomplish nothing more, would at least bring this idiotic cycle to a close. If we were invited to imagine Sisyphus struggling for awhile and accomplishing nothing, perhaps eventually falling from exhaustion, so that we might suppose him then eventually turning to something having some sort of promise, then the meaninglessness of that chapter of his life would not be so stark. It would be a dark and dreadful dream, from which he eventually awakens to sunlight and reality. But he does not awaken, for there is nothing for him to awaken to. His repetitive toil is his life and reality, and it goes on forever, and it is without any meaning whatever. Nothing ever comes of what he is doing, except simply, more of the same. Not by one step, nor by a thousand, nor by ten thousand does he even expiate by the smallest token the sin against the gods that led him into this fate. Nothing comes of it, nothing at all.

This ancient myth has always enchanted men, for countless meanings can be read into it. Some of the ancients apparently thought it symbolized the perpetual rising and setting of the sun, and others the repetitious crashing of the waves upon the shore. Probably the commonest interpretation is that it symbolizes man's eternal struggle and unquenchable spirit, his determination always to try once more in the face of overwhelming discouragement. This interpretation is further supported by that version of the myth according to which Sisyphus was commanded to roll the stone *over* the hill, so that it would finally roll down the other side, but was never quite able to make it.

I am not concerned with rendering or defending any interpretation of this myth, however. I have cited it only for the one element it does unmistakably contain, namely, that of a repetitious, cyclic activity that never comes to anything. We could contrive other images of this that would serve just as well, and no myth-makers are needed to supply the materials of it. Thus, we can imagine two persons transporting a stone—or even a precious gem, it does not matter—back and forth, relay style. One carries it to a near or distant point where it is received by the other; it is returned to its starting point, there to be recovered by the first, and the process is repeated over and over. Except in this relay nothing counts as winning, and nothing brings the contest to any close, each step only leads to a repetition of itself. Or we can imagine two groups of prisoners, one of them engaged in digging a prodigious hole in the ground that is no sooner finished than it is filled in again by the other group, the latter then digging a new hole that is at once filled in by the first group, and so on and on endlessly.

Now what stands out in all such pictures as oppressive and dejecting is not that the beings who enact these roles suffer any torture or pain, for it need not be assumed that they do. Nor is it that their labors are great, for they are no greater than the labors commonly undertaken by most men most of the time. According to the original myth, the stone is so large that Sisyphus never quite gets it to the top and must groan under every step, so that his enormous labor is all for nought. But this is not what appalls. It is not that his great struggle comes to nothing, but that his existence itself is without meaning. Even if we suppose, for example, that the stone is but a pebble that can be carried effortlessly, or that the holes dug by the prisoners are but small ones, not the slightest meaning is introduced into their lives. The stone that Sisyphus moves to the top of the hill, whether we think of it as large or small, still rolls back every time, and the process is repeated forever. Nothing comes of it, and the work is simply pointless. That is the element of the myth that I wish to capture.

Again, it is not the fact that the labors of Sisyphus continue forever that deprives them of meaning. It is, rather, the implication of this: that they come to nothing. The image would not be changed by our supposing him to push a different stone up every time, each to roll down again. But if we supposed that these stones, instead of rolling back to their places as if they had never been moved, were assembled at the top of the hill and there incorporated, say, in a beautiful and enduring temple, then the aspect of meaninglessness would disappear. His labors would then have a point, something would come of them all, and although one could perhaps still say it was not worth it, one could not say that the life of Sisyphus was devoid of meaning altogether. Meaningfulness would at least have made an appearance, and we could see what it was.

That point will need remembering. But in the meantime, let us note another way in which the image of meaninglessness can be altered by making only a very slight change. Let us suppose that the gods, while condemning Sisyphus to the fate just described, at the same time, as an afterthought, waxed perversely merciful by implanting in him a strange and irrational impulse; namely, a compulsive impulse to roll stones. We may if we like, to make this more graphic, suppose they accomplish this by implanting in him some substance that has this effect on his character and drives. I call this perverse, because from our point of view there is clearly no reason why anyone should have a persistent and insatiable desire to do something so pointless as that. Nevertheless, suppose that is Sisyphus' condition. He has but one obsession, which is to roll stones, and it is an obsession that is only for the moment appeased by his rolling them—he no sooner gets a stone rolled to the top of the hill than he is restless to roll up another.

Now it can be seen why this little afterthought of the gods, which I called perverse, was also in fact merciful. For they have by this device managed to give Sisyphus precisely what he wants—by making him want precisely what they inflict on him. However it may appear to us, Sisyphus' fate now does not appear to him as a condemnation, but the very reverse. His one desire in life is to roll stones, and he is absolutely guaranteed its endless fulfillment. Where otherwise he might profoundly have wished surcease, and even welcomed the quiet of death to release him from endless boredom and meaninglessness, his life is now filled with mission and meaning, and he seems to himself to have been given an entry to heaven. Nor need he even fear death, for the gods have promised him an endless opportunity to indulge his single purpose, without concern or frustration. He will be able to roll stones *forever*.

What we need to mark most carefully at this point is that the picture with which we began has not really been changed in the least by adding this supposition. Exactly the same things happen as before. The only change is in Sisyphus' view of them. The picture before was the image of meaningless activity and existence. It was created precisely to be an image of that. It has not lost that meaninglessness, it has now gained not the least shred of meaningfulness. The stones still roll back as before, each phase of Sisyphus' life still exactly resembles all the others, the task is never completed, nothing comes of it, no temple ever begins to rise, and all this cycle of the same pointless thing over and over goes on forever in this picture as in the other. The *only* thing that has happened is this: Sisyphus has been reconciled to it, and indeed more, he has been led to embrace it.

Not, however, by reason or persuasion, but by nothing more rational than the potency of a new substance in his veins.

THE MEANINGLESSNESS OF LIFE

I believe the foregoing provides a fairly clear content to the idea of meaninglessness and, through it, some hint of what meaningfulness in this sense, might be. Meaninglessness is essentially endless pointlessness, and meaningfulness is therefore the opposite. Activity, and even long, drawn-out and repetitive activity, has a meaning if it has some significant culmination, some more or less lasting end that can be considered to have been the direction and purpose of the activity. But the descriptions so far also provide something else; namely, the suggestion of how an existence that is objectively meaningless, in this sense, can nevertheless acquire a meaning for him whose existence it is.

Now let us ask: Which of these pictures does life in fact resemble? And let us not begin with our own lives, for here both our prejudices and wishes are great, but with the life in general that we share with the rest of creation. We shall find, I think, that it all has a certain pattern, and that this pattern is by now easily recognized.

We can begin anywhere, only saving human existence for our last consideration. We can, for example, begin with any animal. It does not matter where we begin, because the result is going to be exactly the same.

Thus, for example, there are caves in New Zealand, deep and dark, whose floors are quiet pools and whose walls and ceilings are covered with soft light. As one gazes in wonder in the stillness of these caves it seems that the Creator has reproduced there in microcosm the heavens themselves, until one scarcely remembers the enclosing presence of the walls. As one looks more closely, however, the scene is explained. Each dot of light identifies an ugly worm, whose luminous tail is meant to attract insects from the surrounding darkness. As from time to time one of these insects draws near it becomes entangled in a sticky thread lowered by the worm, and is eaten. This goes on month after month, the blind worm lying there in the barren stillness waiting to entrap an occasional bit of nourishment that will only sustain it to another bit of nourishment until. . . . Until what? What great thing awaits all this long and repetitious effort and makes it worthwhile? Really nothing. The larva just transforms itself finally to a tiny winged adult that lacks even mouth parts to feed and lives only a day or two. These adults, as soon as they have mated and laid eggs, are themselves caught in the threads and are devoured by the cannibalist worms, often without having ventured into the day, the only point to their existence having now been fulfilled. This has been going on for millions of years, and to no end other than that the same meaningless cycle may continue for another millions of years.

All living things present essentially the same spectacle. The larva of a certain cicada burrows in the darkness of the earth for seventeen years, through season after season, to emerge finally into the daylight for a brief flight, lay its eggs, and die—this all to repeat itself during the next seventeen years, and so on to eternity. We have already noted, in another connection, the struggles of fish, made only that others may do the same after them and that this cycle, having no other point than itself, may never cease. Some birds span an entire side of the globe each year and then return, only to insure that others may follow the same incredibly long path again and again. One is led to wonder what the point of it all is, with what great triumph this ceaseless effort, repeating itself through millions of years, might finally culminate, and why it should go on and on for so long, accomplishing nothing, getting nowhere. But then one realizes that there is no point to it at all, that it really culminates in nothing, that each of these cycles, so filled with toil, is to be followed only by more of the same. The point of any living thing's life is, evidently, nothing but life itself.

This life of the world thus presents itself to our eyes as a vast machine, feeding on itself, running on and on forever to nothing. And we are part of that life. To be sure, we are not just the same, but the differences are not so great as we like to think; many are merely invented, and none really cancels the kind of meaninglessness that we found in Sisyphus and that we find all around, wherever anything lives. We are conscious of our activity. Our goals, whether in any significant sense we choose them or not, are things of which we are at least partly aware and can therefore in some sense appraise. More significantly, perhaps, men have a history, as other animals do not, such that each generation does not precisely resemble all those before. Still, if we can in imagination disengage our wills from our lives and disregard the deep interest each man has in his own existence, we shall find that they do not so little resemble the existence of Sisyphus. We toil after goals, most of them—indeed every single one of them—of transitory significance and, having gained one of them, we immediately set forth for the next, as if that one had never been, with this next one being essentially more of the same. Look at a busy street any day, and observe the throng going hither and thither. To what? Some office or shop, where the same things will be done today as were done yesterday, and are done now so they may be repeated tomorrow. And if we think that, unlike Sisyphus, these labors do have a point, that they culminate in something lasting and, independently of our own deep interests in them, very worthwhile, then we simply have not considered the thing closely enough. Most such effort is directed only to the establishment and perpetuation of home and family; that is, to the begetting of others who will follow in our steps to do more of the same. Each man's life thus resembles one of Sisyphus' climbs to the summit of his hill, and each day of it one of his steps; the difference is that whereas Sisyphus himself returns to push the stone up again, we leave this to our children. We at one point imagined that the labors of Sisyphus finally culminated in the creation of a temple, but for this to make any difference it had to be a temple that would at least endure, adding beauty to the world for the remainder of time. Our achievements, even though they are often beautiful, are mostly bubbles; and those that do last, like the sand-swept pyramids, soon become mere curiosities while around them the rest of mankind continues its perpetual toting of rocks, only to see them roll down. Nations are built upon the bones of their founders and pioneers, but only to decay and crumble before long, their rubble then becoming the foundation for others directed to exactly the same fate. The picture of Sisyphus is the picture of existence of the individual man, great or unknown, of nations, of the race of men, and of the very life of the world.

On a country road one sometimes comes upon the ruined hulks of a house and once extensive buildings, all in collapse and spread over with weeds. A curious eye can in imagination reconstruct from what is left a once warm and thriving life, filled wtih purpose. There was the hearth, where a family once talked, sang, and made plans; there were the rooms, where people loved, and babes were born to a rejoicing mother; there are the musty remains of a sofa, infested with bugs, once bought at a dear price to enhance an ever-growing comfort, beauty, and warmth. Every small piece of junk fills the mind with what once, not long ago, was utterly real, with children's voices, plans made, and enterprises embarked upon. That is how these stones of Sisyphus were rolled up, and that is how they became incorporated into a beautiful temple, and that temple is what now lies before you. Meanwhile other buildings, institutions, nations, and civilizations spring up all around, only to share the same fate before long. And if the question "What for?" is now asked, the answer is clear: so that just this may go on forever.

The two pictures—of Sisyphus and of our own lives, if we look at them from a distance—are in outline the same and convey to the mind the same image. It is not surprising, then, that men invent ways of denying it, their religions proclaiming a heaven that does not crumble, their hymnals and prayer books declaring a significance to life of which our eyes provide no hint whatever.[1] Even our philosophies portray some permanent and lasting good at which all may aim, from the changeless forms invented by Plato to the beatific vision of St. Thomas and the ideals of permanence contrived by the moderns. When these fail to convince, then earthly ideals such as universal justice and brotherhood are conjured up to take their places and give meaning to man's seemingly endless pilgrimage, some final state that will be ushered in when the last obstacle is removed and the last stone pushed to the hilltop. No one believes, of course, that any such state will be final, or even wants it to be in case it means that human existence would then cease to be a struggle; but in the meantime such ideas serve a very real need.

THE MEANING OF LIFE

We noted that Sisyphus' existence would have meaning if there were some point to his labors, if his efforts ever culminated in something that was not just an occasion for fresh labors of the same kind. But that is precisely the meaning it lacks. And human existence resembles his in that respect. Men do achieve things—they scale their towers and raise their stones to their hilltops—but every such accomplishment fades, providing only an occasion for renewed labors of the same kind.

But here we need to note something else that has been mentioned, but its significance not explored, and that is the state of mind and feeling with which such labors are undertaken. We noted that if Sisyphus had a keen and unappeasable desire to be doing just what he found himself doing, then, although his life would in no way be changed, it would nevertheless have a meaning for him. It would be an irrational one, no doubt, because the desire itself would be only the product of the substance in his veins, and not any that reason could discover, but a meaning nevertheless.

And would it not, in fact, be a meaning incomparably better than the other? For let us examine again the first kind of meaning it could have. Let us suppose that, without having any interest in rolling stones, as such, and finding this, in fact, a galling toil, Sisyphus did nevertheless have a deep interest in raising a temple, one that would be beautiful and lasting. And let us suppose he succeeded in this, that after ages of dreadful toil, all directed at this final result, he did at last complete his temple, such that now he could say his work was done, and he could rest and forever enjoy the result. Now what? What picture now presents itself to our minds? It is precisely the picture of infinite boredom! Of Sisyphus doing nothing ever again, but contemplating what he has already wrought and can no longer add anything to, and contemplating it for an eternity! Now in this picture we have a meaning for Sisyphus' existence, a point for his prodigious labor, because we have put it there; yet, at the same time, that which is really worthwhile seems to have slipped away entirely. Where before we were presented with the nightmare of eternal and pointless activity, we are now confronted with the hell of its eternal absence.

Our second picture, then, wherein we imagined Sisyphus to have had inflicted on him the irrational desire to be doing just what he found himself doing, should not have been dismissed so abruptly. The meaning that picture lacked was no meaning that he or anyone could crave, and the strange meaning it had was perhaps just what we were seeking.

At this point, then, we can reintroduce what has been until now, it is hoped, resolutely pushed aside in an effort to view our lives and human existence with objectivity; namely, our own wills, our deep interest in what we find ourselves doing. If we do this we find that our lives do indeed still resemble that of Sisyphus, but that the meaningfulness they thus lack is precisely the meaningfulness of infinite boredom. At the same time, the strange meaningfulness they possess is that of the inner compulsion to be doing just what we were put here to do, and to go on doing it forever. This is the nearest we may hope to get to heaven, but the redeeming side of that fact is that we do thereby avoid a genuine hell.

If the builders of a great and flourishing ancient civilization could somehow return now to see archaeologists unearthing the trivial remnants of what they had once accomplished with such effort—see the fragments of pots and vases, a few broken statues, and such tokens of another age and greatness—they could indeed ask themselves what the point of it all was, if this is all it finally came to. Yet, it did not seem so to them then, for it was just the building, and not what was finally built, that gave their life meaning. Similarly, if the builders of the ruined home and farm that I described a short while ago could be brought back to see what is left, they would have the same feelings. What we construct in our imaginations as we look over these decayed and rusting pieces would reconstruct itself in their very memories, and certainly with unspeakable sadness. The piece of a sled at our feet would revive in them a warm Christmas. And what rich memories would there be in the broken crib? And the weed-covered remains of a fence would reproduce the scene of a great herd of livestock, so laboriously built up over so many years. What was it all worth, if this is the final result? Yet, again, it did not seem so to them through those many years of struggle and toil, and they did not imagine they were building a Gibraltar. The things to which they bent their backs day after day, realizing one by one their ephemeral plans, were precisely the things in which their wills were deeply involved, precisely the things in which their interests lay, and there was no need then to ask questions. There is no more need of them now—the day was sufficient to itself, and so was the life.

This is surely the way to look at all of life—at one's own life, and each day and moment it contains; of the life of a nation; of the species; of the life of the world; and of everything that breathes. Even the glow worms I described, whose cycles of existence over the millions of years seem so pointless when looked at by us, will seem entirely different to us if we can somehow try to view their existence from within. Their endless activity, which gets nowhere, is just what it is their will to pursue. This is its whole justification and meaning. Nor would it be any salvation to the birds who span the globe every year, back and forth, to have a home made for them in a cage with plenty of food and protection, so that they would not have to migrate any more. It would be their condemnation, for it is the doing that counts for them, and not what they hope to win by it. Flying these prodigious distances, never ending, is what it is in their veins to do, exactly as it was in Sisyphus' veins to roll stones, without end, after the gods had waxed merciful and implanted this in him.

A human being no sooner draws his first breath than he responds to the will that is in him to live. He no more asks whether it will be worthwhile, or whether anything of significance will come of it, than the worms and the birds. The point of his living is simply to be living, in the manner that it is his nature to be living. He goes through his life building his castles, each of these beginning to fade into time as the next is begun; yet, it would be no salvation to rest from all this. It would be a condemnation, and one that would in no way be redeemed were he able to gaze upon the things he has done, even if these were beautiful and absolutely permanent, as they never are. What counts is that one should be able to begin a new task, a new castle, a new bubble. It counts only because it is there to be done and he has the will to do it. The same will be the life of his children, and of theirs; and if the philosopher is apt to see in this a pattern similar to the unending cycles of the existence of Sisyphus, and to despair, then it is indeed because the meaning and point he is seeking is not there—but mercifully so. The meaning of life is from within us, it is not bestowed from without, and it far exceeds in both its beauty and permanence any heaven of which men have ever dreamed or yearned for.

Note

1. A popular Christian hymn, sung often at funerals and typical of many hymns, expresses this thought:

> Swift to its close ebbs out life's little day;
> Earth's joys grow dim, its glories pass away;
> Change and decay in all around I see:
> O thou who changest not, abide with me.

R. M. Hare is perplexed by the conclusions reached by such thinkers as Camus. Hare refers specifically to the conclusion in Camus' novel *The Stranger* that *nothing matters*. Hare begins by asking "What does it mean to say that something *matters*, or *does not matter?*" After an attempt to clarify this notion, he concludes that Camus and others have been mistaken to look to the universe for rationality and meaning. That something *matters*, he thinks can only be found in setting our own objectives and in making our own choices. It is our own concern about something that makes it matter, in Hare's view; any other alternative he finds a "meaningless" alternative.

R. M. Hare

'NOTHING MATTERS' *

I

I want to start by telling you a story about something which once happened in my house in Oxford—I cannot remember now all the exact details, but will do my best to be accurate. It was about nine years ago, and we had staying with us a Swiss boy from Lausanne; he was about 18 years old and had just left school. He came of a Protestant family and was both sincerely religious and full of the best ideals. My wife and I do not read French very well, and so we had few French books in the house; but those we had we put by his bedside; they included one or two anthologies of French poetry, the works of Villon, the confessions of Rousseau and, lastly, *L'Etranger* by Camus. After our friend had been with us for about a week, and we thought we were getting to know him as a cheerful, vigorous, enthusiastic young man of a sort that anybody is glad to know, he surprised us one morning by asking for cigarettes—he had not smoked at all up till then—and retiring to his room, where he smoked them one after the other, coming down hurriedly to meals, during which he would say nothing at all. After dinner in the evening, at which he ate little, he said he would go for a walk. So he went out and spent the next three hours—as we learnt from him later—tramping round and round Port Meadow (which is an enormous, rather damp field beside the river Thames on the outskirts of Oxford). Since we were by this time rather worried about what could be on his mind, when he came back at about eleven o'clock we sat him down in an armchair and asked him what the trouble was. It appeared that he had been reading Camus's novel, and had become convinced that *nothing matters*. I do not remember the novel very well; but at the end of it, I think, the hero, who is about to be executed for a murder in which he saw no particular point even when he committed it, shouts, with intense conviction, to the priest who is trying to get him to confess and receive absolution, 'Nothing matters'. It

---

* The original English version of a paper contributed to the Cercle Culturel de Royaumont in 1957. The French version is published with a report of the subsequent discussion and the other proceedings of the Cercle's conference, under the title *La Philosophie Analytique* (Cahiers de Royaumont, no. iv, Editions de Minuit, 1959). Extract reprinted by permission of the author.

was this proposition of the truth of which our friend had become convinced:
Rien, rien n'avait d'importance.

Now this was to me in many ways an extraordinary experience. I have
known a great many students at Oxford, and not only have I never known
one of them affected in this way, but when I have told this story to English
people they have thought that I was exaggerating, or that our Swiss friend
must have been an abnormal, peculiar sort of person. Yet he was not; he
was about as well-balanced a young man as you could find. There was,
however, no doubt at all about the violence with which he had been
affected by what he had read. And as he sat there, it occurred to me that
as a moral philosopher I ought to have something to say to him that would
be relevant to his situation.

Now in Oxford, moral philosophy is thought of primarily as the study
of the concepts and the language that we use when we are discussing moral
questions: we are concerned with such problems as 'What does it mean to
say that something *matters, or does not matter?*' We are often accused of
occupying ourselves with trivial questions about words; but this sort of
question is not really trivial; if it were, philosophy itself would be a trivial
subject. For philosophy as we know it began when Socrates refused to
answer questions about, for example, what *was* right or wrong before he
had discussed the question '*What is it to be* right or wrong?'; and it does
not really make any difference if this question is put in the form 'What is
rightness?' or 'What is the meaning of the word "right"?' or 'What is its
use in our language?' So, like Socrates, I thought that the correct way to
start my discussion with my Swiss friend was to ask what was the meaning
or function of the word 'matters' in our language; what is it to be important?

He very soon agreed that when we say something matters or is important what we are doing, in saying this, is to express concern about that
something. If a person is concerned about something and wishes to give
expression in language to this concern, two ways of doing this are to say
'This is important' or 'It matters very much that so and so should happen
and not so and so'. Here, however, I must utter a warning lest I be mis-
understood. The word 'express' has been used recently as a technical term
by a certain school of moral philosophers known as the Emotivists. The
idea has therefore gained currency that if a philosopher says that a certain
form of expression is used to *express* something, there must be something
a bit shady or suspicious about that form of expression. I am not an
emotivist, and I am using the word 'express' as it is normally used outside
philosophical circles, in a perfectly neutral sense. When I say that the
words 'matters' and 'important' are used to express concern, I am no more
committed to an emotivist view of the meaning of those words than I would

be if I said 'The word "not" is used in English to express negation' or 'Mathematicians use the symbol "+" to express the operation of addition'.

Having secured my friend's agreement on this point, I then pointed out to him something that followed immediately from it. This is that when somebody says that something matters or does not matter, we want to know *whose* concern is being expressed or otherwise referred to. If the function of the expression 'matters' is to express concern, and if concern is always *somebody's* concern, we can always ask, when it is said that something matters or does not matter, 'Whose concern?' The answer to these questions is in most cases obvious from the context. In the simplest cases it is the speaker who is expressing his own concern. If we did not know what it meant in these simple cases to say that something matters, we should not be able to understand what is meant by more complicated, indirect uses of the expression. We know what it is to be concerned about something and to express this concern by saying that it matters. So we understand when anybody else says the same thing; he is then expressing his own concern. But sometimes we say things like 'It matters (or doesn't matter) to *him* whether so and so happens'. Here we are not expressing our own concern; we are referring indirectly to the concern of the person about whom we are speaking. In such cases, in contrast to the more simple cases, it is usual to give a clear indication of the person whose concern is being referred to. Thus we say, 'It doesn't matter to *him*'. If we said 'It doesn't matter', and left out the words 'to him', it could be assumed in ordinary speech, in the absence of any indication to the contrary, that the speaker was expressing his *own* unconcern.

II

With these explanations made, my friend and I then returned to the remark at the end of Camus's novel, and asked whether we really understood it. 'Nothing matters' is printed on the page. So somebody's unconcern for absolutely everything is presumably being expressed or referred to. But whose? As soon as we ask this question we see that there is something funny, not indeed about the remark as made by the character in the novel, in the context in which he is described as making it (though there is something funny even about that, as we shall see), but about the effect of this remark upon my friend. If we ask whose unconcern is being expressed, there are three people to be considered, one imaginary and two real: the character in the novel, the writer of the novel, and its reader, my Swiss friend. The idea that Camus was expressing his *own* unconcern about everything can be quickly dismissed. For to produce a work of art as good as this novel is something which cannot be done by someone who is not most deeply concerned, not only with the form of the work, but with its content. It is quite obvious that it mattered very much to Camus to say as clearly and tellingly as possible what he had to say; and this argues a concern not only for the work, but for its readers.

As for the character in the novel, who thus expresses his unconcern, a writer of a novel can put what sentiments he pleases in the mouths of his characters—subject to the limits of verisimilitude. By the time we have read this particular novel, it seems to us not inappropriate that the character who is the hero of it should express unconcern about absolutely everything. In fact, it has been pretty clear right from the beginning of the novel that he has not for a long time been deeply concerned about anything; that is the sort of person he is. And indeed there are such people. I do not mean to say that there has ever been anybody who has literally been concerned about *nothing*. For what we are concerned about comes out in what we choose to *do;* to be concerned about something is to be disposed to make certain choices, certain efforts, in the attempt to affect in some way that about which we are concerned. I do not think that anybody has ever been *completely* unconcerned about *everything,* because everybody is always doing something, choosing one thing rather than another; and these choices reveal what it is he thinks matters, even if he is not able to express this in words. And the character in Camus's novel, though throughout the book he is depicted as a person who is rather given to unconcern, is depicted at the end of it, when he says these words, as one who is spurred by something—it is not clear what: a sense of conviction, or revelation, or merely irritation—to seize the priest by the collar of his cassock with such violence, while saying this to him, that they had to be separated by the warders. There is something of a contradiction in being so violently concerned to express unconcern; if nothing *really* mattered to him, one feels, he would have been too bored to make this rather dramatic scene.

Still, one must allow writers to portray their characters as their art seems to require, with all their inconsistencies. But why, because an imaginary Algerian prisoner expressed unconcern for the world which he was shortly to leave, should my friend, a young Swiss student with the world before him, come to share the same sentiments? I therefore asked him whether it was really true that nothing mattered to him. And of course it was not true. He was not in the position of the prisoner but in the position of most of us; he was concerned not about nothing, but about many things. His problem was not to find something to be concerned about—something that mattered—but to reduce to some sort of order those things that were matters of concern to him; to decide which mattered most; which he thought worth pursuing even at the expense of some of the others—in short, to decide what he really wanted.

III

The values of most of us come from two main sources; our own wants and our imitation of other people. If it be true that to imitate other people is, especially in the young, one of the strongest desires, these two sources of our values can be seen to have a common head. What is so difficult about growing up is the integration into one stream of these two kinds of values. In the end, if we are to be able sincerely to say that something matters for *us,* we must ourselves be concerned about it; other people's concern is not enough, however much in general we may want to be like them. Thus, to take an aesthetic example, my parents may like the music of Bach, and I may want to be like my parents; but this does not mean that I can say sincerely that I like the music of Bach. What often happens in such cases is that I *pretend* to like Bach's music; this is of course in fact *mauvaise foi*— hypocrisy; but none the less it is quite often by this means that I come in the end to like the music. Pretending to like something, if one does it in the right spirit, is one of the best ways of getting really to like it. It is in this way that nearly all of us get to like alcohol. Most developed art is so complex and remote from what people like at the first experience, that it would be altogether impossible for new generations to get to enjoy the developed art of their time, or even that of earlier generations, without at least some initial dishonesty.

Nevertheless, we also often rebel against the values of our elders. A young man may say, 'My parents think it matters enormously to go to church every Sunday; but *I* can't feel at all concerned about it'. Or he may say, 'Most of the older generation think it a disgrace not to fight for one's country in time of war; but isn't it more of a disgrace not to make a stand against the whole murderous business by becoming a pacifist?' It is by reactions such as these that people's values get altered from generation to generation.

Now to return to my Swiss friend. I had by this time convinced him that many things did matter for him, and that the expression 'Nothing matters' in his mouth could only be (if he understood it) a piece of play-acting. Of course he didn't actually understand it. It is very easy to assume that all words work in the same way; to show the differences is one of the chief ways in which philosophers can be of service to mankind. My friend had not understood that the function of the word 'matters' is to express concern; he had thought mattering was something (some activity or process) that things did, rather like chattering; as if the sentence 'My wife matters to me' were similar in logical function to the sentence 'My wife chatters to me'. If one thinks that, one may begin to wonder what this activity is, called mattering; and one may begin to observe the world closely (aided perhaps by the clear cold descriptions of a novel like that of Camus) to see if one can catch anything doing something that could be called 'mattering'; and when we can observe nothing going on which seems to correspond to this name, it is easy for the novelist to persuade us that after all *nothing matters*. To which the answer is, ' "Matters" isn't that sort of word; it isn't intended to *describe* something that things do, but to express our concern about what they do; so of course we can't *observe* things mattering; but that doesn't mean that they don't matter (as we can be readily assured if, as I told my friend to do, we follow Hume's advice and "turn our reflexion into our own breast" [1])'.

There are real struggles and perplexities about what matters most; but alleged worries about whether anything matters at all are in most cases best dispelled by Hume's other well-known remedy for similar doubts about the possibility of causal reasoning—a good game of backgammon.[2] For people who (understanding the words) say that nothing matters are, it can safely be declared, giving but one example of that hypocrisy or *mauvaise foi* which Existentialists are fond of castigating.

I am not saying that no *philosophical* problem arises for the person who is perplexed by the peculiar logical character of the word 'matters': there is one, and it is a real problem. There are no pseudo-problems in philosophy; if anything causes philosophical perplexity, it is the philosopher's task to find the cause of this perplexity, and so remove it. My Swiss friend was not a hypocrite. His trouble was that, through philosophical naïveté, he took for a real moral problem what was not a moral problem at all, but a philosophical one—a problem to be solved, not by an agonising struggle with his soul, but by an attempt to understand what he was saying.

I am not denying, either, that there may be people who can sincerely say that very little matters to them, or even almost nothing. We should say that they are psychologically abnormal. But for the majority of us to become like this is a contingency so remote as to excite neither fear nor attraction; we just are not made like that. We are creatures who feel concern for things—creatures who think one course of action better than another and act accordingly. And I easily convinced my Swiss friend that he was no exception.

So then, the first thing I want to say in this talk is that you cannot annihilate values—not values as a whole. As a matter of empirical fact, a man is a valuing creature, and is likely to remain so. What may happen is that one set of values may get discarded and another set substituted; for indeed our scales of values are always changing, sometimes gradually, sometimes catastrophically. The suggestion that *nothing* matters naturally arises at times of perplexity like the present, when the claims upon our concern are so many and conflicting that we might indeed wish to be delivered from all of them at once. But this we are unable to do. The suggestion may have one of two opposite effects, one good and one bad. On the one hand, it may make us scrutinise more closely values to which we have given habitual allegiance, and decide whether we really prize them as much as we have been pretending to ourselves that we do. On the other, it may make us stop thinking seriously about our values at all, in the belief that nothing is to be preferred to anything else. The effect of this is not, as might be thought, to overthrow our values altogether (that, as I have said, is impossible); it merely introduces a shallow stagnation into our thought about values. We content ourselves with the appreciation of those things, like eating, which most people can appreciate without effort, and never learn to prize those things whose true value is apparent only to those who have fought hard to reach it.

Notes

1. *Treatise*, III I i.
2. *Treatise*, I 4 vii.

In the following selection from the work of Thomas Nagel questions of the significance of life and death are explored through an analysis of the notion of absurdity. While Nagel does believe that life is worth living even when the bad elements of experience outweigh the good elements, he does find a certain plausibility in the claim that life is absurd. The absurdity is said to rest on the clash of perspectives from which human existence can be viewed—that of purposeful actors creating meaning in our lives and that of disinterested spectators of those same lives. While he does locate absurdity in this situation, he does not adopt either Camus' "heroic" position or a cosmic scepticism.

Thomas Nagel

THE ABSURD *

Most people feel on occasion that life is absurd, and some feel it vividly and continually. Yet the reasons usually offered in defense of this conviction are patently inadequate: they *could* not really explain why life is

* Excerpted from "The Absurd" by Thomas Nagel, *Journal of Philosophy,* LXVIII, no. 20 (October 21, 1971), 716–22, 725–27. Reprinted by permission of the publisher and author.

absurd. Why then do they provide a natural expression for the sense that
it is?

I

Consider some examples. It is often remarked that nothing we do now
will matter in a million years. But if that is true, then by the same token,
nothing that will be the case in a million years matters now. In particular,
it does not matter now that in a million years nothing we do now will matter.
Moreover, even if what we did now *were* going to matter in a million years,
how could that keep our present concerns from being absurd? If their
mattering now is not enough to accomplish that, how would it help if they
mattered a million years from now?

Whether what we do now will matter in a million years could make
the crucial difference only if its mattering in a million years depended on
its mattering, period. But then to deny that whatever happens now will
matter in a million years is to beg the question against its mattering, period;
for in that sense one cannot know that it will not matter in a million years
whether (for example) someone now is happy or miserable, without knowing that it does not matter, period.

What we say to convey the absurdity of our lives often has to do with
space or time: we are tiny specks in the infinite vastness of the universe;
our lives are mere instants even on a geological time scale, let alone a
cosmic one; we will all be dead any minute. But of course none of these
evident facts can be what *makes* life absurd, if it is absurd. For suppose
we lived forever; would not a life that is absurd if it lasts seventy years be
infinitely absurd if it lasted through eternity? And if our lives are absurd
given our present size, why would they be any less absurd if we filled the
universe (either because we were larger or because the universe was
smaller)? Reflection on our minuteness and brevity appears to be intimately
connected with the sense that life is meaningless; but it is not clear what
the connection is.

Another inadequate argument is that because we are going to die,
all chains of justification must leave off in mid-air: one studies and works
to earn money to pay for clothing, housing, entertainment, food, to sustain
oneself from year to year, perhaps to support a family and pursue a career
—but to what final end? All of it is an elaborate journey leading nowhere.
(One will also have some effect on other people's lives, but that simply
reproduces the problem, for they will die too.)

There are several replies to this argument. First, life does not consist
of a sequence of activities each of which has as its purpose some later
member of the sequence. Chains of justification come repeatedly to an end
within life, and whether the process as a whole can be justified has no
bearing on the finality of these end-points. No further justification is needed

to make it reasonable to take aspirin for a headache, attend an exhibit of the work of a painter one admires, or stop a child from putting his hand on a hot stove. No larger context or further purpose is needed to prevent these acts from being pointless.

Even if someone wished to supply a further justification for pursuing all the things in life that are commonly regarded as self-justifying, that justification would have to end somewhere too. If *nothing* can justify unless it is justified in terms of something outside itself, which is also justified, then an infinite regress results, and no chain of justification can be complete. Moreover, if a finite chain of reasons cannot justify anything, what could be accomplished by an infinite chain, each link of which must be justified by something outside itself?

Since justifications must come to an end somewhere, nothing is gained by denying that they end where they appear to, within life—or by trying to subsume the multiple, often trivial ordinary justifications of action under a single, controlling life scheme. We can be satisfied more easily than that. In fact, through its misrepresentation of the process of justification, the argument makes a vacuous demand. It insists that the reasons available within life are incomplete, but suggests thereby that all reasons that come to an end are incomplete. This makes it impossible to supply any reasons at all.

The standard arguments for absurdity appear therefore to fail as arguments. Yet I believe they attempt to express something that is difficult to state, but fundamentally correct.

II

In ordinary life a situation is absurd when it includes a conspicuous discrepancy between pretension or aspiration and reality: someone gives a complicated speech in support of a motion that has already been passed; a notorious criminal is made president of a major philanthropic foundation; you declare your love over the telephone to a recorded announcement; as you are being knighted, your pants fall down.

When a person finds himself in an absurd situation, he will usually attempt to change it, by modifying his aspirations, or by trying to bring reality into better accord with them, or by removing himself from the situation entirely. We are not always willing or able to extricate ourselves from a position whose absurdity has become clear to us. Nevertheless, it is usually possible to imagine some change that would remove the absurdity— whether or not we can or will implement it. The sense that life as a whole is absurd arises when we perceive, perhaps dimly, an inflated pretension or aspiration which is inseparable from the continuation of human life and which makes its absurdity inescapable, short of escape from life itself.

Many people's lives are absurd, temporarily or permanently, for conventional reasons having to do with their particular ambitions, circumstances, and personal relations. If there is a philosophical sense of absurdity, however, it must arise from the perception of something universal—some respect in which pretension and reality inevitably clash for us all. This condition is supplied, I shall argue, by the collision between the seriousness with which we take our lives and the perpetual possibility of regarding everything about which we are serious as arbitrary, or open to doubt.

We cannot live human lives without energy and attention, nor without making choices which show that we take some things more seriously than others. Yet we have always available a point of view outside the particular form of our lives, from which the seriousness appears gratuitous. These two inescapable viewpoints collide in us, and that is what makes life absurd. It is absurd because we ignore the doubts that we know cannot be settled, continuing to live with nearly undiminished seriousness in spite of them.

This analysis requires defense in two respects: first as regards the unavoidability of seriousness; second as regards the inescapability of doubt.

We take ourselves seriously whether we lead serious lives or not and whether we are concerned primarily with fame, pleasure, virtue, luxury, triumph, beauty, justice, knowledge, salvation, or mere survival. If we take other people seriously and devote ourselves to them, that only multiplies the problem. Human life is full of effort, plans, calculation, success and failure: we *pursue* our lives, with varying degrees of sloth and energy.

It would be different if we could not step back and reflect on the process, but were merely led from impulse to impulse without self-consciousness. But human beings do not act solely on impulse. They are prudent, they reflect, they weigh consequences, they ask whether what they are doing is worth while. Not only are their lives full of particular choices that hang together in larger activities with temporal structure: they also decide in the broadest terms what to pursue and what to avoid, what the priorities among their various aims should be, and what kind of people they want to be or become. Some men are faced with such choices by the large decisions they make from time to time; some merely by reflection on the course their lives are taking as the product of countless small decisions. They decide whom to marry, what profession to follow, whether to join the Country Club, or the Resistance; or they may just wonder why they go on being salesmen or academics or taxi drivers, and then stop thinking about it after a certain period of inconclusive reflection.

Although they may be motivated from act to act by those immediate needs with which life presents them, they allow the process to continue by adhering to the general system of habits and the form of life in which such motives have their place—or perhaps only by clinging to life itself. They spend enormous quantities of energy, risk, and calculation on the details. Think of how an ordinary individual sweats over his appearance, his health, his sex life, his emotional honesty, his social utility, his self-knowledge, the quality of his ties with family, colleagues and friends, how well he does his job, whether he understands the world and what is going on in it. Leading a human life is a full-time occupation, to which everyone devotes decades of intense concern.

This fact is so obvious that it is hard to find it extraordinary and important. Each of us lives his own life—lives with himself twenty-four hours a day. What else is he supposed to do—live someone else's life? Yet humans have the special capacity to step back and survey themselves, and the lives to which they are committed, with that detached amazement which comes from watching an ant struggle up a heap of sand. Without developing the illusion that they are able to escape from their highly specific and idiosyncratic position, they can view it *sub specie aeternitatis*—and the view is at once sobering and comical.

The crucial backward step is not taken by asking for still another justification in the chain, and failing to get it. The objections to that line of attack have already been stated; justifications come to an end. But this is precisely what provides universal doubt with its object. We step back to find that the whole system of justification and criticism, which controls our choices and supports our claims to rationality, rests on responses and habits that we never question, that we should not know how to defend without circularity, and to which we shall continue to adhere even after they are called into question.

The things we do or want without reasons, and without requiring reasons—the things that define what is a reason for us and what is not—are the starting points of our skepticism. We see ourselves from outside, and all the contingency and specificity of our aims and pursuits become clear. Yet when we take this view and recognize what we do as arbitrary, it does not disengage us from life, and there lies our absurdity: not in the fact that such an external view can be taken of us, but in the fact that we ourselves can take it, without ceasing to be the persons whose ultimate concerns are so coolly regarded.

III

One may try to escape the position by seeking broader ultimate concerns, from which it is impossible to step back—the idea being that absurdity results because what we take seriously is something small and insignificant and individual. Those seeking to supply their lives with meaning usually envision a role or function in something larger than themselves. They therefore seek fulfillment in service to society, the state, the revolution, the progress of history, the advance of science, or religion and the glory of God.

But a role in some larger enterprise cannot confer significance unless that enterprise is itself significant. And its significance must come back to what we can understand, or it will not even appear to give us what we are seeking. If we learned that we were being raised to provide food for other creatures fond of human flesh, who planned to turn us into cutlets before we got too stringy—even if we learned that the human race had been developed by animal breeders precisely for this purpose—that would still not give our lives meaning, for two reasons. First, we would still be in the dark as to the significance of the lives of those other beings; second, although we might acknowledge that this culinary role would make our lives meaningful to them, it is not clear how it would make them meaningful to us.

Admittedly, the usual form of service to a higher being is different from this. One is supposed to behold and partake of the glory of God, for example, in a way in which chickens do not share in the glory of coq au vin. The same is true of service to a state, a movement, or a revolution. People can come to feel, when they are part of something bigger, that it is part of them too. They worry less about what is peculiar to themselves, but identify enough with the larger enterprise to find their role in it fulfilling.

However, any such larger purpose can be put in doubt in the same way that the aims of an individual life can be, and for the same reasons. It is as legitimate to find ultimate justification there as to find it earlier, among the details of individual life. But this does not alter the fact that justifications come to an end when we are content to have them end—when we do not find it necessary to look any further. If we can step back from the purposes of individual life and doubt their point, we can step back also from the progress of human history, or of science, or the success of a society, or the kingdom, power, and glory of God,[1] and put all these things into question in the same way. What seems to us to confer meaning, justification, significance, does so in virtue of the fact that we need no more reasons after a certain point.

What makes doubt inescapable with regard to the limited aims of individual life also makes it inescapable with regard to any larger purpose that encourages the sense that life is meaningful. Once the fundamental doubt has begun, it cannot be laid to rest.

Camus maintains in *The Myth of Sisyphus* that the absurd arises because the world fails to meet our demands for meaning. This suggests that the world might satisfy those demands if it were different. But now we can see that this is not the case. There does not appear to be any conceivable world (containing us) about which unsettlable doubts could not arise. Consequently the absurdity of our situation derives not from a collision between our expectations and the world, but from a collision within ourselves. . . .

VI

In viewing ourselves from a perspective broader than we can occupy in the flesh, we become spectators of our own lives. We cannot do very much as pure spectators of our own lives, so we continue to lead them, and devote ourselves to what we are able at the same time to view as no more than a curiosity, like the ritual of an alien religion.

This explains why the sense of absurdity finds its natural expression in those bad arguments with which the discussion began. Reference to our small size and short lifespan and to the fact that all of mankind will eventually vanish without a trace are metaphors for the backward step which permits us to regard ourselves from without and to find the particular form of our lives curious and slightly surpising. By feigning a nebula's-eye view, we illustrate the capacity to see ourselves without presuppositions, as arbitrary, idiosyncratic, highly specific occupants of the world, one of countless possible forms of life.

Before turning to the question whether the absurdity of our lives is something to be regretted and if possible escaped, let me consider what would have to be given up in order to avoid it.

Why is the life of a mouse not absurd? The orbit of the moon is not absurd either, but that involves no strivings or aims at all. A mouse, however, has to work to stay alive. Yet he is not absurd, because he lacks the capacities for self-consciousness and self-transcendence that would enable him to see that he is only a mouse. If that *did* happen, his life would become absurd, since self-awareness would not make him cease to be a mouse and would not enable him to rise above his mousely strivings. Bringing his new-found self-consciousness with him, he would have to return to his meagre yet frantic life, full of doubts that he was unable to answer, but also full of purposes that he was unable to abandon.

Given that the transcendental step is natural to us humans, can we avoid absurdity by refusing to take that step and remaining entirely within our sublunar lives? Well, we cannot refuse consciously, for to do that we would have to be aware of the viewpoint we were refusing to adopt. The only way to avoid the relevant self-consciousness would be either never to attain it or to forget it—neither of which can be achieved by the will.

On the other hand, it is possible to expend effort on an attempt to destroy the other component of the absurd—abandoning one's earthly, individual, human life in order to identify as completely as possible with that universal viewpoint from which human life seems arbitrary and trivial. (This appears to be the ideal of certain Oriental religions.) If one succeeds, then one will not have to drag the superior awareness through a strenuous mundane life, and absurdity will be diminished.

However, insofar as this self-etiolation is the result of effort, willpower, asceticism, and so forth, it requires that one take oneself seriously as an individual—that one be willing to take considerable trouble to avoid being creaturely and absurd. Thus one may undermine the aim of unworldliness by pursuing it too vigorously. Still, if someone simply allowed his individual, animal nature to drift and respond to impulse, without making the pursuit of its needs a central conscious aim, then he might, at considerable dissociative cost, achieve a life that was less absurd than most. It would not be a meaningful life either, of course; but it would not involve the engagement of a transcendent awareness in the assiduous pursuit of mundane goals. And that is the main condition of absurdity—the dragooning of an unconvinced transcendent consciousness into the service of an immanent, limited enterprise like a human life.

The final escape is suicide; but before adopting any hasty solutions, it would be wise to consider carefully whether the absurdity of our existence truly presents us with a *problem*, to which some solution must be found —a way of dealing with prima facie disaster. That is certainly the attitude with which Camus approaches the issue, and it gains support from the fact that we are all eager to escape from absurd situations on a smaller scale.

Camus—not on uniformly good grounds—rejects suicide and the other solutions he regards as escapist. What he recommends is defiance or scorn. We can salvage our dignity, he appears to believe, by shaking a fist at the world which is deaf to our pleas, and continuing to live in spite of it. This will not make our lives un-absurd, but it will lend them a certain nobility.[2]

This seems to me romantic and slightly self-pitying. Our absurdity warrants neither that much distress nor that much defiance. At the risk of falling into romanticism by a different route, I would argue that absurdity is one of the most human things about us: a manifestation of our most advanced and interesting characteristics. Like skepticism in epistemology, it is possible only because we possess a certain kind of insight—the capacity to transcend ourselves in thought.

If a sense of the absurd is a way of perceiving our true situation (even though the situation is not absurd until the perception arises), then what reason can we have to resent or escape it? Like the capacity for epistemological skepticism, it results from the ability to understand our human limitations. It need not be a matter for agony unless we make it so. Nor need it evoke a defiant contempt of fate that allows us to feel brave or proud. Such dramatics, even if carried on in private, betray a failure to appreciate the cosmic unimportance of the situation. If *sub specie aeternitatis* there is no reason to believe that anything matters, then that doesn't matter either, and we can approach our absurd lives with irony instead of heroism or despair.

Notes

1. Cf. Robert Nozick, "Teleology," *Mosaic*, xii, 1 (Spring 1971), 27–28.
2. "Sisyphus, proletarian of the gods, powerless and rebellious, knows the whole extent of his wretched condition: it is what he thinks of during his descent. The lucidity that was to constitute his torture at the same time crowns his victory. There is no fate that cannot be surmounted by scorn" (*The Myth of Sisyphus*, Vintage edition, p. 90).

In the following article Joseph Margolis contends that it is difficult to talk about the significance and evil of death itself, since it is goods or opportunities of which we are deprived rather than death *simpliciter* that accounts for its being evil. Margolis argues that actual death is neither good nor evil, even though death may deprive one of a treasured value (and hence be evil) or may remove a painful condition (and hence be good). Margolis concludes that death is an evil only *relative to* one's personal, ongoing objectives. This leads him to the view that to take death itself as an evil is both arbitrary and doctrinaire. He believes all such views ignore personal concerns relative to which we find death to be a good or an evil. Margolis concludes by providing five different perspectives from which significance may be found in death.

Joseph Margolis

DEATH *

Unless privileged articles of faith are invoked, we are all moved by death essentially in accord with the view of Epicurus: "When we are, death is not; and when death is, we are not." Dying is living in a specially diminished way, but death is not a process or an act: it is the limit of life. We ask what its significance is simply because our animal vitality is manifested in what we are pleased to call the significance of life: our devotion to the one obliges us to ask whether there is some continuity of purpose

* From *Negativities: The Limits of Life*. Copyright © 1975, Charles E. Merrill Publishing Company, pp. 9–16 (edited). Reprinted by permission.

involving the other, and perhaps what lies beyond the other. It is psychologically disruptive to have been persuaded that there *is* a point to living, and then merely and in a bland way to be unpuzzled by the ubiquity of death. Projects undertaken are cut short too soon, allegiances are wasted, promises are left unfulfilled, and all hopes and fears are affected by an apparently senseless factor.

But death is only an extreme instance of a family of conditions that invite the same speculation. For instance, a man may be in an irreversible coma for an interval in which he continues to "live" only if nourished by the deliberate efforts of other human beings. To mention the possibility is to draw attention to a normative use of the verb "live" that we favor: men are said to live not only when the minimal metabolic processes of biological survival obtain but also when they are *capable,* so surviving, of pursuing any of an indefinitely wide variety of purposeful ways of life that conform, as nontendentiously as we please, to the norms of *rational, civilized,* or *personal* life. Hence we say, "That's no life," "He's as good as dead," "He's no more than a vegetable," "That's a living death." The point is that, even admitting the intelligibility of one's own death, it is difficult to talk about the significance of death *simpliciter:* irresistibly, speculation takes the form of thinking about the permanent and irreversible *deprivation* of doctrinally favored values of life or about the significance of one's life summed up. On the condition that we have not yet succeeded in confirming the "true" values of life, and on the condition that it may well be impossible to do so, we may fairly take it that such speculation is inherently partisan.

Death is an evil because and only because *we* suppose we lose thereby some *prospectively* favored condition or opportunity; actual death is neither good nor evil. The counterpart for those who deny death or construe it as a temporary discontinuity is that the favored state is still accessible and that, after apparent death, *we* may be ranked and graded with respect to it. Both views fail to come to terms with Epicurus' maxim: to admit death in the relevant sense is to preclude ascriptions to continuing persons.

In death, there is no sense in which *you* can still be deprived of this or that opportunity; or, in which *you* can still aspire or lose hope, whether in Hell or at some point in the cycle of karma. To speak of the interests of the dead, for instance, as formulated in a will, is to speak of constraints on the living, not on what the dead can still take an interest in. Remembering someone, we speak of what *he* would have wished, were he alive. There is no literal sense in which his continuing interests can be served,[1] though we equivocate in speaking of his "interests." In fact, we equivocate in another respect with regard to his will, shifting between what the dead man has avowed in a formal way or in a final moment (no matter how silly or pointless, within limits) and what, were he rational, competent, and informed in the circumstances, he would have chosen (no matter how remote or unlikely). The same ellipsis informs Solon's maxim: "Count that man happy whose life is done," by which we are invited to consider the terrible reversals that may befall a man during his life, certainly not that the end of life is the point of life. So it is a confusion between life and death or a privileged doctrine about what goes on beyond apparent death that leads us to think of death as a *personal state* of some sort inviting appraisal in the same terms that obtain for life itself.

The required distinctions are clear enough but easily confused. A man, living on, sees death as threatening an important and worthwhile venture or as threatening life itself, which he savors. Prospectively, *he* sees death as an evil. But, of course, anything may deflect him from his project; so it is only relative to his personal, ongoing objectives that death may be said to be an evil. If the project is important to others, then death is only accidentally an evil to them; and if it was important only to the man who died, then the project is no longer important because it is no longer important to him. Only if life is a good in itself, not good merely because it is cherished, does the radical claim have any plausibility. It is not that death is normal or inevitable that it is not an evil. That poses no difficulty: men still count it, in prospect, an evil. It is rather that it excludes the very condition of life on which the personal appraisal of good and evil depends. It may be that the condition of dying is to be counted an evil, but the empirical evidence fails to support even this thesis very strongly.[2] To count dying or aging or suffering or ailing or the like as inherent evils is, effectively, to take the human condition as evil; it is more like taking life as an evil than death. But to count mere death as an evil is an utterly arbitrary or doctrinaire view. It ignores just those contingent and personal concerns relative to which it is normally so judged when it is so judged at all, or it imposes a thesis about the inherent evil of the world. Actual death cannot be an evil to the dead; and to the living, it signifies contingent deprivation within the boundaries of life itself. Construing the alternatives thus, those who hold mere death to be an evil are implicitly committed to regarding the world, on balance, as evil; and those who view death as an evil relative to their ongoing objectives fail to assess death itself, except accidentally.

What, then, is the significance of death?

First of all, it is significant that it is significant only for living human beings. Only men, as we understand the matter at present, have the full capacity to use language and, therefore, only men have the full capacity to refer to themselves and to formulate thoughts of counterfactual conditions or remote possibilities or the like. To think of one's death is to think of a world in which, though one obviously still exists, one no longer exists. Whatever may be true of one's speculations about birth, which depend on the same distinction, only men must make their commitments with the knowledge that they will die. Even if they deny it, they must consider the matter. To fail to do so seems incompatible with the very concession of a sustained ability to refer to oneself and the hazards of realizing that, whatever one undertakes, one may not live long enough to complete a venture or to undertake a new one. A minimal rationality, embodied in the capacity to use language and to refer to oneself, must, faced with the hazards of life, reflect on the prospect of one's death.

We are quite naturally led to a second consideration. Birth focuses our extraordinary dependence on the antecedent activities of others and the arbitrary "selection" of our personal setting, our talents, and our opportunities. Death does not seem so arbitrary, unless it is the time or place of death or unless a special theory decides the issue: on the first view, we retreat to deprivation again; on the second, to privileged doctrine. Even Gilgamesh is more perceptive, for he comes to understand the "meaninglessness" of death. The significance of death, then, lies in its having no discoverable significance, no ulterior meaning in terms of the values the dead are deprived of, or in terms of a secret plan that, living and dying, we somehow serve. The meaning of death is just that it is the natural limit of life—natural, since we have no evidence of an animal stock that is immortal. The span of human life is somewhat less than a hundred years. Exceptionally, some Ecuadorian Indian or some peasant from Soviet Azerbaijan lives to the age of one hundred and thirty-five. But we are not tempted by the prospect of immortality, at least on empirical grounds; the best we can visualize is a significant extension of life itself, which is to say that our science is Faustian. But to concede that much is to concede that the question of mortality remains the same—its urgency sometimes postponed, its poignancy inevitably heightened.

Third, the significance of death lies in its affecting whatever we take to be significant in life itself. Being the limit of life, death colors every serious engagement. The point has been beautifully put by Don Juan, the Yaqui sorcerer:

> "Look at me," he said, "I have no doubts or remorse. Everything I do is my decision and my responsibility. The simplest thing I do, to take you for a walk in the desert, for instance, may very well mean my death. Death is stalking me. Therefore, I have no room for doubts or remorse. If I have to die as a result of taking you for a walk, then I must die.
> "You, on the other hand, feel that you are immortal, and the decisions of an immortal man can be canceled or regretted or doubted. In a world where death is the hunter, my friend, there is no time for regrets or doubts. There is only time for decisions." [3]

The imminence of death, then, disqualifies certain beliefs and attitudes for the rational man. Under no circumstances does he have unlimited time to do whatever he may suppose to be important to undertake.

The concept of immortality, however, is a complex one. Sometimes, it signifies unending life—not eternity, which, if intelligible at all, signifies a shift in one's frame of reference or a shift in "levels of being." Immortality would eliminate death but not, for that reason, the problem of the meaning of life; and in fact, in some mythologies, immortality does not even preclude death: the immortals are simply reborn unendingly, which provides the meaning of the cycle or else generates the same question. But immortality may also signify, as it obviously does in Don Juan's analysis, the opportunity to undo whatever one has at an earlier moment undertaken. Hence, immortality is often naively seen as magical power capable of completing all one's ventures indefinitely extended. Not that men actually believe themselves to be immortal; only that, failing to take cognizance of death, they act as if they were immortal.

So the significance of death lies in our appreciation, living, that we pass through the successive moments of our life but once (which, alternatively put, comes to an appreciation of the directionality of time) and that that sequence has a distinctly short, finite limit. In this sense, the significance of death is simply the finitude of life self-consciously infecting action and reflection. Needless to say, the fact of death cannot be merely acknowledged as a fact among others; it must be articulately linked to one's vision of the positive values of life. According to Nietzsche, the wisdom of Silenus teaches us that it is best not to be born at all and, failing that, to end one's life. We need a positive doctrine even to make suicide rational; and suicide, like its repudiation, acknowledges the inevitability of death. So there is a sense in which the bare fact of death has the same significance for all, even though no man can consider death an isolated fact unrelated to his personal convictions. We cannot consider impending death alone, since to do so is psychologically incompatible with the commitments of ongoing life; but the mere fact of death has a significance for all men alike and, minimally, the same significance.

Fourth, the significance of death lies in the reminder, conveyed by another's death, of one's own mortality. Here is the double edge of bereavement: a significant loss to the living, and a reminder that others will inevitably be confronted with one's own death. The fact has a personal force through every ceremony of grief, however austere or baroque it may be. Also, against Heidegger, there need be no equivocation on "death" in speaking of one's own and another's death: we attend to the death of other persons; and our own, in prospect, entails the dissolution of the body.[4] It is perhaps a natural extension to consider the mortality of aggregates and the metaphorical mortality of collective entities, like nations and civilizations. Sometimes, the connection is explicit, as in Spengler; sometimes, implicit, as in Ecclesiastes. It makes no difference. The essential point remains the same, the ubiquity of the import of death, the end of individuals and the reduction of the aggregates of which they are a part.

There is nothing that men may undertake that is not touched with the sense of their mortality. But its pressure is inescapably personal as well as social, simply because it collects the race, reflectively, in terms of an undeniably universal condition of the greatest importance. Birth collects us, too; but since it precedes the very sense of self-identity, it has an alien ring. Death is what every man faces in every encounter, regardless of whatever else may be at stake. Birth is more remotely connected with our lives, linked as it is with social history and the past. Death is directly implicated in every venture. Both murder and war, on the one hand, and the service and care of humanity and one's own intimates, on the other, are uniquely informed by the fact of mortality. Murder cuts down those whose existence interferes with the personal plans of other mortals; war pits mortal aggregates against one another in terms of the metaphorical immortality of their collective lives; and humanity to man, both near and far, is premised on sharing more or less equally and fairly, for the small interval we have, the very goods of life. It is possible that the murderer rages against his own finitude or that the samaritan and philanthropist comfort themselves. In any case, we recognize ourselves and one another as the mortal victims and beneficiaries of analogous acts, the neutral and original insight of every ideology and creed. "The slayer and the slain are one," so seen, simply projects an exalted myth from a homely truth. The ease that infects our lives, confronted with the immanence of death, largely depends on the effectiveness with which we share the comforting doctrines our own society provides.

Finally, the significance of death lies in its not invalidating the significance of life. The race does not suicide simply because it becomes aware of its own mortality. On the contrary, it endlessly invents a conceptual rule for the acceptance of death. Extravagance is possible—perhaps, even necessary. But human life cannot ignore its own end, and even the most flat and apparently neutral acknowledgement is premised on the positive quality of life itself. In fact, the celebration of death can be nothing if not the celebration of life. We are forced to consider the merit of life. To construe it as a "gift" is to theorize about birth and about its inherent worth. But no sustained tradition has been capable of tolerating any and all uses of the putative gift. Directions are laid down for the proper use of life, inevitably for the end of life as well. The right way to die is simply a distinction within the general account of the right way to live. The point is that it cannot be ignored: since dying is a form of living, death provides no threatening complication. The trouble is that we are unable to *discover,* except subscribing to varied and incompatible higher Truths, what the proper use of life is. For that reason, death marks not only the significance of life, whatever we may allege it is, but also that life's significance lies in inventing and "discovering" again and again this or that significance.

There is a point to be pressed here. Otherwise, the fivefold significance of death would be a dubious contribution. Wisdom literature has plagued and comforted the world for ages. What we wish to know are the ineliminable implications of the fact that man knows he will die. Only in this way can we escape tendentious and partisan commitments, which we may well undertake for other reasons, and appreciate the force of the most powerful traditions addressed to the very fact of death. The point is simply this: every effort to specify the significance of death construes it in strictly formal terms, unless we presuppose, by some privileged access, that we already know its true significance. Death is significant to men alone. It has no significance except as the end of life. Its significance lies in affecting whatever is taken to be significant in life itself. Death is significant in that the death and mortality of others compel us to acknowledge our own, and our own compels us to acknowledge that of every other creature. Whatever its significance may be, it does not invalidate but is subsumed under the significance of life. We may say, then, that the significance of death is purely formal, has no doctrinal content at all. Or, we may say that death has no significance.

What is absolutely crucial to understand is that *no internally coherent policy or commitment whatsoever is rationally precluded by man's understanding that he must die.* Human beings can do anything at all consistently with the acknowledgement of mortality. Death forces us to shore up, personally and aggregatively, the convictions of life; that we persist and survive, as at least minimally rational creatures, confirms the pragmatic adequacy of our beliefs. And though the amplified doctrines to which we subscribe may forbid or permit this or that way of living or this or that way of dying, nothing whatsoever of such constraints may be derived from the ubiquity of death. Hence, the flowering of a thousand cultures. In this sense, death is not a morally significant fact: there are no rules that derive from it alone. In another sense, of course, it is the most momentous fact confronting every man.

Notes

1. Contrast Thomas Nagel, "Death," reprinted (somewhat enlarged) in James Rachels, ed., *Moral Problems* (New York: Harper & Row, 1971).
2. See Robert Kastenbaum and Ruth Aisenberg *The Psychology of Death* (New York: Springer, 1972). Perhaps the most intimate account of dying appears in Elisabeth Kübler-Ross, *On Death and Dying* (New York: Macmillan, 1969). The thesis that death is an evil appears in Nagel, "Death"; also, in Paul Ramsey, "The Indignity of 'Death with Dignity,'" *The Hastings Center Studies*, 2 (1974), 47–62. Ramsey tends to blend the conceptual aspects of death, dying, and mortality with normatively satisfactory responses to these conditions. Thus, he rejects the consolation provided by the Epicurean finding that death is not a part of life, the finding by the "death with dignity" move-

ment that dying is a part of living, and Wittgenstein's finding that living has no experienced limit. But the consolation offered rests on discoveries that are in themselves normatively neutral; also, Ramsey fails to demonstrate that it is, in some sense, *invalid* or how a valid mode of consolation could be provided. He urges us, merely as a partisan, to regard death as "evil," "the enemy," "the final indignity," so that some sense can be given to "overcoming" or "conquering" death; he also fears that his own conception is slowly being replaced. Cf. Leon R. Kass, "Averting One's Eyes, or Facing the Music?—on Dignity in Death," *The Hastings Center Studies,* 2 (1974), 67–80; and his "A Plea for Beneficient Euthanasia," *The Humanist,* 34 (1974), 4–5.

3. Carlos Castaneda, *Journey to Ixtlan* (New York: Simon and Schuster, 1972), p. 62. See also Edith Wyschogrod, "Sport, Death, and the Elemental," in Edith Wyschogrod, ed., *The Phenomenon of Death* (New York: Harper & Row, 1973).

4. Cf. Paul Edwards' article, "My Death," in Paul Edwards, ed., *The Encyclopedia of Philosophy,* vol. 5 (New York: Macmillan, 1967), pp. 416–19.

SUGGESTED READINGS FOR CHAPTER 5

Books and Articles

BAIER, KURT. *The Meaning of Life.* Canberra, Australia: Canberra University Press, 1957.

BEAUCHAMP, TOM L., BLACKSTONE, WILLIAM T., and FEINBERG, JOEL, eds. *Philosophy and the Human Condition.* Encino, Calif.: Dickenson Publishing Co., 1978. Chap. 9. With an Introduction by Joel Feinberg.

BRITTON, KARL. *Philosophy and the Meaning of Life.* Cambridge: Cambridge University Press, 1969.

EDWARDS, PAUL. "Life, Meaning and Value of" and "My Death," in *Encyclopedia of Philosophy,* ed. Paul Edwards. New York: The Macmillan Company, 1967.

HADAS, MOSES, ed. *The Essential Works of Stoicism.* New York: Bantam Books, 1961.

HEPBURN, RONALD. *Christianity and Paradox.* New York: Pegasus, 1958.

HOCHBERG, HERBERT. "Albert Camus and the Ethic of Absurdity," *Ethics,* 75 (1964–65), 87–102.

HYDE, WILLIAM DeWITT. *The Five Great Philosophies of Life.* New York: The Macmillan Company, 1952.

JOSKE, W. D. "Philosophy and the Meaning of Life." *Australasian Journal of Philosophy,* 52 (August 1974), 93–104.

KAUFMANN, WALTER, ed. *Existentialism from Dostoievsky to Sartre.* New York: Meridian Books, 1957.

KOESTENBAUM, PETER. "The Vitality of Death." *The Journal of Existentialism* 5 (1964), 139–66.

LEWIS, C. S. "De Futilitate," in *Christian Reflections.* Grand Rapids, Mich.: William Eerdmans, 1967. Pp. 57–71.

NAGEL, THOMAS. "Death." *Nous IV,* no. 1 (1971).

NORTON, DAVID L. *Personal Destinies: A Philosophy of Ethical Individualism.* Princeton, N.J.: Princeton University Press, 1977.

RUSSELL, BERTRAND. "A Free Man's Worship." *Mysticism and Logic.* London: George Allen & Unwin, 1917. Pp. 46–57.

SANDERS, STEVEN M., and CHENEY, DAVID R., eds. *The Meaning of Life: Answers and Analysis.* Encino, Calif.: Dickenson Publishing Co., 1978.

SANTAYANA, GEORGE. *Dialogues in Limbo* (Ann Arbor, Mich.: The University of Michigan Press, 1957), esp. Dialogues I–V.

SCHOPENHAUER, ARTHUR. *The Will to Live, Selected Writings,* ed. Richard Taylor. Garden City, N.Y.: Doubleday Anchor Books, 1962.

WHITE, R. C. "The Meaning of Life." *Australasian Journal of Philosophy,* 53 (August 1975), 148–50.

Bibliography

SANDERS and CHENEY (above) contains the most complete bibliography and also the most complete set of individual selections on the subject.

Encyclopedia of Bioethics Articles

DEATH: Eastern Thought—FRANK REYNOLDS

DEATH: Western Philosophical Thought—JAMES GUTTMAN

DEATH: Western Religious Thought—LLOYD BAILEY, SEYMOUR SIEGEL, MILTON MCGATCH

DEATH: ATTITUDES—RICHARD KALISH

LIFE: Value of Life—PETER SINGER

MAN: IMAGES OF—JULIAN N. HARTT

PROVIDENCE—DAVID TRACY

PURPOSE IN THE UNIVERSE—PATRICK A. HEELAN

BIBLIOGRAPHY OF BOOKS
ON OTHER ASPECTS
OF DEATH AND DYING

[Editors' Note: This list of books has been compiled to aid those readers who wish to explore problems in death and dying other than those explored in this book. This final bibliography has been limited to a few useful books, and an attempt has been made to exclude entries listed previously in the bibliographies at the end of each chapter.]

I. Anthologies

FEIFEL, HERMAN. *The Meaning of Death.* New York: McGraw-Hill, 1977.

KÜBLER-ROSS, ELISABETH. *Death: The Final Stage of Growth.* Englewood Cliffs, N.J.: Prentice-Hall, 1975.

SHNEIDMAN, EDWIN S. *Death: Current Perspectives.* Palo Alto, Calif.: Mayfield, 1976.

STEINFELS, PETER, and VEATCH, ROBERT M. *Death Inside Out.* New York: Harper & Row, 1975.

WYSCHOGROD, EDITH. *The Phenomenon of Death: Faces of Mortality.* New York: Harper & Row, 1973.

II. Original Texts

BECKER, ERNEST. *The Denial of Death.* New York: Free Press, 1973.

CHORON, JACQUES. *Death and Western Thought.* New York: Collier Books, 1963.

HINTON, JOHN. *Dying.* Baltimore: Penguin Books, 1967.

KÜBLER-ROSS, ELISABETH. *On Death and Dying.* New York: The Macmillan Company, 1969.

KÜBLER-ROSS, ELISABETH. *Questions and Answers on Death and Dying.* New York: Collier Books, 1974.

III. Supplementary Materials

ARIES, PHILIPPE. *Western Attitudes Towards Death: From the Middle Ages to the Present.* Translated by Patricia Ranum. Balitmore: Johns Hopkins University Press, 1974.

BRIM, ORVILLE G., JR., ET AL. *The Dying Patient.* New York: Russell Sage Foundation, 1970.

CHORON, JACQUES. *Death and Modern Man.* New York: Collier Books, 1972.

GLASER, BARNEY G., and STRAUSS, ANSELM L. *Awareness of Dying.* Chicago: Aldine Publishing Co., 1965.

KASTENBAUM, ROBERT and AISENBERG, RUTH. *The Psychology of Death.* New York: Springer-Verlag, 1972.

PARKES, COLIN MURRAY. *Bereavement: Studies of Grief in Adult Life.* New York: International Universities Press, 1973.

SAUNDERS, CICELY. *Care of the Dying.* London: The Macmillan Company, 1959.

SUDNOW, DAVID. *Passing On: The Social Organization of Dying.* Englewood Cliffs, N.J.: Prentice-Hall, 1967.

WEISMAN, AVERY D. *On Dying and Denying: A Psychiatric Study of Terminality.* New York: Behavioral Publications, 1972.

WEISMAN, AVERY D., and KASTENBAUM, ROBERT. *The Psychological Autopsy.* New York: Behavioral Publications, 1968.

IV. Bibliographies

KALISH, RICHARD A. "Death and Dying: A Briefly Annotated Bibliography." In *The Dying Patient,* ed. Orville G. Brim, Jr., et al. New York: Russell Sage Foundation, 1970. Pp. 323–80.

VEATCH, ROBERT M. *Death, Dying, and the Biological Revolution.* New Haven: Yale University Press, 1976.

VERNICK, JOEL J. *Selected Bibliography on Death and Dying.* Washington, D.C.: National Institutes of Health, Public Health Service.